Clinical Assessment and Treatment of Multiple Sclerosis

Clinical Assessment and Treatment of Multiple Sclerosis

Editor: Alfred Galswells

hayle medical

New York

Hayle Medical,
750 Third Avenue, 9th Floor,
New York, NY 10017, USA

Visit us on the World Wide Web at:
www.haylemedical.com

ISBN 978-1-64647-578-0 (Hardback)

Cataloging-in-Publication Data

Clinical assessment and treatment of multiple sclerosis / edited by Alfred Galswells.
p. cm.
Includes bibliographical references and index.
ISBN 978-1-64647-578-0
1. Multiple sclerosis. 2. Multiple sclerosis--Diagnosis. 3. Multiple sclerosis--Treatment.
4. Neurology. I. Galswells, Alfred.
RC377 .C55 2023
616.834--dc23

Contents

Preface

Over the recent decade, advancements and applications have progressed exponentially. This has led to the increased interest in this field and projects are being conducted to enhance knowledge. The main objective of this book is to present some of the critical challenges and provide insights into possible solutions. This book will answer the varied questions that arise in the field and also provide an increased scope for furthering studies.

Multiple Sclerosis (MS) is a form of demyelinating disease that affects the central nervous system (CNS). A patient with this disease can experience neurological symptoms such as autonomic, visual, motor and sensory problems. Some common symptoms associated with MS are ataxia, nystagmus, muscle spasms, problems with speech or swallowing, optic neuritis, pain and Uhthoff's phenomenon. The three prominent features of multiple sclerosis are formation of lesions in the CNS, inflammation, and the destruction of myelin sheaths of neurons and the blood-brain barrier (BBB). These characteristics coordinate in a complex manner to induce the breakdown of nerve tissues. The clinical assessment or diagnosis of multiple sclerosis is based on differential diagnosis, a method to rule out other conditions that might generate similar signs and symptoms. There are certain treatments available for managing multiple sclerosis which include medications that modify the progression of MS. These medications can be in the form of injectable medications, oral medications and infusion medications. This book contains some path-breaking studies related to the assessment and treatment of multiple sclerosis. It will serve as a reference to a broad spectrum of readers.

I hope that this book, with its visionary approach, will be a valuable addition and will promote interest among readers. Each of the authors has provided their extraordinary competence in their specific fields by providing different perspectives as they come from diverse nations and regions. I thank them for their contributions.

Editor

1

The Use of the Central Vein Sign in the Diagnosis of Multiple Sclerosis

Marco Castellaro [1,*], Agnese Tamanti [1,†], Anna Isabella Pisani [1,†], Francesca Benedetta Pizzini [2], Francesco Crescenzo [1,‡] and Massimiliano Calabrese [1,‡]

1 Department of Neurosciences, Biomedicine and Movement Sciences, University of Verona, 37134 Verona, Italy; agnese.tamanti@univr.it (A.T.); annaisabella.pisani@univr.it (A.I.P.); francescocrescenzo89@gmail.com (F.C.); massimiliano.calabrese@univr.it (M.C.)

2 Department of Diagnostics and Public Health, University of Verona, 37134 Verona, Italy; francescabenedetta.pizzini@univr.it

* Correspondence: marco.castellaro@gmail.com

† These authors equally contributed to the work.

‡ These authors shared the last-co authorship.

Abstract: ***Background***: The central vein sign (CVS) is a radiological feature proposed as a multiple sclerosis (MS) imaging biomarker able to accurately differentiate MS from other white matter diseases of the central nervous system. In this work, we evaluated the pooled proportion of the CVS in brain MS lesions and to estimate the diagnostic performance of CVS to perform a diagnosis of MS and propose an optimal cut-off value. ***Methods***: A systematic search was performed on publicly available databases (PUBMED/MEDLINE and Web of Science) up to 24 August 2020. Analysis of the proportion of white matter MS lesions with a central vein was performed using bivariate random-effect models. A meta-regression analysis was performed and the impact of using particular sequences (such as 3D echo-planar imaging) and post-processing techniques (such as FLAIR*) was investigated. Pooled sensibility and specificity were estimated using bivariate models and meta-regression was performed to address heterogeneity. Inclusion and publication bias were assessed using asymmetry tests and a funnel plot. A hierarchical summary receiver operating curve (HSROC) was used to estimate the summary accuracy in diagnostic performance. The Youden index was employed to estimate the optimal cut-off value using individual patient data. ***Results:*** The pooled proportion of lesions showing a CVS in the MS population was 73%. The use of the CVS showed a remarkable diagnostic performance in MS cases, providing a pooled specificity of 92% and a sensitivity of 95%. The optimal cut-off value obtained from the individual patient data pooled together was 40% with excellent accuracy calculated by the area under the ROC (0.946). The 3D-EPI sequences showed both a higher pooled proportion compared to other sequences and explained heterogeneity in the meta-regression analysis of diagnostic performances. The 1.5 Tesla (T) scanners showed a lower (58%) proportion of MS lesions with a CVS compared to both 3T (74%) and 7T (82%). ***Conclusions:*** The meta-analysis we have performed shows that the use of the CVS in differentiating MS from other mimicking diseases is encouraged; moreover, the use of dedicated sequences such as 3D-EPI and the high MRI field is beneficial.

Keywords: multiple sclerosis; MS; central vein sign; perivenular; lesion; imaging; MRI; biomarker

1. Introduction

Multiple sclerosis (MS) is one of the most common autoimmune disorders of the central nervous system (CNS), characterized by diffuse inflammatory/demyelinating and neurodegenerative alterations [1]. Magnetic resonance imaging (MRI) is one of the most powerful technological aids supporting MS diagnosis which can be used to demonstrate the distinctive dissemination in space and time of the disease. Over time, the diagnostic criteria, also implementing MRI in the diagnostic process, have increased their sensitivity, allowing an even earlier MS diagnosis, after a first/isolated event suggestive of acute CNS demyelination [2]. However, their specificity remains limited, especially in the presence of atypical history, and this could result in misdiagnosis and initiation/delay of inappropriate/approved disease-modifying treatment [3]. Brain MRI findings in conventional T2-weighted sequences in patients with different morbidities, such as vasculopathies, migraine and non-MS CNS demyelinating or autoimmune disorders, may be mistakenly suggestive of MS lesions [4]. Therefore, more MS-specific MRI criteria to rule out MS-mimicking disorders are needed.

The central vein sign (CVS), a recent radiological feature developed initially in ultra-high field MRI studies [5,6], relying on the pathological specificity of perivenular distribution of MS lesions [7], has been proposed as an MS imaging biomarker able to accurately differentiate MS from other white matter (WM) diseases of the CNS.

Although a definition of the CVS has been provided by an expert consensus, briefly as a distinct vein centrally located in a clearly visible MS lesion > 3 mm in diameter irrespective of its location in supratentorial brain white matter [8], and criteria based on both *proportion lesion threshold* [9,10] or *lesion number threshold* [11,12] have been proposed to discriminate MS from its MRI mimics, the lack of both a standardized imaging acquisition protocol and an accurate (and routinely suitable) CVS evaluation approach in suspected MS cases currently still prevent the applicability of this potential biomarker.

Imaging of a central vein in MS lesions can be achieved by exploiting the ability of susceptibility (T2*-"T2-star")-based MRI sequences to highlight in vivo paramagnetic properties of deoxyhemoglobin in venous blood flow [13]. By combining both magnitude and phase images acquired using T2*-weighted (T2*w) gradient echo (GRE) pulse sequences, it is possible to exploit susceptibility-weighted imaging (SWI) that can reveal the presence of blood vessels in MS lesions [14,15]. Even though the core protocol always includes a GRE sequence, a great variety of MRI parameters can be utilized to obtain SWI [14]. For instance, some studies introduced the use of echo-planar imaging (EPI) that allows for the retrieval of high-resolution images while reducing the scan time [16]. Further heterogeneity in the studies is introduced by the post-processing implementation. The first processing step required to compute SWI is the removal of artifacts from phase images. Several different phase processing approaches have been tested where high-pass filters are applied directly to phase images or following phase unwrapping [17]. Besides obtaining SWI from the combination of both magnitude and phase from the same GRE acquisition, another strategy consists of multiplying a T2*-weighted sequence with the fluid-attenuated inversion recovery (FLAIR) sequence to obtain a FLAIR* image [18]. This approach combines the sensibility of FLAIR in detecting WM lesions and the ability of susceptibility-based imaging to highlight the presence of the vein (Figure 1).

In this meta-analytic study, we aim to systematically review the proportion of MS white matter lesions which show the CVS (MSL Vein+) and estimate the performance diagnostic value, in terms of specificity, sensitivity and accuracy, in discriminating MS from its common radiological differential diagnosis, aiming to endorse its usefulness in clinical practice. Moreover, we further investigate the impact of using different field strengths, specific sequences (i.e., 3D echo-planar imaging) and post-processing techniques (i.e., SWI, FLAIR*).

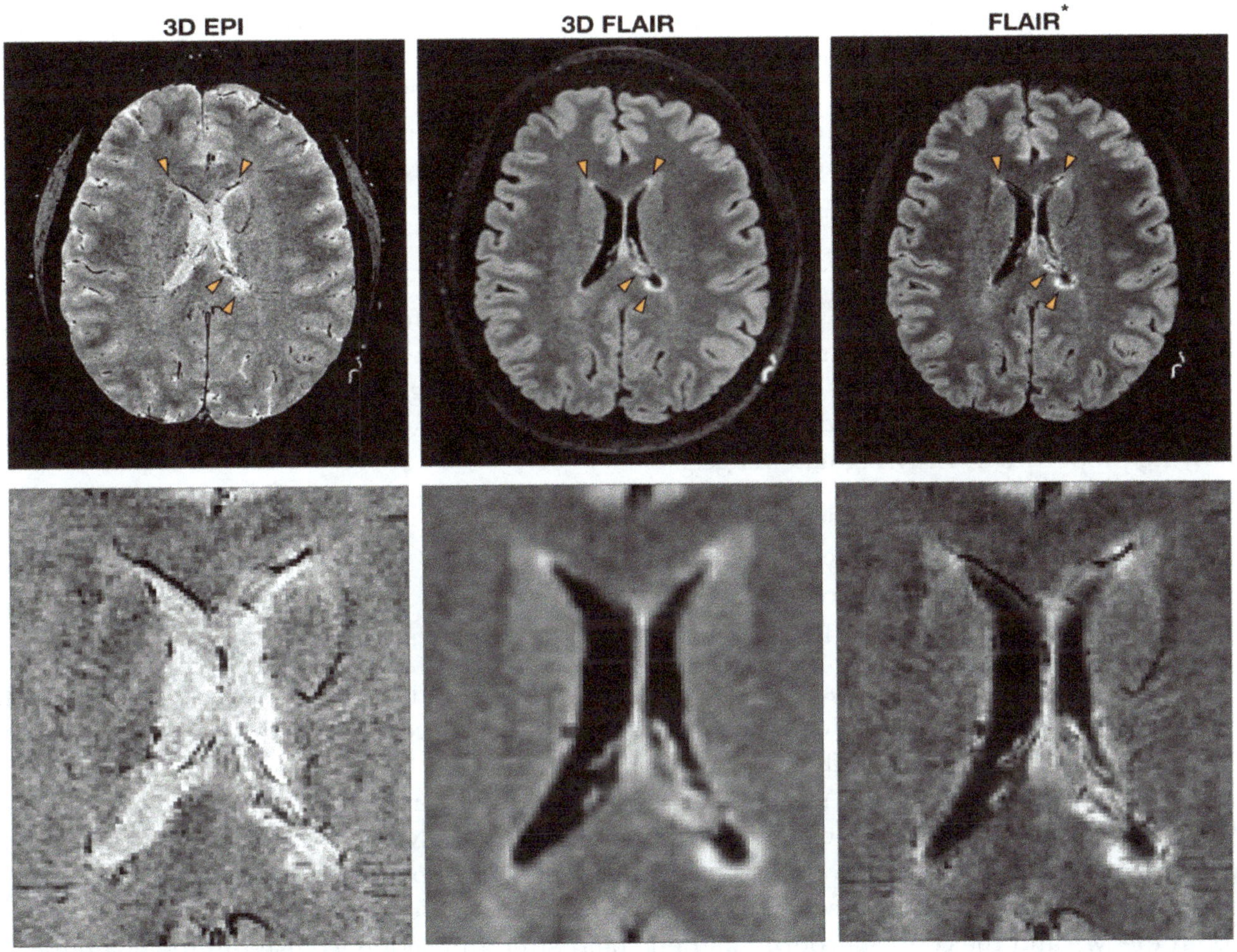

Figure 1. Example of multiple sclerosis (MS) patient MRI images obtained with sequences to detect the central vein sign (CVS). T2*-weighted 3D echo-planar imaging (EPI), 3D fluid-attenuated inversion recovery (FLAIR) and FLAIR*, a post-processing technique that combines the EPI sequence [or more generally a T2*w sequence (used to detect CVS)] and FLAIR. The orange arrowheads indicate MS lesions with the characteristic CVS. A zoomed-in version of the same image is reported to highlight the CVS feature for each modality.

2. Materials and Methods

The systematic review and meta-analysis were performed following the Preferred Reporting Items for a Systematic Review and Meta-analysis of Diagnostic Test Accuracy (PRISMA-DTA) statement [19,20]. The methodological framework used in this review is consistent with a previously published review and meta-analysis on the topic [21,22].

2.1. Literature Search: Databases and Search Phrase

Systematic research over two major databases was conducted following a recent systematic review and meta-analysis guideline [23]. PUBMED/MEDLINE and Web of Science were selected to look for articles using the CSV criteria to strengthen the MS diagnosis capability. The search string used in both databases was: (((“multiple sclerosis”) AND ((“central vein”) OR ((“vein”) AND (“lesion”)) OR (“perivenular”))). The literature research included only papers written in English and published up to 24 August 2020. The management of the literature research was conducted with Zotero (v 5.0.90).

2.2. Eligibility Criteria

Among studies retrieved from searched databases, we selected only published peer-reviewed studies that met all the following criteria: studies including patients with MS; studies evaluating the

CSV. Furthermore, we included studies that provided either the prevalence of the CSV in white matter lesions or true positives (TPs), false negatives (FNs), true negatives (TNs) and false positives (FPs) in diagnosing MS using the CVS.

We excluded from the review and from the meta-analysis any paper that met any of the following criteria: conference proceedings; animal-based studies; reviews; case reports and papers with fewer than five cases; editorial notes, surveys and guidelines.

2.3. Paper Summary and Data Extraction

The prevalence of the CVS in MS lesions and its diagnostic performance in differentiating MS from other diseases were separately summarized for each article included in the review. The CVS has been recently defined by the guidelines of the North American Imaging in Multiple Sclerosis Cooperative (NAIMS Cooperative) [8]. Accordingly, in this review, a central vein was defined as exhibiting the following properties in T2*-weighted images:

- Appears as a thin hypointense line or small hypointense dot;
- Has a small apparent diameter;
- Runs partially or entirely through the lesion;
- Is positioned centrally in the lesion, regardless of the lesion's shape.

Some studies (i.e., those published before the NAIMS Cooperative consensus paper) were included in this review, although the exclusion criteria for scoring the CVS according to the NAIMS Cooperative consensus were fulfilled (i.e., confluent lesion evaluation).

Diagnostic performances in terms of TP, FN, TN and FP for each study were recorded when available or were derived if not explicitly stated in the paper. Moreover, for each study, we also reported: study design (prospective/retrospective), the number of patients in the MS cohort and in the control group; sub-division between MS phenotypes; differential diagnosis; age (mean and interval) of both the MS and the control group; magnetic field strength; sequence used in the evaluation of the CVS; use of contrast agent; the number of readers and their background and blindness to the reference standard; institution and type of study (mono-/multi-centric); cut-off for the prevalence of the CVS in MS lesions and rule used (if multiple thresholds/criteria/rules were used, only the overall best diagnostic performance, in terms of the maximum sum of specificity and sensitivity, was retained).

2.4. Statistical Analysis

Estimations of pooled incidence of the central vein sign in T2*-based MRI acquisition in patients with MS were carried out using a random-effects meta-analysis weighted with the inverse variance supporting DerSimonian–Laird's method [24]. Heterogeneity between studies was quantified by the Higgins inconsistency test through the I^2 index which is not directly influenced by the number of the studies included in the analysis. The I^2 index lies between 0% and 100%. A value of 0% implies no observed heterogeneity, while larger values indicate increasing heterogeneity (25, 50 and 75% indicate low, medium and high heterogeneity, respectively). Publication bias was detected by funnel plots and the asymmetry was assessed by Egger's test. To explain the effects of study heterogeneity, a meta-regression analysis was performed using the study design (prospective study vs. others), post-processing image technique (FLAIR* vs. others), MRI sequence (3D-EPI vs. others), reader (radiologist vs. other), patient age (age median $\leq$ average age weighted on patient number vs. age median > age weighted on patient number), use of the contrast agent before the acquisition of the T2*-weighted sequence (used vs. not used) and blindness to the reference standard as covariates. Sub-group analysis was performed to test the single effect of the scanner magnetic strength (1.5 Tesla (T) vs. 3T vs. 7T), type of post-processing employed (FLAIR* vs. others) and MRI sequence employed (3D-EPI vs. others). The proportional meta-analysis conducted on both the complete set of studies included in this work and separately for each sub-group was preceded by an influence analysis to identify outliers in each set or subset [25].

The bivariate random-effects model was made in order to calculate the pooled sensitivity and specificity for the diagnostic accuracy of the central vein sign for differentiating MS from other common differential diagnoses. The estimated sensitivity and specificity and the credible intervals for each study were reported in a forest plot. The hierarchical summary receiver operating characteristic (HSROC) curve with 95% confidence and prediction regions was plotted. The extent of heterogeneity was assessed using the Cochran Q-test, the Higgins I^2 test and the Spearman correlation coefficient (rho) between sensitivity and false positive rate. Possible publication bias was evaluated by Deeks' funnel plot and assessed with a regression test on the diagnostic odds ratio. A p-value < 0.05 was considered as indicative of statistical significance.

A bivariate meta-regression model was applied to evaluate the effects of study heterogeneity using the following seven covariates: study design (prospective study vs. others), post-processing technique (FLAIR* vs. others), MRI sequence (3D-EPI vs. others), reader (radiologist vs. other), patient age (age median ≤ average age weighted on patient number vs. age median > age weighted on patient number), use of the contrast agent before the acquisition of the T2*-weighted sequence (used vs. not used) and blindness to the reference standard. Finally, subgroup analysis was performed using the proportion of lesions with the central vein sign as a cut-off value on those studies providing individual patient data. The individual data were extracted from the text of the articles or estimated from the plots indicating the proportion of lesions with the central vein sign using Web Plot Digitizer v. 4.3 (https://automeris.io/WebPlotDigitizer/) when data were not reported. The optimal threshold in ROC analysis was defined using the Youden index method [26]. Specifically, the Youden index was applied to estimate the optimal cut-off value for the proportion of lesions with the central vein sign and the corresponding sensitivity and specificity (95% CI). The Youden index is defined as sensitivity + specificity -1, with it having a minimum value of −1 and a maximum value of + 1, with a value of + 1 indicating the optimal value for an algorithm. Statistical analysis was performed using the "metafor", "mada" and "meta4diag" packages in R v. 3.5 and the "metandi" and "midas" modules in STATA 16.1.

3. Results

3.1. Literature Review

A total of 278 studies were screened according to the Preferred Reporting Items for a Systematic Review and Meta-analysis of Diagnostic Test Accuracy (PRISMA-DTA) (Figure 2). For subsequent qualitative and quantitative analysis, a total of 35 studies were considered eligible. A total of 1047 patients, including clinically isolated syndrome (CIS; $n = 256$) or definite multiple sclerosis (MS; $n = 791$), were included in the analysis.

3.2. Features of the Eligible Studies

Eleven studies used a prospective design [9,27–36], while ten reported a retrospective one [11,12,37–44]. The remaining fourteen did not mention the design type or the studied cohort was partially collected prospectively and retrospectively [10,38,45–56]. The mean number ± standard deviation of MS patients included in each study was 45.3 ± 70.78 (range: 5–323).

Five studies used a 1.5T scanner [27,38,39,42,43], twenty-one a 3T scanner [11,12,28–33,35–37,40, 46–48,51–55,57] and six a 7T scanner [10,34,41,45,50,58]. The remaining studies used images acquired at multiple field strengths: one study used either 1.5T or 3T but did not provide the proportion of CVS lesions for each scanner and thus was excluded from the sub-group analysis based on the scanner field strength [9]; two studies used both 3T and 7T scanners, however, in our meta-analysis, only the results from the highest field strength were reported as they provided the best performance [49,56].

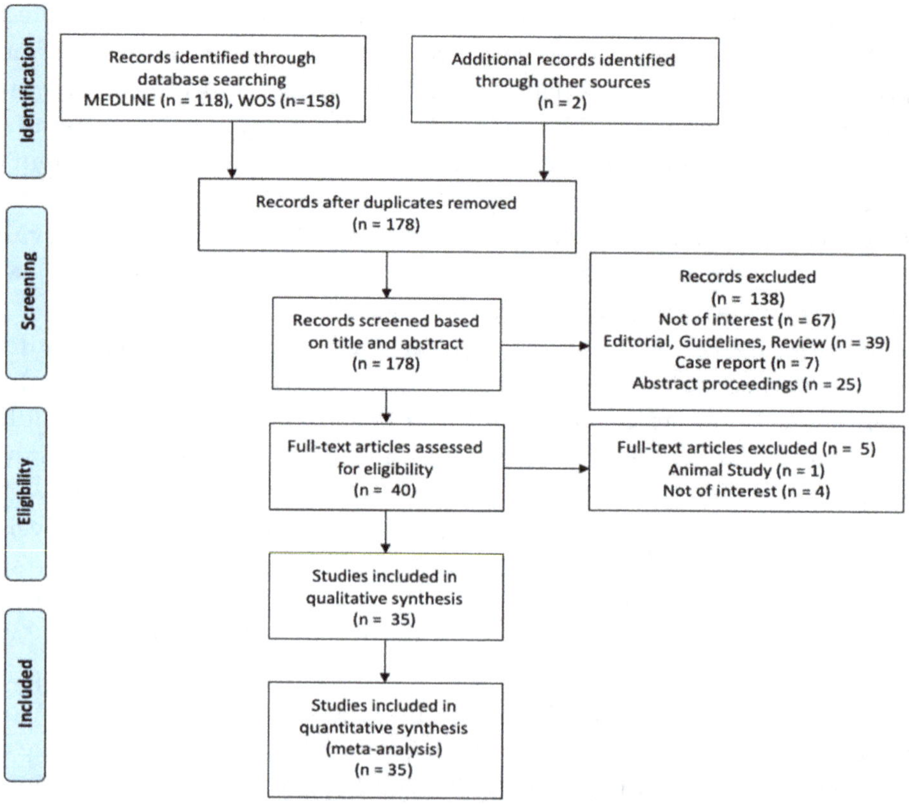

Figure 2. Preferred Reporting Items for a Systematic Review and Meta-analysis of Diagnostic Test Accuracy (PRISMA-DTA) flow diagram to select studies to be included in the subsequent meta-analysis.

Even though all the eligible studies included a susceptibility-based sequence (either susceptibility-weighted images, SWI; T2*-weighted gradient echo, T2*w; or T2*-weighted 3D echo-planar imaging, 3D-EPI), several protocols and processing techniques have been reported. Of the three studies detecting the CVS in T2*w images [45,50,58], one selected contrast-enhancing lesions using post-contrast images [45]. Of the fifteen studies using SWI [27,30,32,35,37–43,47,48,52,54] to identify the central vein sign, one added to the MRI protocol post-contrast sequences to select contrast-enhancing lesions [39], eight added a FLAIR sequence [30,35,40,42,47,48,52,54], one added a conventional T2-weighted acquisitions [32] and four added both FLAIR and conventional T2-weighted acquisitions [27,37,38,43], to delineate white matter lesions. Six studies employed a T2*w EPI sequence [10,11,33,34,46,57] and eight studies acquired both EPI and FLAIR sequences [9,12,28,29,36,49,53] that were combined to obtain FLAIR* images in seven of these studies [9,12,28,29,31,36,53]. Of the remaining studies, one retrieved FLAIR* images from the post-processing of a 3T FLAIR and the phase of a 7T SWI sequence [56], one used multiple susceptibility-weighted qualitative and quantitative images (SWI and R2*, respectively) [55] and one was a multicentric study including a heterogeneous set of MRI sequences [51]. In ten of the eligible studies, the susceptibility-based sequence was acquired during or after the injection of the contrast agent [9,12,28,30,31,39,40,47,53].

3.3. MS Lesions with Central Vein Pooled Proportion

Among the studies included, twenty-nine provided information on the proportion of MS lesions with the central vein sign [10–12,27–30,32–40,42,43,47–52,54–56,58,59]. The proportion of lesions with a central vein sign ranged from 0.4 up to 0.92. The pooled proportion of central vein signs in MS lesions considering all the studies included was 0.73 (95% CI, 0.67–0.79 (Figure 3). Influence analysis to detect outliers did not find any study that largely impacted on the pooled proportion. The Higgins inconsistency test showed high heterogeneity (I^2 = 98%). The meta-regression carried out to describe this heterogeneity did not find any statistical significance among the modeled covariates.

The publication bias assessment performed with the funnel plot showed no asymmetry (Supplementary Figure S1) and Egger's test showed no statistically significant asymmetry ($p = 0.074$).

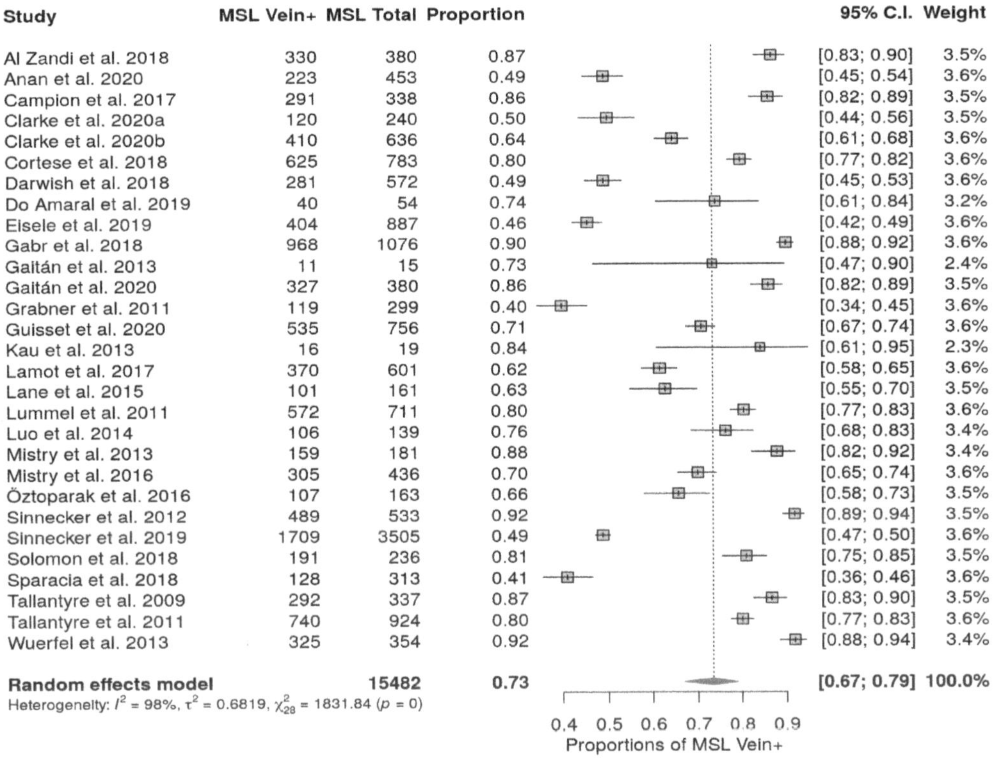

Figure 3. Forest plot showing the proportion of MS lesions with central vein sign (MSL Vein+) and the weight in the Random effect model for each study considered. Proportions are reported with estimated 95% confidence intervals (C.I.). In bold are reported the total number of MS lesions, the pooled proportions and the pooled C.I. and the total weights.

Regarding the effect of the scanner magnetic strength (1.5T vs. 3T vs. 7T), we did not find any study largely driving any subgroup. Moreover, the pooled proportion of central veins obtained with 1.5T MRI scanners was 0.58 (95% CI, 0.47–0.68). It was statistically different compared to the proportion obtained with both 3T (0.74 - 95% CI, 0.66–0.81, $p = 0.011$) and 7T (0.82 - 95% CI, 0.67–0.91, $p = 0.011$) scanners (Supplementary Figure S2). There was no statistically significant difference in the pooled proportion between 3T and 7T ($p = 0.32$).

The type of the post-processing employed (FLAIR* vs. others) did not show any influential study nor any statistically significant difference in the pooled proportion, that was 0.77 (95% CI, 0.61–0.87) when employing the FLAIR* and 0.74 (95% CI, 0.66–0.80) when it was not used (Supplementary Figure S3).

The MRI sequence used in the acquisition (3D-EPI vs. others) showed a study influencing the pooled proportion in the 3D-EPI sub-group [48], that was excluded from further sub-group analysis. After removing this outlying study, the proportion of lesions showing a central vein when using 3D-EPI was 0.82 (95% CI, 0.76–0.87) and it was statistically significantly higher ($p = 0.018$) compared to the use of other sequences (0.71 - 95% CI, 0.62–0.78, Supplementary Figure S4).

3.4. MS Diagnostic Accuracy Measured by Pooled Sensitivity and Specificity

Eighteen studies [9–12,27,28,32–35,41,44,47,48,51–53] provided the data to perform a pooled diagnostic accuracy meta-analysis. The pooled sensitivity and pooled specificity were 95% (95% CI, 90–99%) and 92% (95% CI, 87–97%), respectively (Figure 4, Figure 5). The area under the HSROC curve was 0.98 (95% CI, 0.96–0.99%) (Figure 6). Both the Q-test ($Q = 18.915$, $p = 0.333$) and the Higgins I^2 (10.12) suggested low heterogeneity across the studies. Both the forest plots and the Spearman correlation (rho = −0.18, 95% CI, −0.595–0.316) coefficient revealed no evidence of a threshold effect. Publication bias was detected by Deeks' funnel plot ($p < 0.001$, Supplementary Figure S5).

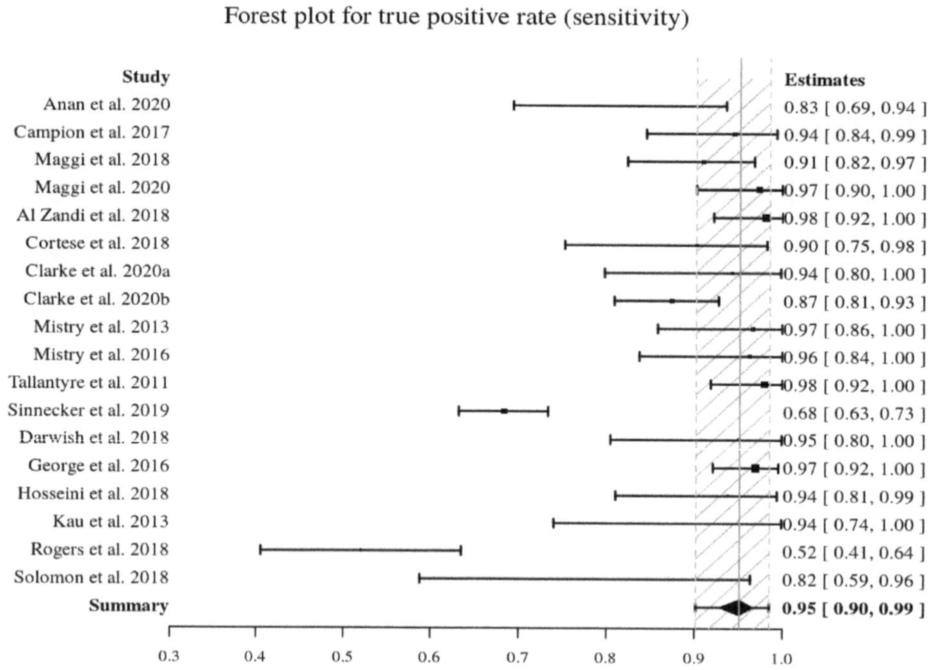

Figure 4. Forest plot of pooled sensitivity (in bold) of the central vein sign in T2*-weighted images for differentiating MS from other mimicking diseases. Sensitivity values are reported with estimated 95% confidence intervals (CIs) for each study included.

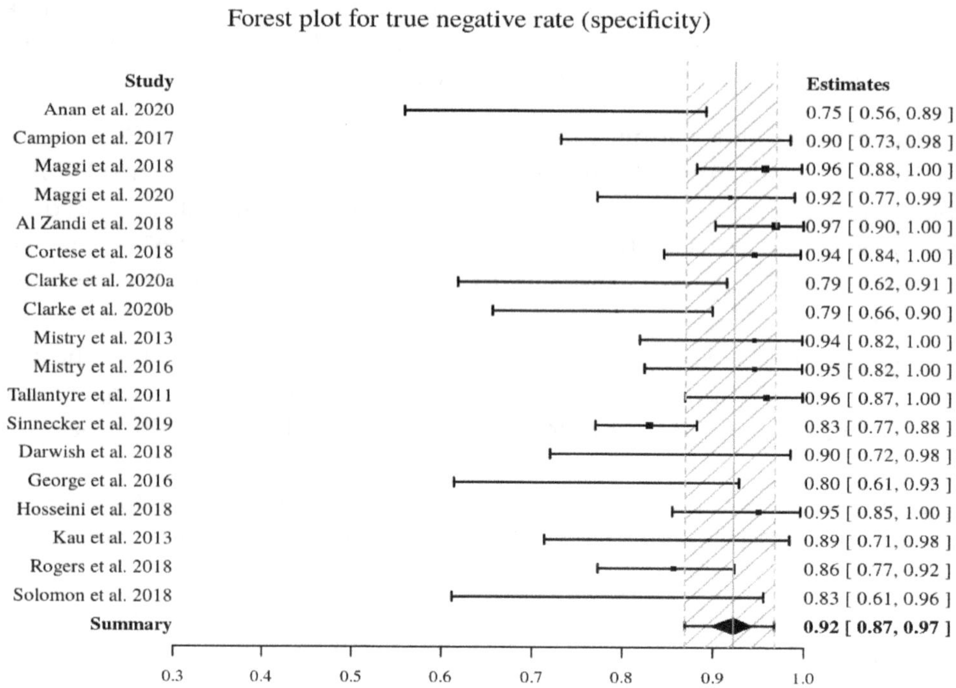

Figure 5. Forest plot of pooled specificity (in bold) of the central vein sign in T2*-weighted images for differentiating MS from other mimicking diseases. Specificity values are reported with estimated 95% confidence intervals (CIs) for each study included.

In the meta-regression, among the covariates, only the MRI sequence (p = 0.04) significantly affected the heterogeneity. Other covariates, including study design (p = 0.24), reader blindness to the reference standard ($p = 0.48$), age ($p = 0.06$), reader ($p = 0.48$) and post-processing technique ($p = 0.20$), did not show statistical differences.

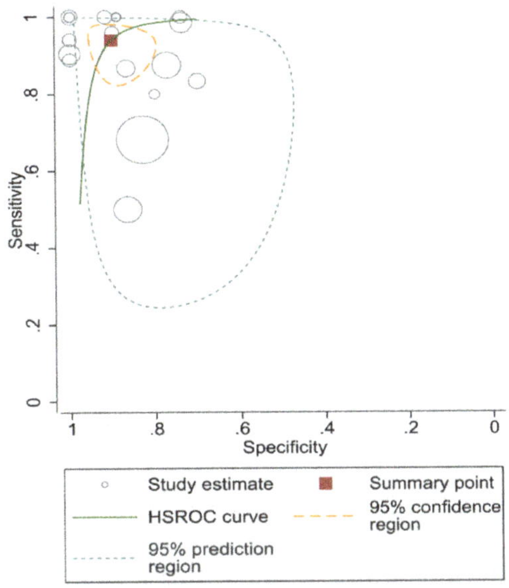

Figure 6. Hierarchical summary receiver operating characteristic (HSROC) curve of the diagnostic performance of the central vein sign in T2*-based images for differentiating MS from other mimicking diseases.

3.5. Diagnostic Performance using Distinct Patient Data

Fifteen studies reported the single patient percentage of lesions with a central vein [9–11,27,28,32, 34,36,41,46,48,50,52,57,58]. The number of considered MS patients was 284, while 178 were patients with other diseases or healthy controls (58% of MS patients). The cut-off values among the considered distinct patients ranged from 0 to 100 with a median value of 54%. The area under the ROC curve of the proportion of lesions with the central vein sign for the diagnosis of MS was 0.946 (95% CI, 0.924–0.967) (Figure 7). The optimal cut-off value identified by the Youden approach was 40%, with a sensitivity of 90% (95% CI, 81–95%) and a specificity of 89% (95% CI, 82%–96%).

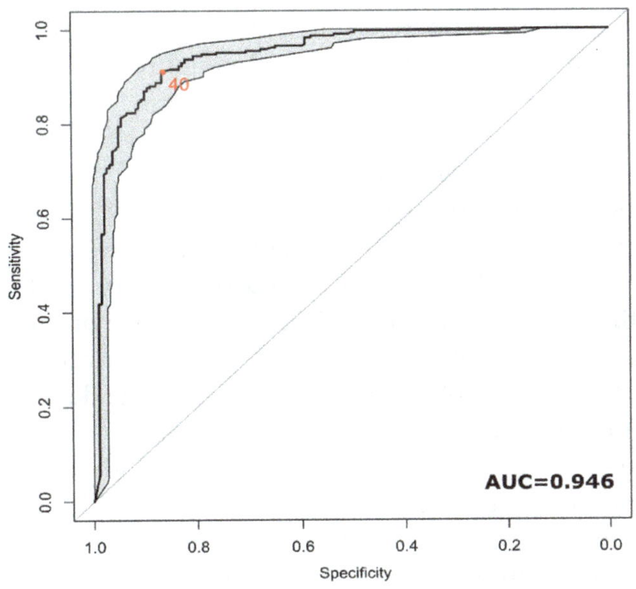

Figure 7. ROC curve of the diagnostic performance of central vein sign in T2*-based images for differentiating MS from other mimicking diseases at an individual level. The red dot indicates the optimal cut-off identified (40%).

4. Discussion

Evaluating the role of more specific magnetic resonance imaging (MRI) features of multiple sclerosis (MS) lesions, such as the central vein sign (CVS), is considered a high-priority area for research according to The International Panel on Diagnosis of MS, which produced the 2017 revised diagnostic criteria [60].

The systematic review and meta-analysis we performed aimed to assess the prevalence of the CVS in white matter (WM) MS brain lesions with respect to other WM diseases, as well as to investigate the use of the CVS in the differential diagnosis of MS by suggesting an optimal cut-off to differentiate MS from other conditions with MRI T2 hyperintensities and analyze the diagnostic performance measured with pooled sensitivity and specificity.

In this regard, the pooled proportion analysis revealed a high proportion (73%) of lesions showing a CVS in MS. Moreover, the use of the CVS reported a notable diagnostic performance, providing a pooled specificity of 92% and sensitivity of 95%. The pooled diagnostic performances in differentiating MS from other diseases estimated with the area under the HSROC of 0.98 (95% CI, 0.96–0.99%) revealed an excellent performance in this task. The optimal cut-off value obtained from the single patient data pooled together was 40% with an excellent value of the accuracy calculated by the area under the ROC (0.946). The heterogeneity in the dataset is high and this can be explained by the various features and settings of the eligible studies in terms of sequence, scanner field strength, post-processing technique and control group (both MS mimics and healthy control groups were considered). Nevertheless, the analysis conducted supports the potential role of the CVS in the diagnostic work-up of MS. Among several neuropathological features that characterize MS lesions, despite their different and asynchronous evolutive aspects over time, the vasocentricity is one of the most specific [61], in line with the generally accepted pathogenic theory that the early formation of a demyelinating focal area—an MS lesion—depends on the entry of lymphocytes and other inflammatory cells from the systemic circulation into the central nervous system across the blood–brain barrier [1]. WM lesions in MS, following the parenchymal venous topography (mainly at the level of small and medium veins), are commonly found in periventricular, infratentorial and medullary areas (deep venous system), as well as in juxtacortical regions (superficial venous system) and within the optic nerve (central retinal vein). Therefore, the careful evaluation of WM lesion distribution is certainly helpful in distinguishing MS from its MRI mimics, although some of them can involve the same areas, leading to image misinterpretation [62]. An elevated concentration of deoxyhemoglobin—higher oxygen consumption—and increased venous diameters—increased venous flow—at the inflamed site could be some of the reasons for peculiar vessel evidence by MR venography in MS lesions [63], even though this is still a topic of investigation.

One of the goals of our study was to investigate the optimal cut-off for WM lesions showing the CVS to differentiate between MS and other diseases. The cut-off values for the proportion of lesions with the CVS for the diagnosis of MS at the single-patient level ranged from 0 to 100. We found an optimal threshold of 40%, that has been reported in several single studies [9,10,27,31,33,34,46,48,53], confirming this threshold as an excellent value with a sensitivity of 90% and a specificity of 89%. However, manually counting and visually detecting the presence of the CVS for each lesion is very time consuming, influenced by both intra- and inter-observer variability and prone to error due to repetitiveness and the tiredness of the observer performing the task. Therefore, reliable and robust complete automatic detection and counting are highly desirable. A few attempts have been made based on classical machine learning and novel deep learning methods [64,65] but further studies to validate these promising methods are needed. A portion of the studies included in this review used the FLAIR* approach [18], but the analyses included in this study did not provide any difference in the proportion of detectable CVS-positive lesions when using this approach with respect to others. The limited number of studies employing this method available for this review might have influenced this result, however, this approach might be rarely accessible in a clinical setting since to produce FLAIR* images, processing steps such as coregistration and multiplication, often not implemented directly in

MRI scanners, are necessary. Another interesting aspect highlighted by this examination is that both the choice of the sequence as well as the scanner field strength play an important role in the identification of the CVS. As expected, the higher signal-to-noise ratio and contrast-to-noise ratio of high-field MRI scanners do contributes to better delineate and detect the CVS (0.82), however, we found that the use of 3T scanner might be sufficient in this regard (0.74), whereas the use of 1.5T scanners showed a statistically significant reduction in CSV detection (0.58). Among sequences, we found a statistically significant improvement of the CVS proportion detected in MS lesions using a 3D-EPI sequence versus all other sequences (0.82 vs. 0.71) regardless of the field strength. However, this particular sequence is not routinely used, perhaps due to the unavailability of a standard product sequence from some manufacturers. Therefore, a standardization and a larger study on this aspect should be envisaged. Another aspect that should be better investigated is the use of the contrast agent with this particular sequence. A quantitative evaluation of the beneficial use of the contrast agent in the detection of the CVS has not yet been performed, nevertheless, some studies [16,66,67] reported a notable improvement in this regard.

Two meta-analyses of using the CVS in MS were performed recently [21,22]. Our results are in agreement with Suh et al. [21], showing a similar proportion of lesions with the CVS and a slightly lower optimal cut-off value of 40% compared to 45%, even if this does not include the largest European multicenter study on the diagnostic value of the CVS in MS to date [51]. We further provide insight on the use of the 3D-EPI sequence and we also found a significantly different proportion of MS lesions with the CVS by comparing 1.5T and 3T scanners, suggesting that 3T scanners might provide a better performance. A more recent meta-analysis [22] was performed only with 1.5T and 3T and provided a lower proportion of MS lesions with the CVS than our findings, suggesting a threshold of 45% for the differentiation of MS from radiological mimics, however, this study included only a small portion of the articles included in our review.

Nevertheless, this work has some limitations. Regarding publication bias, we verified that the proportional analysis did not show any significant publication bias effect, while the pooled specificity and sensitivity analysis reported a publication bias assessed by Deeks' funnel plot and the regression test on the diagnostic odds ratio ($p < 0.001$), suggesting that the diagnostic performances could have been overestimated. We have included studies with a control population composed of heterogeneous mimicking disease spectra and also healthy controls that are vulnerable to selection bias. The studies included are even more heterogeneous in terms of the number of subjects (range: 5–323) as well as scanner field strength, sequence and post-processing technique used. Taking together the above reported limitations, special care should be taken when using the CSV in routine clinical practice.

5. Conclusions

Despite the high heterogeneity of the studies included in this meta-analysis, the CVS in differentiating MS lesions from other confounding disease could be used. We do highlight that the minimum scanner field strength needed to better exploit the CVS specificity is 3T, and the T2*-weighted 3D-EPI sequence could be suggested as a preferable image acquisition strategy.

Author Contributions: Conceptualization: M.C. (Marco Castellaro); Methodology: M.C. (Marco Castellaro), A.T., A.I.P., F.B.P., F.C., M.C. (Massimiliano Calabrese); Software: M.C. (Marco Castellaro), A.I.P.; Validation: M.C. (Marco Castellaro), A.T.; Formal Analysis: M.C. (Marco Castellaro), A.I.P.; Investigation: M.C. (Marco Castellaro), F.C., A.T.; Data Curation: M.C. (Marco Castellaro), F.C., A.T.; Writing—original draft preparation: M.C. (Marco Castellaro), F.C.; Writing—review and editing: M.C. (Marco Castellaro), F.C., A.T., A.I.P., F.B.P., M.C. (Massimiliano Calabrese); Visualization, M.C. (Marco Castellaro), A.I.P.; Supervision: F.C., M.C. (Massimiliano Calabrese); Project administration: M.C. (Marco Castellaro), F.C., M.C. (Massimiliano Calabrese); funding acquisition: M.C. (Massimiliano Calabrese). All authors have read and agreed to the published version of the manuscript.

References

1. Reich, D.S.; Lucchinetti, C.F.; Calabresi, P.A. Multiple sclerosis. *N. Engl. J. Med.* **2018**, *378*, 169–180. [CrossRef]

2. Schwenkenbecher, P.; Wurster, U.; Konen, F.F.; Gingele, S.; Sühs, K.-W.; Wattjes, M.P.; Stangel, M.; Skripuletz, T. Impact of the mcdonald criteria 2017 on early diagnosis of relapsing-remitting multiple sclerosis. *Front. Neurol.* **2019**, *10*, 188. [CrossRef]
3. Solomon, A.J.; Corboy, J.R. The tension between early diagnosis and misdiagnosis of multiple sclerosis. *Nat. Rev. Neurol.* **2017**, *13*, 567–572. [CrossRef]
4. Calabrese, M.; Gasperini, C.; Tortorella, C.; Schiavi, G.; Frisullo, G.; Ragonese, P.; Fantozzi, R.; Prosperini, L.; Annovazzi, P.; Cordioli, C.; et al. "Better explanations" in multiple sclerosis diagnostic workup: A 3-year longitudinal study. *Neurology* **2019**, *92*, e2527–e2537. [CrossRef]
5. Hammond, K.E.; Metcalf, M.; Carvajal, L.; Okuda, D.T.; Srinivasan, R.; Vigneron, D.; Nelson, S.J.; Pelletier, D. Quantitative in vivo magnetic resonance imaging of multiple sclerosis at 7 Tesla with sensitivity to iron. *Ann. Neurol.* **2008**, *64*, 707–713. [CrossRef]
6. Tallantyre, E.C.; Brookes, M.J.; Dixon, J.E.; Morgan, P.S.; Evangelou, N.; Morris, P.G. Demonstrating the perivascular distribution of ms lesions in vivo with 7-tesla mri. *Neurology* **2008**, *70*, 2076–2078. [CrossRef]
7. Lassmann, H. Multiple sclerosis pathology: Evolution of pathogenetic concepts. *Brain Pathol.* **2006**, *15*, 217–222. [CrossRef] [PubMed]
8. Sati, P.; Oh, J.; Constable, R.T.; Evangelou, N.; Guttmann, C.R.G.; Henry, R.G.; Klawiter, E.C.; Mainero, C.; Massacesi, L.; McFarland, H.; et al. The central vein sign and its clinical evaluation for the diagnosis of multiple sclerosis: A consensus statement from the North American imaging in multiple sclerosis cooperative. *Nat. Rev. Neurol.* **2016**, *12*, 714–722. [CrossRef] [PubMed]
9. Maggi, P.; Absinta, M.; Grammatico, M.; Vuolo, L.; Emmi, G.; Carlucci, G.; Spagni, G.; Barilaro, A.; Repice, A.M.; Emmi, L.; et al. Central vein sign differentiates Multiple Sclerosis from central nervous system inflammatory vasculopathies. *Ann. Neurol.* **2018**, *83*, 283–294. [CrossRef] [PubMed]
10. Tallantyre, E.C.; Dixon, J.E.; Donaldson, I.; Owens, T.; Morgan, P.S.; Morris, P.G.; Evangelou, N. Ultra-high-field imaging distinguishes MS lesions from asymptomatic white matter lesions. *Neurology* **2011**, *76*, 534–539. [CrossRef]
11. Mistry, N.; Abdel-Fahim, R.; Samaraweera, A.; Mougin, O.; Tallantyre, E.; Tench, C.; Jaspan, T.; Morris, P.; Morgan, P.S.; Evangelou, N. Imaging central veins in brain lesions with 3-T T2*-weighted magnetic resonance imaging differentiates multiple sclerosis from microangiopathic brain lesions. *Mult. Scler. J.* **2016**, *22*, 1289–1296. [CrossRef] [PubMed]
12. Solomon, A.J.; Watts, R.; Ontaneda, D.; Absinta, M.; Sati, P.; Reich, D.S. Diagnostic performance of central vein sign for multiple sclerosis with a simplified three-lesion algorithm. *Mult. Scler. Houndmills Basingstoke Engl.* **2018**, *24*, 750–757. [CrossRef] [PubMed]
13. Reichenbach, J.R.; Venkatesan, R.; Schillinger, D.J.; Kido, D.K.; Haacke, E.M. Small vessels in the human brain: MR venography with deoxyhemoglobin as an intrinsic contrast agent. *Radiology* **1997**, *204*, 272–277. [CrossRef] [PubMed]
14. Haacke, E.M.; Mittal, S.; Wu, Z.; Neelavalli, J.; Cheng, Y.-C.N. Susceptibility-weighted imaging: Technical aspects and clinical applications, part 1. *Am. J. Neuroradiol.* **2009**, *30*, 19–30. [CrossRef]
15. Mittal, S.; Wu, Z.; Neelavalli, J.; Haacke, E.M. Susceptibility-weighted imaging: Technical aspects and clinical applications, part 2. *AJNR Am. J. Neuroradiol.* **2009**, *30*, 232–252. [CrossRef]
16. Sati, P.; Thomasson, D.; Li, N.; Pham, D.; Biassou, N.; Reich, D.; Butman, J. Rapid, high-resolution, whole-brain, susceptibility-based MRI of multiple sclerosis. *Mult. Scler. J.* **2014**, *20*, 1464–1470. [CrossRef]
17. Li, N.; Wang, W.-T.; Sati, P.; Pham, D.L.; Butman, J.A. Quantitative assessment of susceptibility weighted imaging processing methods. *J. Magn. Reson. Imaging JMRI* **2014**, *40*, 1463–1473. [CrossRef]
18. Sati, P.; George, I.C.; Shea, C.D.; Gaitán, M.I.; Reich, D.S. FLAIR*: A combined MR contrast technique for visualizing white matter lesions and parenchymal veins. *Radiology* **2012**, *265*, 926–932. [CrossRef]
19. Frank, R.A.; Bossuyt, P.M.; McInnes, M.D.F. Systematic reviews and meta-analyses of diagnostic test accuracy: The PRISMA-DTA statement. *Radiology* **2018**, *289*, 313–314. [CrossRef]
20. McInnes, M.D.F.; Moher, D.; Thombs, B.D.; McGrath, T.A.; Bossuyt, P.M.; Clifford, T.; Cohen, J.F.; Deeks, J.J.; Gatsonis, C.; PRISMA-DTA Group; et al. Preferred reporting items for a systematic review and meta-analysis of diagnostic test accuracy studies: The prisma-dta statement. *JAMA* **2018**, *319*, 388–396. [CrossRef]

21. Suh, C.H.; Kim, S.J.; Jung, S.C.; Choi, C.G.; Kim, H.S. The "Central Vein Sign" on T2*-weighted Images as a Diagnostic Tool in Multiple Sclerosis: A Systematic Review and Meta-analysis using Individual Patient Data. *Sci. Rep.* **2019**, *9*, 18188. [CrossRef] [PubMed]
22. Bhandari, A.; Xiang, H.; Lechner-Scott, J.; Agzarian, M. Central vein sign for multiple sclerosis: A systematic review and meta-analysis. *Clin. Radiol.* **2020**, *75*, 479.e9–479.e15. [CrossRef] [PubMed]
23. Bramer, W.M.; Rethlefsen, M.L.; Kleijnen, J.; Franco, O.H. Optimal database combinations for literature searches in systematic reviews: A prospective exploratory study. *Syst. Rev.* **2017**, *6*, 245. [CrossRef] [PubMed]
24. DerSimonian, R.; Laird, N. Meta-analysis in clinical trials. *Control. Clin. Trials* **1986**, *7*, 177–188. [CrossRef]
25. Williams, D.A. Generalized linear model diagnostics using the deviance and single case deletions. *Appl. Stat.* **1987**, *36*, 181. [CrossRef]
26. Youden, W.J. Index for rating diagnostic tests. *Cancer* **1950**, *3*, 32–35. [CrossRef]
27. Anan, R.A.; El-Adalany, M.A.; Belal, T.M.I.; Elmogy, S.A.E.-D. Detection of central veins using susceptibility weighted imaging (SWI) for discrimination between lesions in multiple sclerosis (MS) and cerebral small vessel disease (CSVD). *Egypt. J. Radiol. Nucl. Med.* **2020**, *51*, 1–7. [CrossRef]
28. Campion, T.; Smith, R.J.P.; Altmann, D.R.; Brito, G.C.; Turner, B.P.; Evanson, J.; George, I.C.; Sati, P.; Reich, D.S.; Miquel, M.E.; et al. FLAIR* to visualize veins in white matter lesions: A new tool for the diagnosis of multiple sclerosis? *Eur. Radiol.* **2017**, *27*, 4257–4263. [CrossRef]
29. Gabr, R.E.; Pednekar, A.S.; Kamali, A.; Lincoln, J.A.; Nelson, F.M.; Wolinsky, J.S.; Narayana, P.A. Interleaved susceptibility-weighted and FLAIR MRI for imaging lesion-penetrating veins in multiple sclerosis. *Magn. Reson. Med.* **2018**, *80*, 1132–1137. [CrossRef]
30. Gaitán, M.I.; Yañez, P.; Paday Formenti, M.E.; Calandri, I.; Figueiredo, E.; Sati, P.; Correale, J. SWAN-venule: An optimized mri technique to detect the central vein sign in ms plaques. *AJNR Am. J. Neuroradiol.* **2020**, *41*, 456–460. [CrossRef]
31. Maggi, P.; Absinta, M.; Sati, P.; Perrotta, G.; Massacesi, L.; Dachy, B.; Pot, C.; Meuli, R.; Reich, D.S.; Filippi, M.; et al. The "central vein sign" in patients with diagnostic "red flags" for multiple sclerosis: A prospective multicenter 3T study. *Mult. Scler. Houndmills Basingstoke Engl.* **2020**, *26*, 421–432. [CrossRef] [PubMed]
32. Cortese, R.; Magnollay, L.; Tur, C.; Abdel-Aziz, K.; Jacob, A.; De Angelis, F.; Yiannakas, M.C.; Prados, F.; Ourselin, S.; Yousry, T.A.; et al. Value of the central vein sign at 3T to differentiate MS from seropositive NMOSD. *Neurology* **2018**, *90*, e1183–e1190. [CrossRef]
33. Clarke, M.A.; Samaraweera, A.P.; Falah, Y.; Pitiot, A.; Allen, C.M.; Dineen, R.A.; Tench, C.R.; Morgan, P.S.; Evangelou, N. Single Test to ARrive at Multiple Sclerosis (STAR-MS) diagnosis: A prospective pilot study assessing the accuracy of the central vein sign in predicting multiple sclerosis in cases of diagnostic uncertainty. *Mult. Scler. Houndmills Basingstoke Engl.* **2020**, *26*, 433–441. [CrossRef] [PubMed]
34. Mistry, N.; Dixon, J.; Tallantyre, E.; Tench, C.; Abdel-Fahim, R.; Jaspan, T.; Morgan, P.S.; Morris, P.; Evangelou, N. Central veins in brain lesions visualized with high-field magnetic resonance imaging: A pathologically specific diagnostic biomarker for inflammatory demyelination in the brain. *JAMA Neurol.* **2013**, *70*, 623–628. [CrossRef]
35. Kau, T.; Taschwer, M.; Deutschmann, H.; Schönfelder, M.; Weber, J.R.; Hausegger, K.A. The "central vein sign": Is there a place for susceptibility weighted imaging in possible multiple sclerosis? *Eur. Radiol.* **2013**, *23*, 1956–1962. [CrossRef] [PubMed]
36. Guisset, F.; Lolli, V.; Bugli, C.; Perrotta, G.; Absil, J.; Dachy, B.; Pot, C.; Théaudin, M.; Pasi, M.; van Pesch, V.; et al. The central vein sign in multiple sclerosis patients with vascular comorbidities. *Mult. Scler. J.* **2020**, 135245852094378. [CrossRef] [PubMed]
37. Lamot, U.; Avsenik, J.; Šega, S.; Šurlan Popovič, K. Presence of central veins and susceptibility weighted imaging for evaluating lesions in multiple sclerosis and leukoaraiosis. *Mult. Scler. Relat. Disord.* **2017**, *13*, 67–72. [CrossRef] [PubMed]
38. Sparacia, G.; Agnello, F.; Gambino, A.; Sciortino, M.; Midiri, M. Multiple sclerosis: High prevalence of the "central vein" sign in white matter lesions on susceptibility-weighted images. *Neuroradiol. J.* **2018**, *31*, 356–361. [CrossRef] [PubMed]

39. Do Amaral, L.L.F.; Fragoso, D.C.; Nunes, R.H.; Littig, I.A.; da Rocha, A.J. gadolinium-enhanced susceptibility-weighted imaging in multiple sclerosis: Optimizing the recognition of active plaques for different mr imaging sequences. *AJNR Am. J. Neuroradiol.* **2019**, *40*, 614–619. [CrossRef]
40. Eisele, P.; Fischer, K.; Szabo, K.; Platten, M.; Gass, A. Characterization of contrast-enhancing and non-contrast-enhancing multiple sclerosis lesions using susceptibility-weighted imaging. *Front. Neurol.* **2019**, *10*, 1082. [CrossRef]
41. Hosseini, Z.; Matusinec, J.; Rudko, D.A.; Liu, J.; Kwan, B.Y.M.; Salehi, F.; Sharma, M.; Kremenchutzky, M.; Menon, R.S.; Drangova, M. Morphology-specific discrimination between ms white matter lesions and benign white matter hyperintensities using ultra-high-field mri. *AJNR Am. J. Neuroradiol.* **2018**, *39*, 1473–1479. [CrossRef] [PubMed]
42. Lane, J.I.; Bolster, B.; Campeau, N.G.; Welker, K.M.; Gilbertson, J.R. Characterization of multiple sclerosis plaques using susceptibility-weighted imaging at 1.5 T: Can perivenular localization improve specificity of imaging criteria? *J. Comput. Assist. Tomogr.* **2015**, *39*, 317–320. [CrossRef] [PubMed]
43. Öztoprak, B.; Öztoprak, I.; Yıldız, Ö.K. The effect of venous anatomy on the morphology of multiple sclerosis lesions: A susceptibility-weighted imaging study. *Clin. Radiol.* **2016**, *71*, 418–426. [CrossRef] [PubMed]
44. Rogers, D.M.; Shah, L.M.; Wiggins, R.H. 3rd the central vein: Flair signal abnormalities associated with developmental venous anomalies in patients with multiple sclerosis. *AJNR Am. J. Neuroradiol.* **2018**, *39*, 2007–2013. [CrossRef]
45. Gaitán, M.I.; Sati, P.; Inati, S.J.; Reich, D.S. Initial investigation of the blood-brain barrier in MS lesions at 7 tesla. *Mult. Scler. Houndmills Basingstoke Engl.* **2013**, *19*, 1068–1073. [CrossRef]
46. Samaraweera, A.P.R.; Falah, Y.; Pitiot, A.; Dineen, R.A.; Morgan, P.S.; Evangelou, N. The MRI central vein marker; differentiating PPMS from RRMS and ischemic SVD. *Neurol. Neuroimmunol. Neuroinflamm.* **2018**, *5*. [CrossRef]
47. Al-Zandi, S.H.; Fayadh, N.A.H.; Al-Waely, N.K.N. Central vein sign detected by SWI at 3 T MRI as a discriminator between multiple sclerosis and leukoaraiosis. *Egypt. J. Radiol. Nucl. Med.* **2018**, *49*, 158–164. [CrossRef]
48. Clarke, M.A.; Pareto, D.; Pessini-Ferreira, L.; Arrambide, G.; Alberich, M.; Crescenzo, F.; Cappelle, S.; Tintoré, M.; Sastre-Garriga, J.; Auger, C.; et al. Value of 3T Susceptibility-Weighted Imaging in the Diagnosis of Multiple Sclerosis. *AJNR Am. J. Neuroradiol.* **2020**. [CrossRef]
49. Tallantyre, E.C.; Morgan, P.S.; Dixon, J.E.; Al-Radaideh, A.; Brookes, M.J.; Evangelou, N.; Morris, P.G. A comparison of 3T and 7T in the detection of small parenchymal veins within MS lesions. *Investig. Radiol.* **2009**, *44*, 491–494. [CrossRef]
50. Wuerfel, J.; Sinnecker, T.; Ringelstein, E.B.; Jarius, S.; Schwindt, W.; Niendorf, T.; Paul, F.; Kleffner, I.; Dörr, J. Lesion morphology at 7 Tesla MRI differentiates Susac syndrome from multiple sclerosis. *Mult. Scler. Houndmills Basingstoke Engl.* **2012**, *18*, 1592–1599. [CrossRef]
51. Sinnecker, T.; Clarke, M.A.; Meier, D.; Enzinger, C.; Calabrese, M.; De Stefano, N.; Pitiot, A.; Giorgio, A.; Schoonheim, M.M.; Paul, F.; et al. Evaluation of the central vein sign as a diagnostic imaging biomarker in multiple sclerosis. *JAMA Neurol.* **2019**, *76*. [CrossRef] [PubMed]
52. Darwish, E.A.F.; Ibrahim, Y.A.; Zamzam, D.A. Value of central vein sign in discriminating multiple sclerosis plaques from other white matter lesions. *Egypt. J. Radiol. Nucl. Med.* **2018**, *49*, 165–171. [CrossRef]
53. George, I.C.; Sati, P.; Absinta, M.; Cortese, I.C.; Sweeney, E.M.; Shea, C.D.; Reich, D.S. Clinical 3-tesla FLAIR* MRI improves diagnostic accuracy in multiple sclerosis. *Mult. Scler. Houndmills Basingstoke Engl.* **2016**, *22*, 1578–1586. [CrossRef] [PubMed]
54. Lummel, N.; Boeckh-Behrens, T.; Schoepf, V.; Burke, M.; Brückmann, H.; Linn, J. Presence of a central vein within white matter lesions on susceptibility weighted imaging: A specific finding for multiple sclerosis? *Neuroradiology* **2011**, *53*, 311–317. [CrossRef] [PubMed]
55. Luo, J.; Yablonskiy, D.A.; Hildebolt, C.F.; Lancia, S.; Cross, A.H. Gradient echo magnetic resonance imaging correlates with clinical measures and allows visualization of veins within multiple sclerosis lesions. *Mult. Scler. Houndmills Basingstoke Engl.* **2014**, *20*, 349–355. [CrossRef]

56. Grabner, G.; Dal-Bianco, A.; Schernthaner, M.; Vass, K.; Lassmann, H.; Trattnig, S. Analysis of multiple sclerosis lesions using a fusion of 3.0 T FLAIR and 7.0 T SWI phase: FLAIR SWI. *J. Magn. Reson. Imaging* **2011**, *33*, 543–549. [CrossRef] [PubMed]
57. Samaraweera, A.P.R.; Clarke, M.A.; Whitehead, A.; Falah, Y.; Driver, I.D.; Dineen, R.A.; Morgan, P.S.; Evangelou, N. The central vein sign in multiple sclerosis lesions is present irrespective of the T2* sequence at 3 T. *J. Neuroimaging Off. J. Am. Soc. Neuroimaging* **2017**, *27*, 114–121. [CrossRef]
58. Sinnecker, T.; Dörr, J.; Pfueller, C.F.; Harms, L.; Ruprecht, K.; Jarius, S.; Brück, W.; Niendorf, T.; Wuerfel, J.; Paul, F. Distinct lesion morphology at 7-T MRI differentiates neuromyelitis optica from multiple sclerosis. *Neurology* **2012**, *79*, 708–714. [CrossRef]
59. Gaitán, M.I.; de Alwis, M.P.; Sati, P.; Nair, G.; Reich, D.S. Multiple sclerosis shrinks intralesional, and enlarges extralesional, brain parenchymal veins. *Neurology* **2013**, *80*, 145–151. [CrossRef]
60. Thompson, A.J.; Banwell, B.L.; Barkhof, F.; Carroll, W.M.; Coetzee, T.; Comi, G.; Correale, J.; Fazekas, F.; Filippi, M.; Freedman, M.S.; et al. Diagnosis of multiple sclerosis: 2017 revisions of the McDonald criteria. *Lancet Neurol.* **2018**, *17*, 162–173. [CrossRef]
61. Hickey, W.F. The pathology of multiple sclerosis: A historical perspective1Supported in part by award NS 27321.1. *J. Neuroimmunol.* **1999**, *98*, 37–44. [CrossRef]
62. Liu, S.; Kullnat, J.; Bourdette, D.; Simon, J.; Kraemer, D.F.; Murchison, C.; Hamilton, B.E. Prevalence of brain magnetic resonance imaging meeting Barkhof and McDonald criteria for dissemination in space among headache patients. *Mult. Scler. J.* **2013**, *19*, 1101–1105. [CrossRef] [PubMed]
63. Dal-Bianco, A.; Hametner, S.; Grabner, G.; Schernthaner, M.; Kronnerwetter, C.; Reitner, A.; Vass, C.; Kircher, K.; Auff, E.; Leutmezer, F.; et al. Veins in plaques of multiple sclerosis patients—A longitudinal magnetic resonance imaging study at 7 Tesla. *Eur. Radiol.* **2015**, *25*, 2913–2920. [CrossRef] [PubMed]
64. Maggi, P.; Fartaria, M.J.; Jorge, J.; La Rosa, F.; Absinta, M.; Sati, P.; Meuli, R.; Du Pasquier, R.; Reich, D.S.; Cuadra, M.B.; et al. CVSnet: A machine learning approach for automated central vein sign assessment in multiple sclerosis. *NMR Biomed.* **2020**, *33*, e4283. [CrossRef] [PubMed]
65. Dworkin, J.D.; Sati, P.; Solomon, A.; Pham, D.L.; Watts, R.; Martin, M.L.; Ontaneda, D.; Schindler, M.K.; Reich, D.S.; Shinohara, R.T. Automated integration of multimodal mri for the probabilistic detection of the central vein sign in white matter lesions. *AJNR Am. J. Neuroradiol.* **2018**, *39*, 1806–1813. [CrossRef]
66. Raz, E.; Pontecorvo, S.; Barra, V.; Marincola, B.C.; Morreale, M.; Tinelli, E.; Saba, L.; Di Paolo, P.L.; Aceti, A.; Catalano, C.; et al. MR venography in patients with multiple sclerosis and correlation with clinical and MRI parameters. *J. Neuroimaging Off. J. Am. Soc. Neuroimaging* **2014**, *24*, 492–497. [CrossRef]
67. Maggi, P.; Mazzoni, L.N.; Moretti, M.; Grammatico, M.; Chiti, S.; Massacesi, L. SWI enhances vein detection using gadolinium in multiple sclerosis. *Acta Radiol. Open* **2015**, *4*, 2047981614560938. [CrossRef]

2

Altered PPARγ Expression Promotes Myelin-Induced Foam Cell Formation in Macrophages in Multiple Sclerosis

Elien Wouters [1], Elien Grajchen [1], Winde Jorissen [1], Tess Dierckx [1], Suzan Wetzels [2], Melanie Loix [1], Marie Paule Tulleners [1], Bart Staels [3], Piet Stinissen [1], Mansour Haidar [1], Jeroen F.J. Bogie [1] and Jerome J.A. Hendriks [1,*]

1 Department of Immunology and Infection, Biomedical Research Institute, Hasselt University, 3590 Diepenbeek, Belgium; elien.wouters@uhasselt.be (E.W.); elien.grajchen@uhasselt.be (E.G.); winde.jorissen@gmail.com (W.J.); tess.dierckx@uhasselt.be (T.D.); melanie.loix@uhasselt.be (M.L.); mariepaule.tulleners@uhasselt.be (M.P.T.); piet.stinissen@uhasselt.be (P.S.); mansour.haidar@uhasselt.be (M.H.); Jeroen.Bogie@uhasselt.be (J.F.J.B.)
2 Department of Pathology, CARIM, Maastricht University Medical Center, 6229 HX Maastricht, The Netherlands; suzan.wetzels@gmail.com
3 University of Lille, Inserm, CHU Lille, Institut Pasteur de Lille, U1011-EGID, F-59000 Lille, France; bart.Staels@pasteur-lille.fr
* Correspondence: jerome.hendriks@uhasselt.be

Abstract: Macrophages play a crucial role during the pathogenesis of multiple sclerosis (MS), a neuroinflammatory autoimmune disorder of the central nervous system. Important regulators of the metabolic and inflammatory phenotype of macrophages are liver X receptors (LXRs) and peroxisome proliferator-activated receptors (PPARs). Previously, it has been reported that PPARγ expression is decreased in peripheral blood mononuclear cells of MS patients. The goal of the present study was to determine to what extent *PPAR*γ, as well as the closely related nuclear receptors *PPAR*α and β and *LXR*α and β, are differentially expressed in monocytes from MS patients and how this change in expression affects the function of monocyte-derived macrophages. We demonstrate that monocytes of relapsing-remitting MS patients display a marked decrease in *PPAR*γ expression, while the expression of *PPAR*α and *LXR*α/β is not altered. Interestingly, exposure of monocyte-derived macrophages from healthy donors to MS-associated proinflammatory cytokines mimicked this reduction in *PPAR*γ expression. While a reduced *PPAR*γ expression did not affect the inflammatory and phagocytic properties of myelin-loaded macrophages, it did impact myelin processing by increasing the intracellular cholesterol load of myelin-phagocytosing macrophages. Collectively, our findings indicate that an inflammation-induced reduction in *PPAR*γ expression promotes myelin-induced foam cell formation in macrophages in MS.

Keywords: multiple sclerosis; myelin-loaded macrophages; inflammation; PPARγ

1. Introduction

Multiple sclerosis (MS) is a neurodegenerative autoimmune disease of the central nervous system (CNS) characterized by chronic inflammation, demyelination, and axonal degeneration. During MS, circulating monocytes are recruited to the site of CNS inflammation. At the lesion site, monocyte-derived macrophages (MDMs) mediate demyelination and neurodegeneration [1]. Conversely, MDMs can also stimulate repair by internalizing myelin debris or by producing anti-inflammatory and repair-promoting factors [2–5]. After the internalization of myelin, cholesterol—the main lipid constituent of myelin—is transported out of the cell via ATP-binding cassette transporters (e.g., ABCA1 and ABCG1) [6]. The efflux of cholesterol is essential to maintain intracellular lipid homeostasis and to prevent MDMs from becoming foamy. Nevertheless, a vast number of foamy macrophages containing abundant myelin remnants are found within demyelinating plaques of MS patients, indicating that lipid homeostasis is dysregulated in these cells [5,7].

Previously, we found that myelin uptake by bone marrow-derived mouse macrophages results in the activation of lipid sensing nuclear receptors (NRs), called peroxisome proliferator-activated receptors (PPARs) [8]. PPARs are ligand-activated transcription factors that control both lipid metabolism and inflammation [9]. Three PPAR isoforms have been identified, namely, PPARα (NR1C1), PPARβ/δ (NR1C2), and PPARγ (NR1C3). Upon ligand binding, PPARs form heterodimers with retinoic X receptors (RXRs) and bind to specific DNA regions, called hormone response elements, resulting in the transcriptional regulation of target genes. PPAR activation in macrophages results in the active transcription of genes involved in lipid uptake, transport, synthesis, and efflux, thereby controlling cellular lipid homeostasis [10]. Additionally, PPAR activation inhibits proinflammatory signaling pathways [11].

It is previously reported that PPARγ protein level is decreased in peripheral blood mononuclear cells (PBMCs) of MS patients [12]. Furthermore, stimulation of PBMCs with phytohemagglutinin (PHA), a mitogen that stimulates inflammation, significantly reduces PPARγ protein abundance [12]. In this study, we demonstrate that the expression of *PPARγ* is decreased in monocytes of relapsing-remitting MS (RR-MS) patients and that MS-associated proinflammatory cytokines IFNγ and IL1β reduce *PPARγ* expression. In addition, we find that PPARγ deficiency in myelin-containing macrophages has a significant impact on myelin processing by increasing the intracellular cholesterol load in these cells. Our findings highlight the importance of PPARγ in maintaining the intracellular lipid homeostasis in macrophages.

2. Results

2.1. The Inflammatory Environment in MS Reduces Macrophage PPARγ Expression

We determined to what extent *PPARγ*, as well as the closely related nuclear receptors *PPARα*, *β* and *LXRα*, *β*, are differentially expressed in monocytes from MS patients. For this purpose, CD14 positive cells from age- and gender-matched healthy donors and MS patients were isolated. Our data show that the mRNA expression of *PPARγ*, but not *LXRα*, *LXRβ*, nor *PPARα* was lower in monocytes of RR-MS patients compared to healthy donors (Figure 1A). No correlation of *PPARγ* expression with gender, disease activity, or therapy was observed in our samples. A negative correlation for *LXRβ* and age was found (Supplementary Figure S1). However, given the relatively small sample size, future studies should confirm the latter finding using a larger study cohort and identify possible correlations with other factors. No detectable levels of *PPARβ* were found in control and MS patient-derived monocytes (undetermined Ct values). Interestingly, monocytes from secondary progressive (SP)-MS patients did not display a reduced expression of *PPARγ* (Supplementary Figure S2A). Furthermore, the reduced *PPARγ* expression in monocytes of RR-MS patients was lost upon differentiation into macrophages in vitro (Supplementary Figure S2B). These findings suggest that disease-associated factors present in RR-MS patients, but not in SP-MS patients and in vitro cultures, maintain reduced *PPARγ* expression in myeloid cells.

Given overt systemic inflammation in RR-MS patients compared to SP-MS patients, we next defined whether inflammation impacts the expression of the different *LXR*- and *PPAR*-isoforms. Our data show that the expression of *PPARγ* as well as *PPARα* is suppressed by the inflammatory cytokines IFNγ and IL1β in in vitro differentiated MDMs. In contrast, the expression of *LXRs* was not influenced by inflammatory cytokines (Figure 1B). To investigate the individual effect of both cytokines, cells were treated with either IFNγ or IL1β. Here, we observed that IFNγ most potently decreased *PPARγ* expression (Figure 1C). Taken together, these results strongly suggest that inflammation reduces the expression of $PPAR\alpha$ and $PPAR\gamma$ in myeloid cells of MS patients, and that $PPAR\gamma$ is most susceptible to the inhibitory impact of inflammatory mediators.

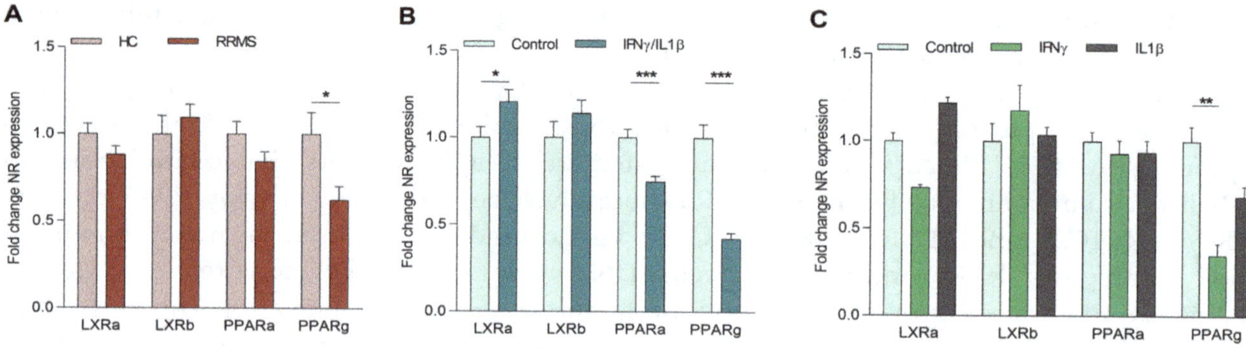

Figure 1. Inflammatory cytokines decrease *PPARγ* expression in macrophages. (**A**) Basal mRNA expression of *LXR*- and *PPAR*-isoforms in monocytes from age- and gender-matched healthy controls and relapsing-remitting multiple sclerosis (MS) patients ($n = 15$). (**B**) Gene expression of *LXR*- and *PPAR*-isoforms in monocyte-derived macrophages (MDMs) from healthy controls stimulated with IFNγ/IL1β ($n = 11$). (**C**) Gene expression of *LXR*- and *PPAR*-isoforms in MDMs from healthy controls stimulated with IFNγ or IL1β compared to nonstimulated cells ($n = 4$). RR-MS = relapsing-remitting MS patient; NR = nuclear receptor. Values represent the mean ± S.E.M. Statistical significance (**A**,**B**; unpaired Student's t-test, and **C**; one-way ANOVA with Dunn's multiple comparison correction) is indicated with asterisks: * $p \leq 0.05$, ** $p \leq 0.01$, and *** $p \leq 0.001$. n represents the total number of donors included in the experiment.

2.2. Myelin Uptake Activates PPARγ in Phagocytes

In the CNS of MS patients, infiltrated monocytes differentiate into macrophages and actively phagocytose myelin [5]. Given that fatty acids are present in myelin and are well-known endogenous ligands of PPARs, we next sought to determine if altered PPARγ activity affects the physiology of myelin-phagocytosing macrophages. For this purpose, we first determined whether myelin internalization activates PPARγ in these cells. To this end, MDMs from healthy donors (HCs) were exposed to isolated human myelin and/or the PPARγ specific agonist (rosiglitazone) and antagonist (GW9662). First, PPARγ activation through its ligand-binding domain was studied using a GAL-4-PPARγ LBD chimera reporter assay in cells treated with myelin for 24 h. As depicted in Figure 2A, myelin treatment resulted in a 2-fold increase in PPARγ activity. Given that in vitro differentiation into macrophages abolishes the reduced *PPARγ* expression observed in monocytes of RR-MS patients (Supplementary Figure S2B), and the fact that monocytes are notoriously inefficient phagocytes, we were unable to study the direct impact of reduced PPAR signaling in MS-derived monocytes on their function. Therefore, we studied if the PPAR antagonist GW9662 altered the macrophage response to myelin. Myelin induced the expression of the PPAR responsive genes *perilipin 2* (*PLIN2*) and *stearoyl-CoA desaturase-1* (*SCD1*). This induction was reduced by GW9662 (Figure 2B). While *ABCG1* expression was also increased upon myelin internalization, this did not depend on PPARγ activation (Figure 2B). Of interest, myelin also increased the expression of *PPARγ* (Figure 2C), suggesting a positive feedback loop that augments PPARγ signaling. The expression of *PLIN2*, *SCD1*, and *ABCG1* was also increased upon rosiglitazone treatment, confirming that these genes are regulated through PPARγ (Figure 2D). Next, we defined if an inflammatory environment and the consequent reduction in *PPARγ* expression impacts the capacity of myelin to induce *PPARγ* and the PPARγ-responsive gene *PLIN2* in MDMs from HCs. Our data demonstrate that myelin does not significantly induce *PPARγ* and *PLIN2* expression under inflammatory conditions (Figure 2E). Collectively, these data illustrate that myelin internalization results in the activation of PPARγ, and that the inflammation-associated reduction in *PPARγ* expression reduces the capacity of myelin to (auto)regulate *PPARγ* and *PLIN2* expression.

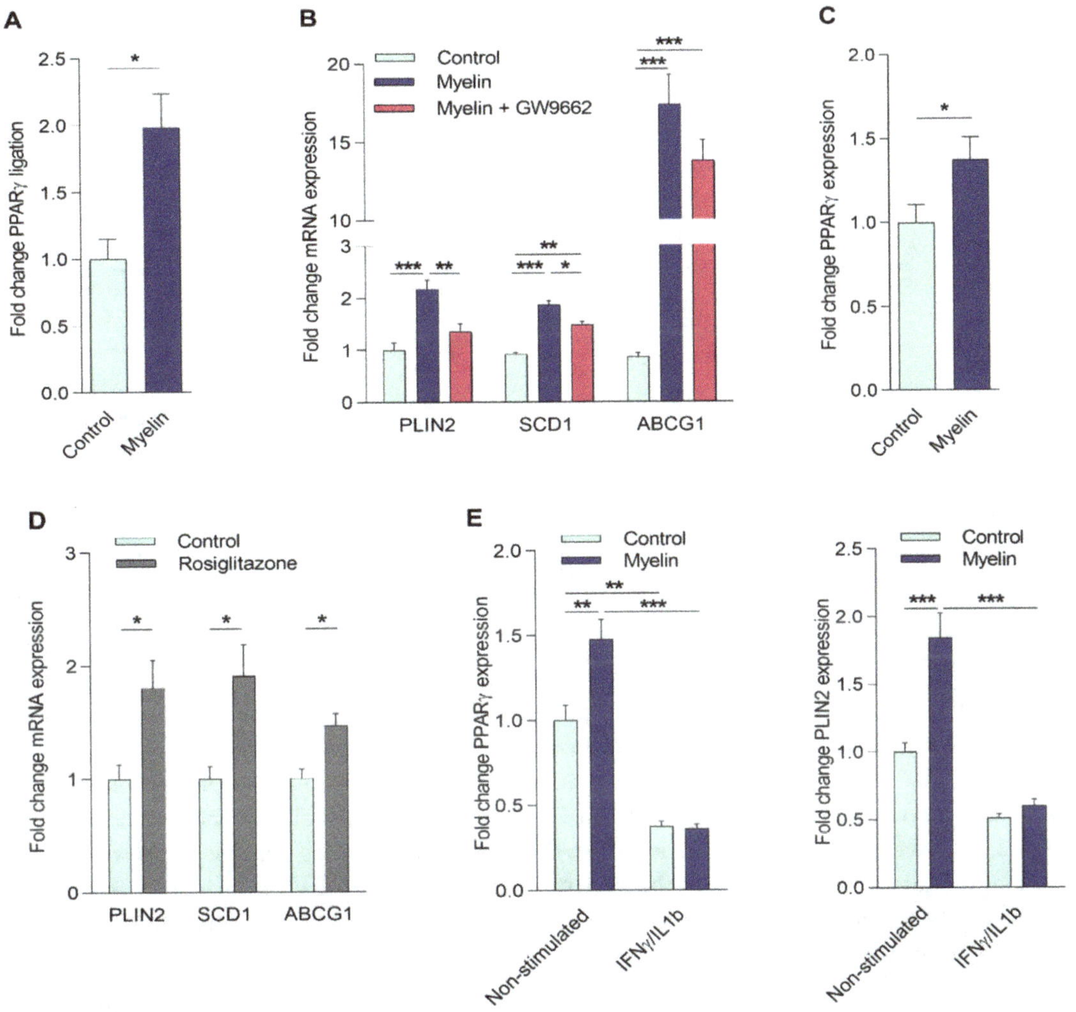

Figure 2. Myelin uptake activates PPARγ in phagocytes. (**A**) CHME3 cells treated with myelin or left untreated. PPARγ ligand-binding activity was determined using the GAL-4-PPARγ chimera assay system ($n = 5$). (**B**) mRNA expression of PPARγ response genes in MDMs from healthy controls (HCs) stimulated with myelin in the presence or absence of GW9662 (25 μM; $n = 8$). (**C**) *PPARγ* mRNA expression in MDMs from HCs treated with myelin compared to non-stimulated cells ($n = 11$). (**D**) mRNA expression of PPARγ response genes in MDMs from HCs stimulated with rosiglitazone (1 μM; $n = 9$). (**E**) *PPARγ* and perilipin 2 (*PLIN2*) expression in MDMs from HCs treated with IFNγ/IL1β, followed with or without stimulation with myelin ($n = 6$). Values represent the mean ± S.E.M. Statistical significance (**A**,**C**,**D**; Mann–Whitney test, **B**; one-way ANOVA with Tukey's multiple comparison correction, and **E**; two-way ANOVA with Sidak's multiple comparison correction) is indicated with asterisks: * $p \leq 0.05$, ** $p \leq 0.01$, and *** $p \leq 0.001$. n represents the total number of biological replicates (**A**) or donors (**B**–**E**) included in the experiment.

2.3. Myelin Controls the Inflammatory Phenotype of Macrophages Independently of PPARγ

Ample evidence indicates that myelin internalization modulates inflammatory gene expression in macrophages [8,13]. As PPARγ is well-known to suppress the inflammatory status of macrophages [11], we next defined whether PPARγ activation impacts the inflammatory phenotype of myelin-containing macrophages (mye-macrophages) [11]. Our data show that myelin uptake decreased TNFα expression, both on mRNA and protein level, in MDMs from healthy donors. However, this decrease did not reach statistical significance. In contrast, the PPARγ agonist rosiglitazone reduced IL6 expression (mRNA and protein), without affecting TNFα expression (Figure 3A,B). These results suggest that PPARγ is not the main regulator of myelin-induced changes in inflammatory gene expression. To confirm that myelin impacts the inflammatory phenotype in a PPARγ-independent manner, myelin-treated MDMs from HCs were exposed to the PPARγ antagonist GW9662. Inhibiting PPARγ activity did not change the expression of *TNFα* and *IL6* in myelin-treated MDMs, providing further evidence for the redundant role of PPARγ in driving the expression of these inflammatory genes in mye-macrophages (Figure 3C). Taken together, these data demonstrate that myelin uptake does not change the inflammatory phenotype of macrophages through the activation of PPARγ.

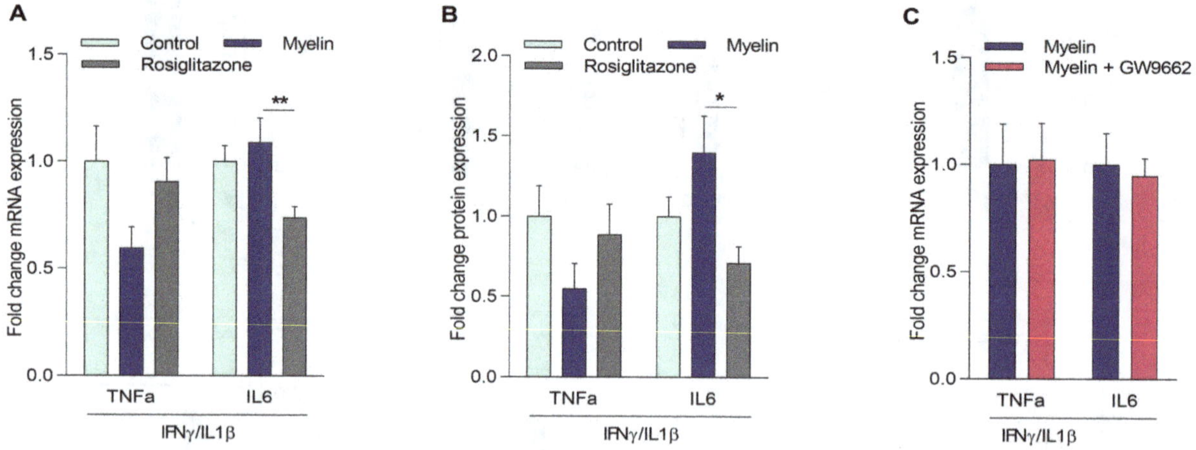

Figure 3. Myelin controls the inflammatory phenotype of mye-macrophages independently of PPARγ. MDMs from HCs treated with myelin, rosiglitazone, or left untreated, followed by incubation with IFNγ/IL1β ($n = 6$). *TNFα* and *IL6* mRNA expression levels (**A**) and protein expression levels (**B**) were detected. (**C**) *TNFα* expression in MDMs from HCs treated with myelin in the presence or absence of GW9662, followed by incubation with IFNγ/IL1β ($n = 4$). Values represent the mean ± S.E.M. Statistical significance (**A**,**B**; one-way ANOVA with Dunn's multiple comparison correction, and **C**; Mann–Whitney test) is indicated with asterisks: * $p \leq 0.05$, and ** $p \leq 0.01$. n represents the total number of donors included in the experiment.

2.4. Reduced PPARγ Activity Does Not Impact Myelin Phagocytosis but Hampers Intracellular Lipid Processing

MDMs of MS patients have a reduced capacity to phagocytose myelin [14]. As PPARs control the expression of phagocytic receptors involved in the uptake of myelin such as cluster of differentiation 36 (CD36) and scavenger receptor-A1 (SR-A1) [15,16], we assessed whether PPARγ controls myelin phagocytosis. First, we examined whether myelin-induced PPARγ activation increases the expression of *CD36* or *SR-A1*. By treating MDMs from healthy donors with myelin in the absence or presence of the PPARγ antagonist, we show that PPARγ did not significantly influence *CD36* or *SR-A1* mRNA expression in MDMs upon myelin uptake (Figure 4A). Next, the effect of PPARγ deficiency on the phagocytosis of myelin was determined. For this purpose, MDMs from HCs were exposed to DiI-labeled myelin in the presence or absence of GW9662. No change in DiI myelin phagocytosis was observed when PPARγ was inhibited (Figure 4B). These findings indicate that PPARγ does not regulate myelin internalization. A vast number of foamy macrophages containing abundant myelin remnants are found within demyelinating plaques of MS patients. Since PPARγ has been reported to be a crucial mediator of lipid processing [17,18], we next determined the effect of a reduced PPARγ activity on lipid storage after myelin uptake. By means of the Amplex^{TM} Red Cholesterol Assay, more cholesteryl esters (CEs) were detected inside mye-macrophages from HCs when PPARγ was inhibited (Figure 4C). In line with these results, an increased amount of lipid droplets (LDs) was observed in cells treated with the PPARγ antagonist after myelin uptake (Figure 4D). Similar as before, inefficient phagocytosis by monocytes and the negating effect of monocyte differentiation into macrophages on PPARγ expression did not allow us to confirm these findings directly in MS patient-derived monocytes and macrophages. Collectively, these data indicate that a reduced PPARγ activity promotes the formation of foamy macrophages without affecting the uptake of myelin.

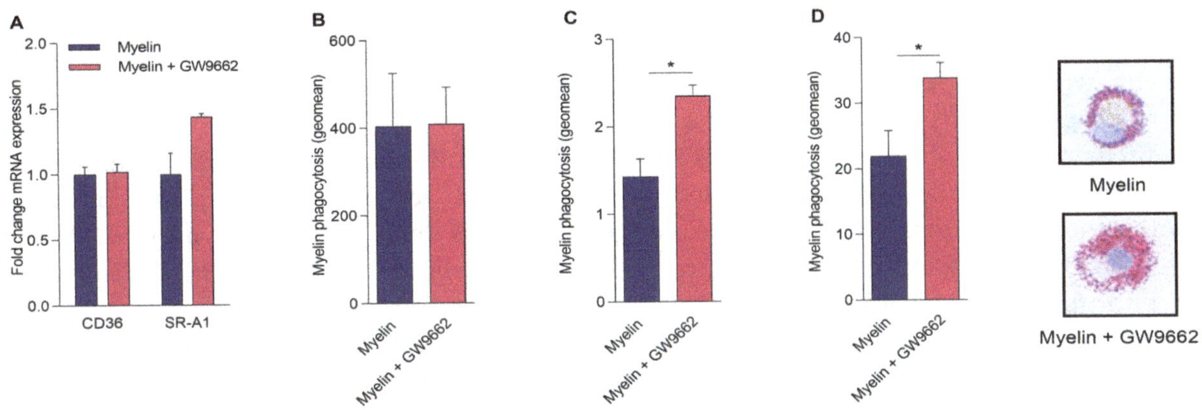

Figure 4. PPARγ controls the formation of lipid droplets in mye-macrophages but does not impact myelin phagocytosis. (**A**) cluster of differentiation 36 (*CD36*) and scavenger receptor-A1 (*SR-A1*) expression in MDMs from HCs pretreated with GW9662 or DMSO, followed by an incubation with myelin ($n = 5$). (**B**) DiI myelin phagocytosis by MDMs from HCs preincubated with GW9662 or DMSO ($n = 4$). (**C**) MDMs from HCs incubated with myelin in the absence or presence of GW9662. Cholesteryl esters (CE) load was measured using the Amplex™ Red Cholesterol Assay ($n = 4$). (**D**) MDMs from HCs incubated with myelin in the absence or presence of GW9662. Neutral lipids were stained and quantified using Oil red O (ORO) ($n = 5$). Values represent the mean ± S.E.M. Statistical significance (Mann–Whitney test) is indicated with asterisks: * $p \leq 0.05$. n represents the total number of donors included in the experiment.

3. Discussion

The activation of NRs such as LXRs and PPARs suppresses neuroinflammation by changing the metabolic and inflammatory properties of immune cells. Here, we show that an inflammation-induced reduction in *PPARγ* expression promotes myelin-induced foam cell formation in macrophages, which may negatively impact MS lesion progression.

Diverse studies demonstrated that inflammatory cytokine levels in biological fluids correlate with disease activity and the occurrence of relapses in MS patients [19,20]. Interestingly, our findings show that MS-associated inflammatory mediators reduce the expression of *PPARγ*, mimicking the *PPARγ* expression profile of monocytes in RR-MS patients. More specifically, IFNγ most prominently reduced *PPARγ* expression. IFNγ is secreted by activated immune cells, including Th1-cells, and is highly elevated in the serum and cerebrospinal fluid (CSF) of MS patients, as well as inside MS lesions [21,22]. Genetic ablation of IFNγ aggravates the disease course in experimental autoimmune encephalomyelitis (EAE), a well-established animal model of MS [23]. However, when IFNγ administration was tested as a clinical drug in MS patients, it resulted in an exacerbation of the disease activity [24,25]. Considering the protective impact of PPARγ activation on neuroinflammation, it is tempting to speculate that IFNγ partially promotes disease severity by reducing monocytic *PPARγ* expression. Our findings are in line with a previous study that showed that PPARγ expression is decreased in PBMCs of MS patients [12]. Collectively, our data show that the proinflammatory environment that is typically associated with MS decreases *PPARγ*, thereby potentially promoting MS disease progression.

PPARγ agonists are well-known to ameliorate disease activity in mice with EAE. In these animals, PPARγ activation reduces CNS inflammation by decreasing the expression of proinflammatory cytokines, including TNFα and IL6 [26–28]. In macrophages, PPARγ activation results in the retention of the NCoR corepressor complex at the promotor region of NF-kB target genes, keeping the expression of inflammatory genes in a repressed state [11]. Here, we demonstrate that myelin internalization increases the transcriptional activity of PPARγ in human macrophages. Nonetheless, phenotypic analysis showed that myelin impacts the inflammatory features of mye-macrophages in a PPARγ-independent manner. Based on these findings, the activation of other NRs likely explains the observed effects of myelin on the inflammatory phenotype of macrophages in our study. With respect to the latter, in a previous study we reported that myelin suppresses the inflammatory properties of myelin-containing mouse macrophages in a PPARβ/δ- and LXR-dependent manner [6,8,29]. Collectively, these findings indicate that myelin activates PPARγ but that this activation does not impact the inflammatory phenotype of human macrophages.

Inefficient clearance of myelin debris inhibits oligodendrocyte precursor cell differentiation. Hence, adequate uptake of myelin debris is essential for remyelination to occur [3,30]. Macrophages phagocytose myelin via scavenger receptors including CD36 and SR-A1 [16,31]. Although CD36 and SR-A1 expression is transcriptionally regulated by PPARγ [15,16], we show that myelin uptake does not increase *CD36* or *SR-A1* expression in macrophages, nor did PPARγ inhibition reduce the phagocytosis of myelin. In contrast to our findings, a study by Natrajan et al. demonstrated that PPARγ activation increases the uptake of myelin [32]. However, in the latter study the authors made use of synthetic PPARγ agonists to show that PPARγ activation has an additive effect on myelin phagocytosis. Here, we utilized a PPARγ antagonist to define the role of endogenous PPARγ activity in myelin uptake. Thus, our findings indicate that the reduced myeloid cell expression of PPARγ in RR-MS patients probably does not impact the capacity of these cells to internalize myelin debris.

Alongside controlling the phagocytic and inflammatory features of macrophages, PPARγ mediates the intracellular processing and efflux of lipids. In macrophages present in atherosclerotic plaques, PPARγ activation results in an increase in cholesterol efflux, and ultimately a reduction in foam cell formation [33]. The presence of foamy macrophages is also a characteristic of active MS lesions, indicating dysregulation of lipid metabolism inside these cells. Interestingly, we recently found that sustained intracellular accumulation of myelin debris in macrophages induces a highly inflammatory transcriptional profile [13]. Here, we demonstrate that mye-macrophages display a marked increase in LDs when PPARγ activity is reduced. This increase in LDs could be the result of a decrease in lipid processing or efflux [18]. At the level of lipid processing, PPAR-stimulation induces mitochondrial β-oxidation of fatty acids (FAs) via increasing the expression of carnitine palmitoyl transferase (CPT)1 [34]. A reduction in mitochondrial β-oxidation increases the availability of FAs for neutral lipid synthesis, thereby augmenting lipid droplet formation [35]. Additionally, PPAR activation induces reverse cholesterol transport by increasing the expression of ABCA1, ABCG1, and SR-B1 [18,36,37]. Blocking this efflux will result in the buildup of free cholesterol inside the cell which will be esterified and stored inside LDs to protect the cell from lipotoxicity. However, we did not find a difference in *ABCA1* and *ABCG1* mRNA expression after blocking PPARγ activity. Nevertheless, further research is necessary to study the expression and localization of these transporters at the protein level.

While our findings link decreased *PPARγ* expression to inflammation, levels of PPARγ and PLIN2 have been reported to be elevated in the spinal cord of EAE mice and in the CSF of MS patients [38,39]. This induction in PPARγ expression might reflect an endogenous protective mechanism to counteract the proinflammatory response during MS or an increase in infiltrating macrophages that express high levels of PPARγ. We show that the expression of LD-associated protein *PLIN2* is increased after PPARγ stimulation. PLIN2 is important for the stability of LDs in macrophages. Nevertheless, mye-macrophages display a marked increase in LDs when PPARγ activity is blocked. These findings indicate that either other factors in the lesion environment impact *PLIN2* expression, or that PPARs also control other (unidentified) processes that contribute to LD processing and biogenesis (e.g., β-oxidation and cholesterol efflux). Therefore, more research is warranted to unravel the molecular mechanisms that underlie the impact of PPARγ on the accumulation of LDs in mye-macrophages.

We found that differentiation of monocytes into macrophages in vitro nullifies the reduced *PPARγ* expression observed in monocytes of RR-MS patients. This finding confirms that the inflammatory microenvironment in RR-MS is essential for maintaining reduced PPARγ activation. This indicates that when inflammatory mediator production is resolved in MS lesions, PPAR function in macrophages will be restored. In future studies, it would be of interest to confirm these findings in post-mortem inflammatory and noninflammatory lesions of MS patients, or compare foamy phagocyte physiology in MS patients to individuals affected by non- or less-inflammatory demyelinating disorders such as adrenoleukodystrophy.

In conclusion, we report that PPARγ deficiency in mye-macrophages results in an increased intracellular lipid load. This study brings us closer to understanding the mechanisms by which PPARγ can modulate macrophage function and MS lesion progression, and may help in the development of therapeutic strategies to target MS.

4. Materials and Methods

4.1. Human Subjects

This study was approved by the Medical Ethics Committees of Hasselt University and UZ Leuven (UH-VAISMS-P1/S56441; March 2014). Written informed consent was obtained from all donors. A total of 22 HCs, 15 RR-MS patients, and 7 SP-MS patients were included in the study (Supplementary Table S1). RR-MS patients participating in the study were in remission at the time of sampling. MS patients were included independent of their treatment. Exclusion criteria for HCs and patients were reported hypercholesterolemia, cardiovascular diseases, diabetes, pregnancy, cancer, liver disease, and treatment with cholesterol modifying agents.

4.2. Cell Culture

PBMCs were isolated from whole blood using density gradient centrifugation, as previously described [40]. $CD14^+$ monocytes were collected by positive selection according to the manufacturer's guidelines (Stemcell Technologies, Grenoble, France). MDMs were obtained by culturing isolated monocytes (2×10^6 cells/mL) in MDM culture medium (DMEM-high glucose medium (Sigma-Aldrich, Diegem, Belgium) supplemented with 10% human serum (Sigma-Aldrich), 50 U/mL penicillin, 50 U/mL streptomycin, and 2 mM L-glutamine (Sigma-Aldrich)) at 37 °C, 5% CO_2. After 7 days, MDMs were collected using PBS/EDTA (10 mM) and plated at 0.5×10^6 cells/mL in MDM culture medium.

4.3. Human Myelin Isolation

Myelin was isolated from post-mortem nondemented human brain using sucrose density-gradient centrifugation, as previously described [41]. Briefly, tissue was homogenized in 0.32 M sucrose and layered over 0.85 M sucrose. The homogenate was ultra-centrifuged (75,000× g, 4 °C, 30 min) and crude myelin was collected from the interface. The collected myelin was washed in ddH_2O and subjected to osmotic disintegration. A second sucrose density-gradient centrifugation was carried out by dissolving the pellet in 0.32 M sucrose and layering it on top of 0.85 M sucrose. After ultracentrifugation (75,000× g, 4 °C, 30 min), the myelin-containing interface was collected, washed in ddH_2O, and dissolved in PBS. Myelin protein concentration was measured using the BCA protein assay kit (Thermo Fisher Scientific, Erembodegem, Belgium). The amount of endotoxin was determined using the Chromogenic Limulus Amebocyte Lysate assay kit (Genscript Incorperation, Aachen, Germany). Isolated myelin contained a negligible amount of endotoxin ($\leq 1.8 \times 10^{-3}$ pg/μg myelin) [42].

4.4. Macrophage Stimulation and Pharmacological Treatments

The effect of a proinflammatory environment on mRNA expression was measured by treating cells with IFNγ and/or IL1β (100 ng/mL, PeproTech, London, UK) for 6 h. To study PPARγ expression and activity, MDMs were stimulated with myelin (100 μg/mL), rosiglitazone (PPARγ agonist, 1 μM, Sigma-Aldrich), or dimethylsulfoxide (DMSO; Leuven, Belgium) for 24 h, in the presence or absence of the PPARγ antagonist, GW9662 (25 μM, Sigma-Aldrich) or IFNγ/IL1β (100 ng/mL). Inflammatory gene expression was measured after treating cells with myelin (100 μg/mL) or rosiglitazone (1 μM) for 18 h, followed by incubation with IFNγ/IL1β (100 ng/mL) for 6 h. GW9662 (25 μM) was added to the myelin conditions to study the involvement of PPARγ in myelin-induced suppression of inflammatory gene expression.

4.5. RNA Extraction and Real-Time Quantitative PCR (RT-qPCR)

Total RNA was isolated with Qiazol (Qiagen, Venlo, The Netherlands) and the RNeasy mini kit (Qiagen), according to the manufacturer's guidelines. A NanoDrop spectrophotometer (Isogen Life Science, De Meern, The Netherlands) was used to determine RNA concentration and purity. RNA was reverse-transcribed using qScriptTM cDNA SuperMix (Quanta Biosciences, VWR, Leuven, Belgium) according to the manufacturer's instructions. RT-qPCR was conducted on a Step One Plus detection system (Applied biosystems, Foster City, CA, USA). Cycle conditions were 95 °C for 20 s, followed by 40 cycles of 95 °C for 3 s, and 60 °C for 30 s. The PCR reaction mixture contained SYBR green master mix (Thermo Fisher Scientific), 0.3 μM forward and reverse primer (IDT technologies, Leuven, Belgium), RNase free water, and 12.5 ng cDNA template in a total reaction volume of 10 μL. Relative quantitation of gene expression was accomplished using the comparative Ct method. Data were normalized to the most stable reference genes. Primers used for RT-qPCR are shown in Supplementary Table S2.

4.6. Enzyme-Linked Immunosorbent Assay (ELISA)

MDMs were pretreated for 18 h with myelin (100 μg/mL), rosiglitazone (1 μM), or DMSO, followed by an incubation with IFNγ/IL1β (100 ng/mL) for 24 h. Afterwards, medium was collected, centrifuged at 1400 rpm for 10 min, and diluted 1/10. TNFα and IL6 protein expression was measured using ELISA (eBioscience, San Diego, CA, USA). Absorbance was determined by a microplate reader (BIORAD iMarkTM Microplate Reader, Temse, Belgium) at 450 nm.

4.7. Luciferase Assay

Human CHME3 microglial cells were cultured in DMEM-high glucose medium supplemented with 10% fetal bovine serum (Invitrogen, Merelbeke, Belgium), 50 U/mL penicillin, and 50 U/mL streptomycin at 37 °C, 5% CO_2. CHME3 cells were transfected overnight with plasmids using JetPEI® transfection reagent (Polyplus, Illkirch, France), according to the manufacturer's protocol. Plasmids used for transfection encoded for pG5-TK-GL3 (GAL5), pCMV-Bgal, and PPARγ (kindly provided by Prof. dr. Bart Staels, University of Lille, France). Following transfection, cells were serum starved for 5 h. Afterwards, CHME3 cells were treated with myelin (100 μg/mL, 24 h) and lysed in lysis buffer (25 mM Gly-Gly (Sigma-Aldrich), 1% Triton (Sigma-Aldrich), 15 mM $MgSO_4$ (Sigma-Aldrich), and 4 mM EGTA (Sigma-Aldrich)). Ligation of myelin components to PPARγ was measured using the ONE-Glo™ Luciferase Assay System kit (Promega, Leiden, The Netherlands). Luminescence was determined with the FLUOstar optima microplate reader (BMG Labtech, Ortenberg, Germany). To study transfection efficacy, β-galactosidase was measured using B-gal buffer (80% Buffer Z (100 mM Na_2HPO_4, 10 mM KCl, 1 mM $MgSO_4$, 0.05 mM 2-mercaptoethanol) and 20% ONGP buffer (13.28 mM ONGP, 82 mM Na_2HPO_4, 18 mM NaH_2PO_4). Absorbance was determined at 410 nm by the FLUOstar optima microplate reader.

4.8. Flow Cytometry

To study myelin phagocytosis, isolated myelin (10 mg/mL) was fluorescently labelled with 12.5 μg/mL 1,1″-diotadecyl-3,3,3′,3′,-tetramethylindocarbocyanide perchlorate (DiI; Sigma-Aldrich) for 30 min at 37 °C, as previously described [43]. MDMs were pretreated with GW9662 (25 μM) or DMSO for 30 min, followed by an incubation with DiI-labeled myelin (100 μg/mL, 1.5 h) at 37 °C, 5% CO_2. DiI fluorescence was measured using a FACS Calibur flow cytometer (BD biosciences, Erembodegem, Belgium).

4.9. Cholesteryl Ester (CE) Determination

MDMs were preincubated with GW9662 (25 μM) or DMSO for 30 min, followed by an incubation with myelin (100 μg/mL) for 24 h. CEs were measured using the Amplex™ Red Cholesterol Assay Kit (Thermo Fisher Scientific), according to manufacturer's instructions. Briefly, cells were washed twice with PBS after treatment and lysed in Amplex™ Red reaction buffer. Amplex™ Red working solution, with or without cholesterol esterase was added to the cell lysate and incubated at 37 °C protected from light. After 30 min, fluorescence was measured at an excitation wavelength of 540 nm and an emission wavelength of 590 nm using the FLUOstar optima microplate reader. CE concentration was calculated by subtracting free cholesterol concentration from total cholesterol concentration.

4.10. Oil Red O (ORO) Staining and Quantification

MDMs were preincubated with GW9662 (25 μM) or DMSO for 30 min, followed by an incubation with myelin (100 μg/mL) for 24 h. Cells were fixed in 4% paraformaldehyde (Sigma-Aldrich) for 20 min at RT. Neutral lipids were stained using ORO (Sigma-Aldrich) in 60% isopropanol for 10 min. Following incubation, unbound particles were washed away with deionized water. For the ORO staining, coverslips were counterstained with Mayer's hematoxylin for 60 s to visualize nuclei. Afterwards, cells were rinsed in running tab water and mounted on microscope slides with aqueous mounting solution. Representative images were taken using a Leica DM2000 LED microscope (Leica Microsystems, Wetzlar, Germany). For ORO quantification, ORO was extracted by incubating the cells with isopropanol for 10 min, while shaking. Absorbance was measured using a microplate reader (BIORAD iMark™ Microplate Reader) at 510 nm.

4.11. Statistical Analysis

MS patients were diagnosed based on the 2017 McDonald criteria [44]. Multiple linear regression models for each dependent response variable were fitted using SPSS Statistics 25.0 (SPSS, Chicago, IL, USA). A backward-elimination approach was performed in each multiple linear regression model until all remaining variables had $p < 0.05$. Data were statistically analyzed using GraphPad Prism v6 (GraphPad Software, La Jolla, CA, USA) and are reported as mean ± standard error of the mean (S.E.M.). D'Agostino-Pearson omnibus normality test was used to test normal distribution. One-way analysis of variance (ANOVA) with Tukey's multiple comparison correction, two-way ANOVA with Sidak's multiple comparison correction, or two-tailed unpaired Student's t-test were used for normally distributed data sets. The Mann–Whitney analysis or one-way ANOVA with Dunn's multiple comparison correction was used for data sets which did not pass normality. * $p \leq 0.05$, ** $p \leq 0.01$, and *** $p \leq 0.001$.

Author Contributions: Conceptualization, E.W., J.F.J.B. and J.J.A.H.; formal analysis, E.W.; funding acquisition, P.S., J.F.J.B. and J.J.A.H.; investigation, E.W., E.G., W.J., T.D., S.W., M.L. and M.P.T.; methodology, E.W., J.F.J.B. and J.J.A.H.; project administration, E.W.; resources, B.S. and J.J.A.H.; supervision, J.F.J.B. and J.J.A.H.; validation, E.W.; writing—original draft, E.W.; writing—review and editing, M.H., J.F.J.B. and J.J.A.H. All authors have read and agreed to the published version of the manuscript.

Abbreviations

ABCA1	ATP-binding cassette transporter A1
ABCG1	ATP-binding cassette transporter G1
ANOVA	Analysis of variance
CD36	Cluster of differentiation 36
CE	Cholesteryl ester
CNS	Central nervous system
CPT1	Carnitine palmitoyl transferase 1

CSF	Cerebrospinal fluid
DiI	1,1″-diotadecyl-3,3,3′,3′,-tetramethylindocarbocyanide perchlorate
DMSO	Dimethylsulfoxide
EAE	Experimental autoimmune encephalomyelitis
ELISA	Enzyme-linked immunosorbent assay
FA	Fatty acids
HC	Healthy control
LD	Lipid droplet
LXR	Liver X receptor
MDM	Monocyte-derived macrophage
MS	Multiple sclerosis
NCoR	Nuclear receptor co-repressor
NR	Nuclear receptor
ORO	Oil red O
PBMC	Peripheral blood mononuclear cell
PHA	Phytohemagglutinin
PLIN2	Perilipin 2
PPAR	Peroxisome proliferator-activated receptor
RR-MS	Relapsing-remitting MS
RT-qPCR	Real-time quantitative PCR
RXR	Retinoid X receptor
SCD1	Stearoyl-CoA desaturase-1
S.E.M.	Standard error of the mean
SP-MS	Secondary progressive MS
SR-A1	Scavenger receptor-A1
SR-B1	Scavenger receptor-B1

References

1. Bogie, J.F.; Stinissen, P.; Hendriks, J.J. Macrophage subsets and microglia in multiple sclerosis. *Acta Neuropathol.* **2014**, *128*, 191–213. [CrossRef]
2. Jiang, Z.; Jiang, J.X.; Zhang, G.X. Macrophages: A double-edged sword in experimental autoimmune encephalomyelitis. *Immunol. Lett.* **2014**, *160*, 17–22. [CrossRef] [PubMed]
3. Kotter, M.R.; Zhao, C.; van Rooijen, N.; Franklin, J.M.R. Macrophage-depletion induced impairment of experimental CNS remyelination is associated with a reduced oligodendrocyte progenitor cell response and altered growth factor expression. *Neurobiol. Dis.* **2005**, *18*, 166–175. [CrossRef] [PubMed]
4. Nally, F.K.; De Santi, C.; McCoy, C.E. Nanomodulation of macrophages in multiple sclerosis. *Cells* **2019**, *8*, 543. [CrossRef] [PubMed]
5. Grajchen, E.; Hendriks, J.J.A.; Bogie, J.F.J. The physiology of foamy phagocytes in multiple sclerosis. *Acta Neuropathol. Commun.* **2018**, *6*, 124. [CrossRef]
6. Bogie, J.F.; Timmermans, S.; Huynh-Thu, V.A.; Irrthum, A.; Smeets, J.M.H.; Gustafsson, J.-A.; Steffensen, K.R.; Mulder, M.; Stinissen, P.; Hellings, N. Myelin-derived lipids modulate macrophage activity by liver X receptor activation. *PLoS ONE* **2012**, *7*, e44998. [CrossRef]
7. Kuhlmann, T.; Ludwin, S.; Prat, A.; Antel, J.; Bruck, W.; Lassmann, H. An updated histological classification system for multiple sclerosis lesions. *Acta Neuropathol.* **2017**, *133*, 13–24. [CrossRef]
8. Bogie, J.F.; Jorissen, W.; Mailleux, J.; Nijland, P.G.; Zelcer, N.; Vanmierlo, T.; Van Horssen, J.; Stinissen, P.; Hellings, N.; Hendriks, J.J.A. Myelin alters the inflammatory phenotype of macrophages by activating PPARs. *Acta Neuropathol. Commun.* **2013**, *1*, 43. [CrossRef]
9. Bensinger, S.J.; Tontonoz, P. Integration of metabolism and inflammation by lipid-activated nuclear receptors. *Nature* **2008**, *454*, 470–477. [CrossRef]

10. Rigamonti, E.; Chinetti-Gbaguidi, G.; Staels, B. Regulation of macrophage functions by PPAR-alpha, PPAR-gamma, and LXRs in mice and men. *Arterioscler. Thromb. Vasc. Biol.* **2008**, *28*, 1050–1059. [CrossRef]
11. Bougarne, N.; Weyers, B.; Desemet, S.J.; Deckers, J.; Ray, D.W.; Staels, B.; De Bosscher, K. Molecular actions of PPARalpha in lipid metabolism and inflammation. *Endocr. Rev.* **2018**, *39*, 760–802. [CrossRef] [PubMed]
12. Klotz, L.; Schmidt, M.; Giese, T.; Sastre, M.; Knolle, P.; Klockgether, T.; Heneka, M.T. Proinflammatory stimulation and pioglitazone treatment regulate peroxisome proliferator-activated receptor gamma levels in peripheral blood mononuclear cells from healthy controls and multiple sclerosis patients. *J. Immunol.* **2005**, *175*, 4948–4955. [CrossRef] [PubMed]
13. Bogie, J.F.J.; Grajchen, E.; Wouters, E.; Corales Garcia, A.; Dierckx, T.; Vanherle, S.; Mailleux, J.; Gervois, P.; Wolfs, E.; Dehairs, J.; et al. Stearoyl-CoA desaturase-1 impairs the reparative properties of macrophages and microglia in the brain. *J. Exp. Med.* **2020**, *217*, e20191660. [CrossRef] [PubMed]
14. Healy, L.M.; Ho Jang, J.; Won, S.J.; Lin, H.; Touil, H.; Aljarallah, S.; Bar-Or, A.; Antel, J.P. MerTK-mediated regulation of myelin phagocytosis by macrophages generated from patients with MS. *Neurol. Neuroimmunol. Neuroinflamm.* **2017**, *4*, e402. [CrossRef] [PubMed]
15. Moore, K.J.; Rosen, E.D.; Fitzgerald, M.L.; Randow, F.; Andersson, L.P.; Altshuler, D.; Milstone, D.S.; Mortensen, R.M.; Spiegelman, B.M.; Freeman, M.W. The role of PPAR-gamma in macrophage differentiation and cholesterol uptake. *Nat. Med.* **2001**, *7*, 41–47. [CrossRef] [PubMed]
16. Reichert, F.; Rotshenker, S. Complement-receptor-3 and scavenger-receptor-AI/II mediated myelin phagocytosis in microglia and macrophages. *Neurobiol. Dis.* **2003**, *12*, 65–72. [CrossRef]
17. Argmann, C.A.; Sawyez, C.G.; McNeil, C.J.; Hegele, R.A.; Huff, M.W. Activation of peroxisome proliferator-activated receptor gamma and retinoid X receptor results in net depletion of cellular cholesteryl esters in macrophages exposed to oxidized lipoproteins. *Arterioscler. Thromb. Vasc. Biol.* **2003**, *23*, 475–482. [CrossRef]
18. Chinetti, G.; Lestavel, S.; Bocher, V.; Remaley, A.T.; Neve, B.; Torra, I.P.; Teissier, E.; Minnich, A.; Jaye, M.; Duverger, N.; et al. PPAR-alpha and PPAR-gamma activators induce cholesterol removal from human macrophage foam cells through stimulation of the ABCA1 pathway. *Nat. Med.* **2001**, *7*, 53–58. [CrossRef]
19. Van Boxel-Dezaire, A.H.; Hoff, S.C.; van Oosten, B.W.; Verweij, C.L.; Dräger, A.M.; Adèr, H.J.; van Houwelingen, J.C.; Barkhof, F.; Polman, C.H.; Nagelkerken, L. Decreased interleukin-10 and increased interleukin-12p40 mRNA are associated with disease activity and characterize different disease stages in multiple sclerosis. *Ann. Neurol.* **1999**, *45*, 695–703. [CrossRef]
20. Rieckmann, P.; Albertch, M.; Kitze, B.; Weber, T.; Tumani, H.; Broocks, A.; Luer, W.; Helvig, A.; Poser, S. Tumor necrosis factor-alpha messenger RNA expression in patients with relapsing-remitting multiple sclerosis is associated with disease activity. *Ann. Neurol.* **1995**, *37*, 82–88. [CrossRef]
21. Khaibullin, T.; Ivanova, V. Elevated levels of proinflammatory cytokines in cerebrospinal fluid of multiple sclerosis patients. *Front. Immunol.* **2017**, *8*, 531. [CrossRef] [PubMed]
22. Lees, J.R.; Cross, A.H. A little stress is good: IFN-gamma, demyelination, and multiple sclerosis. *J. Clin. Investig.* **2007**, *117*, 297–299. [CrossRef] [PubMed]
23. Chu, C.Q.; Wittmer, S.; Dalton, D.K. Failure to suppress the expansion of the activated CD4 T cell population in interferon gamma-deficient mice leads to exacerbation of experimental autoimmune encephalomyelitis. *J. Exp. Med.* **2000**, *192*, 123–128. [CrossRef] [PubMed]
24. Panitch, H.S.; Haley, A.S. Exacerbations of multiple sclerosis in patients treated with gamma interferon. *Lancet* **1987**, *1*, 893–895. [CrossRef]
25. Panitch, H.S.; Hirsch, R.L.; Schindler, J.; Johnson, K.P. Treatment of multiple sclerosis with gamma interferon: Exacerbations associated with activation of the immune system. *Neurology* **1987**, *37*, 1097–1102. [CrossRef]
26. Niino, M.; Iwabuchi, K.; Kikuchi, S.; Ato, M.; Morohashi, T.; Ogata, A.; Tashiro, K.; Onoe, K. Amelioration of experimental autoimmune encephalomyelitis in C57BL/6 mice by an agonist of peroxisome proliferator-activated receptor-gamma. *J. Neuroimmunol.* **2001**, *116*, 40–48. [CrossRef]
27. Storer, P.D.; Xu, J.; Chavis, J.; Drew, P.D. Peroxisome proliferator-activated receptor-gamma agonists inhibit the activation of microglia and astrocytes: Implications for multiple sclerosis. *J. Neuroimmunol.* **2005**, *161*, 113–122. [CrossRef]
28. Schett, G. Physiological effects of modulating the interleukin-6 axis. *Rheumatology* **2018**, *57* (Suppl. S2), ii43–ii50. [CrossRef]

29. Mailleux, J.; Vanmierlo, T.; Bogie, J.F.J.; Wouters, E.; Lutjohann, D.; Hendriks, J.J.A.; van Horssen, J. Active liver X receptor signaling in phagocytes in multiple sclerosis lesions. *Mult. Scler.* **2018**, *24*, 279–289. [CrossRef]
30. Kotter, M.R.; Li, W.W.; Zhao, C.; Franklin, R.J.M. Myelin impairs CNS remyelination by inhibiting oligodendrocyte precursor cell differentiation. *J. Neurosci.* **2006**, *26*, 328–332. [CrossRef]
31. Zhu, Y.; Lyapichev, D.H.L.; Motti, D.; Ferraro, N.M.; Zhang, Y.; Yahn, S.; Soderblom, C.; Zha, J.; Bethea, Z.J.R.; Spiller, K.L. Macrophage transcriptional profile identifies lipid catabolic pathways that can be therapeutically targeted after spinal cord injury. *J. Neurosci.* **2017**, *37*, 2362–2376. [CrossRef] [PubMed]
32. Natrajan, M.S.; Komori, M.; Kosa, P.; Johnson, K.R.; Wu, T.; Franklin, R.J.M.; Bielekova, B. Pioglitazone regulates myelin phagocytosis and multiple sclerosis monocytes. *Ann. Clin. Transl. Neurol.* **2015**, *2*, 1071–1084. [CrossRef] [PubMed]
33. Wang, N.; Yin, R.; Liu, Y.; Guangmei, Y.L.; Mao, G.; Xi, F. Role of peroxisome proliferator-activated receptor-gamma in atherosclerosis: An update. *Circ. J.* **2011**, *75*, 528–535. [CrossRef] [PubMed]
34. Chinetti, G.; Lestavel, S.; Fruchart, J.-C.; Clavey, V.; Staels, B. Peroxisome proliferator-activated receptor alpha reduces cholesterol esterification in macrophages. *Circ. Res.* **2003**, *92*, 212–217. [CrossRef] [PubMed]
35. Boren, J.; Brindle, K.M. Apoptosis-induced mitochondrial dysfunction causes cytoplasmic lipid droplet formation. *Cell Death Differ.* **2012**, *19*, 1561–1570. [CrossRef]
36. Chawla, A.; Boisvert, W.A.; Lee, C.-H.; Laffitte, B.A.; Barak, Y.; Joseph, S.B.; Liao, D.; Nagy, L.; Edwards, P.A. A PPAR gamma-LXR-ABCA1 pathway in macrophages is involved in cholesterol efflux and atherogenesis. *Mol. Cell* **2001**, *7*, 161–171. [CrossRef]
37. Chinetti, G.; Gbaguidi, F.C.; Griglio, S.; Mallat, Z.; Antonucci, M.; Poulain, P.; Chapman, J.; Frucgart, J.C.; Tedgui, A.; Fruchart, J.N. CLA-1/SR-BI is expressed in atherosclerotic lesion macrophages and regulated by activators of peroxisome proliferator-activated receptors. *Circulation* **2000**, *101*, 2411–2417. [CrossRef]
38. Diab, A.; Deng, C.; Smith, J.D.; Hussain, R.Z.; Phanavanh, B.; Lovett-Racke, A.E.; Drew, P.D.; Racke, K.M. Peroxisome proliferator-activated receptor-gamma agonist 15-deoxy-Delta(12,14)-prostaglandin J(2) ameliorates experimental autoimmune encephalomyelitis. *J. Immunol.* **2002**, *168*, 2508–2515. [CrossRef]
39. Szalardy, L.; Zadori, D.; Tanzos, E.; Simu, M.; Bencsik, K.; Vecsei, L.; Klivenyi, P. Elevated levels of PPAR-gamma in the cerebrospinal fluid of patients with multiple sclerosis. *Neurosci. Lett.* **2013**, *554*, 131–134. [CrossRef]
40. Jorissen, W.; Wouters, E.; Bogie, J.F.; Vanmierlo, T.; Noben, J.-P.; Sviridov, D.; Hellings, N.; Somers, V.; Valcke, R.; Vanwijmeersch, B. Relapsing-remitting multiple sclerosis patients display an altered lipoprotein profile with dysfunctional HDL. *Sci Rep.* **2017**, *7*, 43410. [CrossRef]
41. Bogie, J.F.; Mailleux, J.; Wouters, E.; Jorissen, W.; Grajchen, E.; Vanmol, J.; Wouters, K.; Hellings, N.; van Horssen, J.; Vanmierlo, T. Scavenger receptor collectin placenta 1 is a novel receptor involved in the uptake of myelin by phagocytes. *Sci. Rep.* **2017**, *7*, 44794. [CrossRef] [PubMed]
42. Bogie, J.F.; Stinissen, P.; Hellings, N.; Hendriks, J.J.A. Myelin-phagocytosing macrophages modulate autoreactive T cell proliferation. *J. Neuroinflam.* **2011**, *8*, 85. [CrossRef] [PubMed]
43. Van der Laan, L.J.; Ruuls, S.R.; Weber, K.S.; Lodder, I.J.; Dopp, E.A.; Dijkstra, C.D. Macrophage phagocytosis of myelin in vitro determined by flow cytometry: Phagocytosis is mediated by CR3 and induces production of tumor necrosis factor-alpha and nitric oxide. *J. Neuroimmunol.* **1996**, *70*, 145–152. [CrossRef]
44. Thompson, A.J.; Banwell, B.L.; Barkof, B.; Caroll, W.M.; Coetzee, T.; Comi, G.; Correale, J.; Fazekas, F.; Filippi, M.; Fujihara, K. Diagnosis of multiple sclerosis: 2017 revisions of the McDonald criteria. *Lancet Neurol.* **2018**, *17*, 162–173. [CrossRef]

3

Assessment and Impact of Cognitive Impairment in Multiple Sclerosis

Miguel Ángel Macías Islas [1,*] and Ethel Ciampi [2]

1 Department of Neurosciences, CUCS. University of Guadalajara and Mexico, Guadalajara 44160, Mexico
2 Neurology, Pontificia Universidad Católica de Chile, Neurology, Hospital Dr. Sótero del Río, Santiago 8320000, Chile; ethelciampi@gmail.com
* Correspondence: miguelangelmacias@hotmail.com;

Abstract: Cognitive impairment affects 40–60% of patients with multiple sclerosis. It may be present early in the course of the disease and has an impact on a patient's employability, social interactions, and quality of life. In the last three decades, an increasing interest in diagnosis and management of cognitive impairment has arisen. Neuropsychological assessment and neuroimaging studies focusing on cognitive impairment are now being incorporated as primary outcomes in clinical trials. However, there are still key uncertainties concerning the underlying mechanisms of damage, neural basis, sensitivity and validity of neuropsychological tests, and efficacy of pharmacological and non-pharmacological interventions. The present article aimed to present an overview of the assessment, neural correlates, and impact of cognitive impairment in multiple sclerosis.

Keywords: multiple sclerosis; demyelinating diseases; cognitive impairment; cognitive dysfunction

1. Introduction

Multiple sclerosis (MS) is a chronic inflammatory demyelinating disease of the central nervous system (CNS). Typically, the disease affects the brain, spinal cord, and optic nerves, with acute inflammation as seen during MS relapses, and variable degrees of chronic inflammation and neurodegenerative processes within the white and gray matter, associated with progressive accumulation of disability. In about 85% of the patients, MS begins as a relapsing-remitting course and secondarily evolves to a progressive stage (secondary-progressive MS) in about 15–30% of patients [1,2]. From the onset, about 15% of the patients will develop a primary progressive course [3].

Most people experience their first symptoms of MS between the ages of 20 and 40. The clinical heterogeneity of MS, as well as the findings of different pathological patterns, suggests that MS may be a spectrum of diseases representing different processes [4–7]. MS can be clinically categorized in different phenotypes, including clinically isolated syndrome (CIS), relapsing/remitting (RRMS), primary progressive and secondary progressive MS (SPMS), and can be subclassified according to its clinical and radiological activity [8]. These phenotypes are related to potentially different pathophysiological disease mechanisms, including acute/chronic inflammation, axonal/neuronal loss and gliosis, and variable degrees of tissue repair, as well as plasticity and clinical recovery, mainly related to each individual [7], although these differences have yet to be demonstrated at the molecular level [2].

Clinical symptoms of MS may include motor dysfunction (pyramidal); tremor, dysmetria, or ataxia (cerebellar); diplopia or nystagmus (brainstem); numbness (sensory); urinary/bowel hesitancy, incontinence, or retention; disturbances in vision and cognitive impairment. The latter functional systems can be measured with the Expanded Disability Status Scale (EDSS), which range from 0 (normal neurological examination), to 10 (death due to MS) [9], and although it is the most widely used disability score worldwide, cognitive impairment related to the disease seems fairly underrepresented, even when cognitive and neuropsychiatric symptoms are a major cause of disability, loss of employment, and poor quality of life of patients and their families [10].

Although more than a century ago J.M. Charcot described "marked enfeeblement of the memory" with "conceptions that are formed slowly" in persons with "sclérose en plaques" [11], this elegant clinical observation was almost forgotten for more than a hundred years as a remarkable symptom of what is now known as MS. In 1991, S. Rao brought renewed attention to cognitive impairment in MS patients [12]. Since then, it has been a topic of clinical and basic research, trying to reveal the precise mechanisms behind its presentation, in order to develop effective treatments that include cognitive impairment as an outcome in clinical trials, many of them with unsatisfactory results [13].

The following manuscript is not a systematic review about the topic, but an overview that aims to raise awareness on the cognitive deficits in MS, including the most affected cognitive domains and related neuropsychological batteries for their assessment, their neural correlates with an emphasis on neuroimaging, and a potential therapeutic approach as well as future perspectives.

2. Cognitive Impairment in Multiple Sclerosis

Cognition represents the function of several neural pathways involved in the processing of information in the brain, including several correlated and interdependent cognitive domains such as executive function, perceptual-motor function, language, learning and memory, complex attention, and social cognition, as defined by the Diagnostic and Statistical Manual of Mental Disorders 5th edition (DSM-5) [14]. Impairment of individual domains may cause dysfunction of the global cognitive performance [15].

Although impairment in cognitive function occurs in different neurologic diseases, the clinical syndromes, the degree of dysfunction, and related disability, depend on the involvement of different brain structures (cortical or subcortical), the extent of neural damage or number of affected domains, and the patient's previous cognitive reserve and performance. In MS, as a heterogeneous disease, all of the aforementioned characteristics makes it even more difficult to study cognition as a single manifestation of the disease [16,17].

Despite advances in knowledge about the neural basis of cognitive function in MS, there are still key uncertainties concerning what it is called 'normal cognition', and consequently with the assessment of cognitive dysfunction, typically defined as a performance below a chosen threshold in a number of cognitive domains, assessed in a specific neuropsychological test (e.g., 1.5–2 standard deviations below normal of a *Z*-score of one or more cognitive domains). In these batteries, results are commonly expressed as "intact/preserved" or "impaired" [18], and prevalent studies usually differ in cognitive impairment definitions.

Almost thirty years ago, in a population-based study performed by S. Rao et al., a 45% frequency of cognitive impairment in MS was found [12]. Other epidemiological studies reported frequencies of cognitive impairment in patients with MS between 40–70% in North America and Europe [19]. Frequencies of 40–60% have been reported in Latin America [20]. Even though a variety of different methodological approaches and neuropsychological batteries have been used, results are very similar across all reported populations.

MS is commonly diagnosed during a patient's most productive life period, and employment years and cognitive impairment supposes a severe impact over a patient's behavior, social functioning, adaptative strategies, and profound functional limitations affecting the activities of daily living and employment [10,21]. A large cross-sectional study carried out in nine European countries showed that only 35.8% of MS patients were employed. Low mood and cognitive impairment affecting domains like memory, attention, and slowed information processing speed were reported as frequent determinants of work-related difficulties, but only working memory impairment was responsible for higher unemployment rates [22]. Employment provides higher quality of life, independence, social participation, personal and professional reaffirmation, monetary income, health insurance, financial support for medication, and in some countries access to work benefits and social security [23], so cognition should be a priority in an era with highly active treatments reducing relapses and new lesions, and even new horizons in preventing accumulation of physical disability with new disease modifying treatments available [2].

A review by Shiavolin et al. concluded that difficulties that people with MS can experience with employment are always secondary outcomes of research, and it is quite difficult to address which factors contribute to reduced work participation. In their review, fatigue, mobility reduction, and cognitive impairment were reported as the main drivers of unemployment, and unemployment was related with worse quality of life scores [21].

In the same line, social cognition has gained relevance as a non-traditional cognitive domain present in MS since early stages of the disease, a domain that has been related to the capability for developing deep social interactions [24]. Recent evidence has shown 20% of social cognition impairment among patients, with a similar distribution for different phenotypes [25], and social cognition deficits show a significant correlation with the performance in other cognitive domains as working memory, processing speed, and executive functions [26–28] and exhibit behavioral impact affecting moral evaluation of other individuals' actions [29].

Finally, cognitive impairment not only affects patients, but also affects their relationship with their families and is a frequent complaint of higher burden for caregivers [21]. Mickens et al. studied the mediational effect on the relationships between MS impairments (neurological, cognitive, behavioral, emotional, and functional), unmet family needs (household information, financial, social, support, and health), and caregiver mental health (satisfaction with life, anxiety, burden, and depression) using a structural equation model. They suggested that intervention research on MS caregivers in Latin America may consider focusing on caregiver mental health problems by addressing unmet family needs and teaching caregivers' ways to manage the impairments of the individual with MS [30].

3. Cognitive Domains

All cognitive domains may be affected in MS, but the most affected ones are episodic memory and information processing speed [17,31]. Working memory, executive function, verbal fluency, and attention have also been widely described [12,32,33], with a recent interest in social cognition impairment [24,34]. Although clinical phenotypes may differ in the prevalence or severity of cognitive impairment, main determinants are physical disability as measured by EDSS, and patients' age [35]. Other individual characteristics such as gender, genetic factors, and cognitive reserve may also play a relevant role [36]. For a summary of the most frequent cognitive domains affected in MS see Table 1.

Table 1. Frequency of cognitive impairment in patients with multiple sclerosis (MS) by cognitive domain.

Cognitive Domain	Frequency
Learning Memory	**40–65%**
Visual Episodic Memory	20–75%
Verbal Episodic Memory	15–80%
Complex Attention	**5–25%**
Information processing Speed	15–50%
Executive Function	**15–25%**
Working Memory	15–60%
Inhibitory control	15–30%
Language	**20–58%**
Verbal Fluency	15–25%
Social Cognition	**20–40%**

MS: Multiple sclerosis. Adapted from Rao et al. 1991 [12], Benedict et al. 2006 [32], Chiaravaloti et al. 2008 [17], Dulau 2017 [25], Cotter et al. 2018 [34], Ciampi et al. 2018 [37], Ntoskou et al. 2018 [38].

3.1. Learning Memory

Long-term memory refers to the ability to learn new information and to recall that information at a later time point [39]. It is the most consistently affected cognitive domain in MS patients. Impaired learning of new information seems to be the primary problem [36], but the encoding, storing, and retrieval from long-term storage processes of memory seems to be affected in MS patients, so there is still controversy about which of these components of memory is the most influential factor for explaining memory deficits [40]. Other factors, such as slow processing speed, susceptibility to interference, executive disfunction, and perceptual deficits can also determine poor learning abilities [41].

3.2. Complex Attention—Information Processing

Complex attention domain involves sustained attention, divided attention, selective attention, and processing speed [42]. MS patients usually present with deficits in information processing efficiency, which refers to the ability to maintain and manipulate information in the brain for a short time period (working memory–executive function) [43] and to the speed with which one can process that information (processing speed–complex attention) [44]. It represents a key cognitive deficit in MS patients and might contribute to the presence of impairment in other cognitive domains [45,46].

3.3. Executive Function

Executive function is a complex domain which involves goal-directed behavior to adapt individuals to changes and demands of the environment, including planning, decision-making, working memory, responding to feedback, inhibition, and flexibility [42], and is affected in around 20% of MS patients. Some studies claim the difficulty to differentiate executive impairment from information processing, due to most of the tests used to evaluate executive function imply integrity of information processing and are affected by emotional affections such as depression. Leavitt et al. [47] studied executive functions and speed tasks (trail making test and Wisconsin card sorting test) in MS patients versus healthy controls. They found that MS patients score worse than controls, but differences decreased when corrected for information processing. They concluded that slow information processing accounts for executive function deficits in MS patients. The difficulty in assessing a specific domain, such as executive function, may be extrapolated to all other domains, as cognitive abilities are assessed individually in optimal environments, but patients usually struggle with managing multiple goals simultaneously [18].

3.4. Language

The language domain includes tasks such as object naming, word finding, fluency, grammar and syntax, and receptive language [42]. In MS, language deficits have been less studied than episodic memories or information processing speed. While some articles show intact functionality [48], more recent studies report frequencies of language impairment between 20% and 58% in RRMS or SPMS, respectively [38]. The most affected tasks seem to be phonological and semantic fluency, although verbal fluency tests are directly influenced by executive functions, thus many of the deficits have been considered as due to a dysfunctional executive syndrome [39].

3.5. Social Cognition

Social cognition, including social perception, empathy and theory of the mind, focuses on how people process, store, and apply information about other people and social situations, guiding social interactions [24]. Therefore, it is the sum of these processes that allow subjects of the same species to interact and exchange social codes to obtain information about another's behavior, and about the environment [49]. Its recent inclusion within the six main cognitive domains of the DSM-5, and its association with quality of life and employment, have raised awareness among MS researchers in the last years [34].

Social perception has been defined as the ability to perceive information about the mental state of other subjects based on behavioral signals [50]. Empathy refers to the generation of an emotional response in the observer to situations affecting other subjects (e.g., same or different emotion), and it is an essential component of human emotional experience and social interaction, because when an observed mental state is understood, and affective responses are generated, prosocial and cooperative behaviors can exist [51,52]. Theory of the mind is the ability to represent the psychological perspective of interacting subjects, requiring an internal theorization about their thoughts and beliefs, emotions, affective states, and feelings [53].

Recent studies have shown 20–40% of social cognition impairment in MS patients, with similar distribution across phenotypes, greater impact in theory of the mind tasks, as well as in the recognition of certain negative facial emotion expressions [25,34]. It also seems that social cognition interacts with other cognitive domains, although a distinct patter of association with an exclusive domain (e.g., executive functions) has not been demonstrated [34,37].

4. Neuropsychological Assessment

Cognitive function assessment in MS patients should become a part of everyday clinical practice and as a constant outcome in clinical trials. Ideally, every patient with a diagnosis of MS should undergo a complete neuropsychological assessment and routinely repeat a standardized and validated battery to detect clinically meaningful changes, as well as start a timely and effective treatment, similar to what the Magnetic Resonance Imaging in MS (MAGNIMS) group has proposed for the MRI protocols in the diagnosis and monitoring of the disease [54,55]. Nonetheless, this desire from the cognitive research community has many obstacles, including key knowledge gaps and methodological limitations related to the understanding and measurement of cognitive deficits, neuroimaging of neural bases and correlations of deficits, as well as the development of effective treatments [18].

Mini-Mental State Examination by Folstein in 1975, which was used for dementia, is not sensitive to MS cognitive disorders [56]. The three most frequently used neurocognitive batteries in MS are: (1) The Brief Repeatable Battery of Neuropsychological tests (BRB-N), also known as Rao's battery [57], (2) the minimal assessment of cognitive function in MS (MACFIMS) introduced by Benedict et al. [32], and (3) the Brief International Cognitive Assessment for Multiple Sclerosis (BICAMS), a shorter version that was developed in 2012 by an expert team, and is recommended for small centers with one or few staff members who may not have neuropsychological training [58]. All these screening batteries allow to establish the presence or absence of cognitive dysfunction and the specific domains affected. All of them have similarities and differences but share the fact that they are sensitive, specific, and cover the most frequently affected cognitive domains, and are also reasonably brief.

It is important to note that BICAMS should not be used within one month of recovery from relapse or within one month of steroid therapy, and the recommended order of administration is first the Symbol Digit Modalities Test (SDMT), then the California Verbal Learning Test (CVLT-II T1-5), and then the Brief Visuospatial Memory Test Revised (BVMT-R T1-3). In most clinical situations, yearly or bi-annual BICAMS evaluations will be appropriate.

Emphasis in testing MS cognitive impairment must be focused on the assessment of the most frequently affected domains, learning/memory, and information processing speed. In this context, experts are encouraging the MS multidisciplinary team (e.g., neurologists, nurses, psychologists, speech therapists, etc.) to be trained to use short MS cognitive assessment batteries, such as the BICAMS [12]. The subtests that compose the structure of domain specific evaluation of these batteries are shown in Table 2.

Table 2. Comparison of the three most used neuropsychological batteries in MS.

Cognitive Domain	BRB-N	MACFIMS	BICAMS
Auditory processing speed and working memory	PASAT	PASAT	-
Visual processing speed and working memory	SDMT	SDMT	SDMT
Auditory or verbal episodic memory	SRT	CVLT-II	CVLT-II
Visual or spatial episodic memory	10/36 Spatial Recall Test	BVMT-R	BVMT-R
Expressive language	COWAT	COWAT	-
Spatial processing	-	JLO	-
Executive function	-	DKEFS sorting	-

MS: Multiple sclerosis, BRB-N: Brief Repeatable Battery of Neuropsychological tests, MACFIMS: Minimal assessment of cognitive function in MS, BICAMS: Brief International Cognitive Assessment for Multiple Sclerosis, PASAT: Paced Auditory Serial Addition, SDMT: Symbol Digit Modalities Test, SRT: Selective Reminding Test, CVLT-II: California Verbal Learning Test, BVMT-R: Brief Visuospatial Memory Test Revised, COWAT: Controlled Oral Word Association Test, JLO: Judgement of Line Orientation test, DKEFS: Delis-Kaplan Executive Function System.

For the purpose of this review, we will describe the components of the BICAMS battery, due to its extensive use and validation in many countries, as well as the PASAT as being included as the cognitive test in MSFC, as well as a brief summary of social cognition tasks.

4.1. *Information Processing Speed: Symbol Digit Modalities Test (SDMT)*

When SDMT was first published in 1982, there were precedents of similar formats since 1927 and was adopted by the United States Army to assess precisely the speed of substitution of symbols by digits. SDMT has been used in almost every MS cognitive assessment battery and found to be exceptionally reliable and sensitive to assess information processing speed. The test consists of single digits paired with abstract symbols, with rows of the nine symbols arranged pseudo-randomly. The patient must say (or write) the number that corresponds with each symbol. The SDMT can be completed within 5 min, including instructions, practice, and testing. The SDMT has a reported sensitivity of 82% and a specificity of 60% [59]. It is the most sensitive task in MS, with good to excellent reliability, well tolerated by patients, has uniformity across languages, with no floor or ceiling effects, and a preliminary clinically meaningful change of 3–4 points [59], so it is recommended for clinical practice and research [18].

4.2. *Episodic Verbal Memory: California Learning Verbal Test (CVLT)*

This comprises of a 16-item word list, with four items belonging to each of the four categories, arranged randomly. The list is read aloud five times in the same order to the patient, at a slightly slower rate than one item per second. Patients are required to recall as many items as possible, in any order, after each reading. The CVLT-II T1-5 [60] can be completed in 5–10 min. It is recommended for clinical use, and it has high sensitivity with good age and sex adjusted normative data [18].

4.3. *Episodic Visuospatial Memory: Brief Visuospatial Memory Test Revised (BVMT-R)*

The BVMT-R T1-3 requires the patient to inspect a 2 × 3 stimulus array of abstract geometric figures. There are three learning trials of 10 s. The array is removed, and the patient is required to draw the array from memory, with the correct shapes in the correct position. It is also recommended for clinical and research use and has high sensitivity, it is time efficient, and is well tolerated by patients. Its main disadvantage is for patients with severe motor impairment [18].

4.4. *Working Memory: Paced Auditory Serial Addition Test (PASAT-3")*

The PASAT is a measure of cognitive function that specifically assesses auditory information processing speed and flexibility, as well as calculation ability [61]. Stimulus presentation rates were adapted for use with MS patients by Rao and colleagues in 1989, and the measure has been widely used in MS studies since then. Single digits are presented either every 3" (or every 2" for the optional PASAT-2", which could be a more accurate assessment of information processing speed) and the patient must add each new digit to the one immediately prior to it. The test score is the number of correct sums given (out of 60 possible sums) in each trial. To minimize familiarity with stimulus items in clinical trials and other serial studies, two alternate forms have been developed; the order of these should be counterbalanced across testing sessions [62,63]. Although it has been widely used in clinical research and clinical trials, and it has been included within the MSFC, there are several disadvantages to this test including a limited reliability due to practice effects, susceptibility to ceiling effect, poor tolerability due to a patient's math ability, and test-related anxiety. Therefore, it is not recommended for cognitive monitoring in clinical practice, nor for clinical trials designed with multiple administrations, but it is better used as a putative cognitive processing task to compare results across previous studies [18].

4.5. Social Cognition

The assessment of social cognition in MS include a myriad of tests used in other neurological disorders, for example the Face and Emotion Recognition (e.g., Ekman faces [64]) for social perception, Faux Pas, or Reading the Mind in the Eyes tests for theory of the mind tasks, or compound batteries previously used in other neurological disorders such as in frontotemporal dementia (e.g., Social Emotion Assessment [65,66]). For example, the mini-Social and Emotional Assessment test (mini-SEA) includes the Faux Pas and the Face Emotion Recognition. The Faux Pas is comprised by ten narrative vignettes or short stories in which a character inadvertently hurts or offends another, using Theory of the Mind tasks to infer another's mental state, making attributions to their knowledge, beliefs, and emotions. Half of the vignette test is control stories and the other half includes a principal character who inadvertently hurts or offends another, the 'victim of the Faux Pas'. The subject is expected to recognize the situations in which a Faux Pas is committed, why the leading character did it (cognitive theory of mind, he did not mean it), and how the victim of the Faux Pas must have felt (affective theory of mind, we expect him to recognize that the victim must have had a negative emotion). The Face Emotion Recognition consists of 35 pictures for face affect recognition of basic emotions among a list presented at the bottom of the screen including happiness, sadness, anger, surprise, fear, disgust, and neutral [66].

There is still the need for a consensus statement from expert groups to select those tests with best sensitivity, specificity, and reliability in MS.

5. Neural Basis of Cognitive Impairment in MS

Underlying neural mechanisms of cognitive damage can be related to the inflammatory and neurodegenerative changes in the MS brain, including grey and white matter structures, both globally and regionally, structurally, and functionally [67]. Although one can appreciate some of these changes at a single-subject level (Figure 1), routine measurements (e.g., brain atrophy) are still not suggested to be used in clinical practice, mainly due to biological changes (e.g., dehydration, pseudo atrophy, etc.), that can exceed the accuracy threshold of current brain analysis software [55]. On the other hand, a myriad of group-analysis studies have been published trying to unveil the neural basis of cognitive impairment in MS. Differences in the results obtained by various studies may represent biased sample selection and differences between the image technology and software utilized in reported studies. Nonetheless, in vivo studies of neural correlations may contribute to early diagnosis, monitoring, and treatment of cognitive impairment in MS.

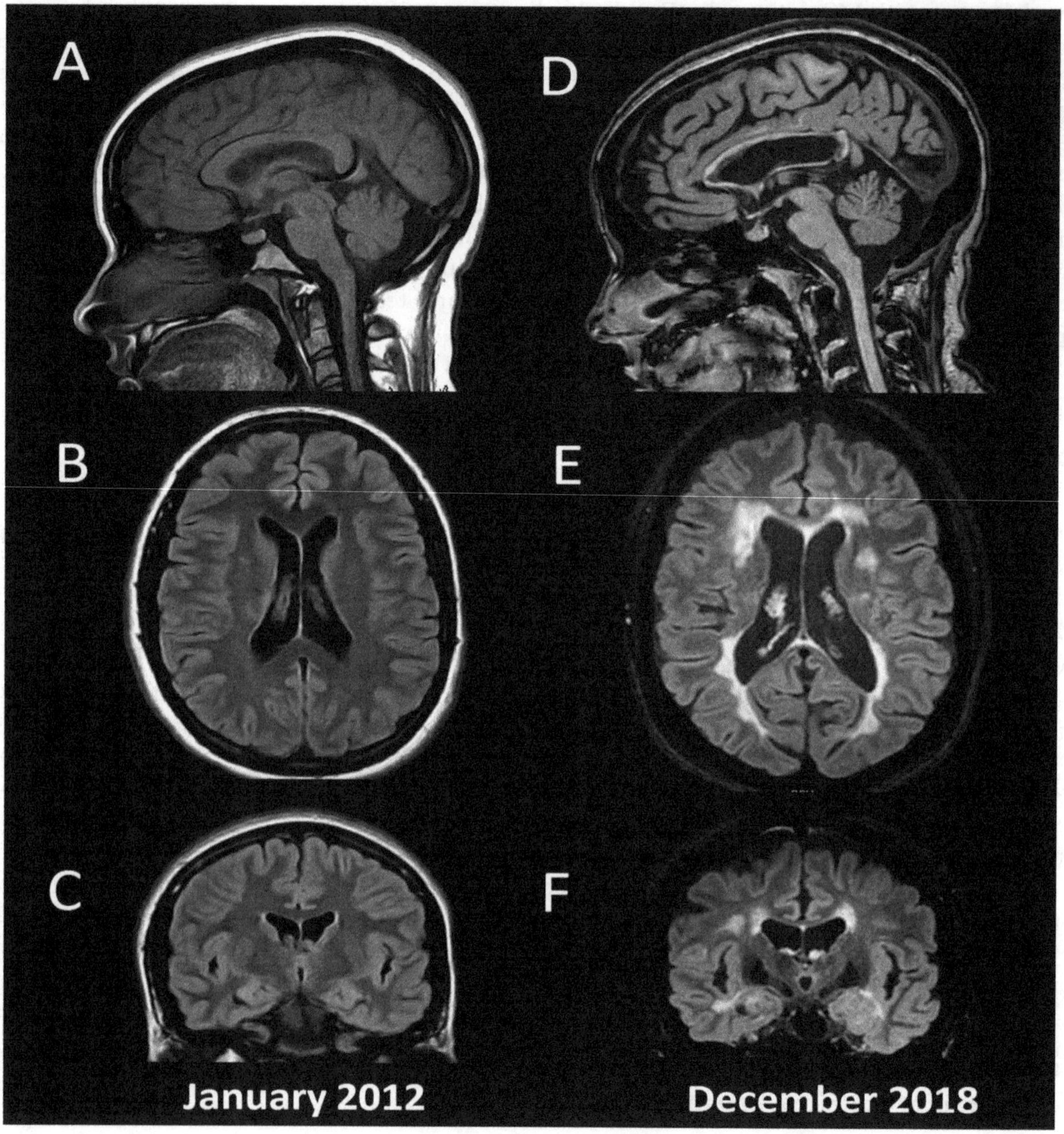

Figure 1. Conventional MRI in a patient with multiple sclerosis and cognitive impairment. Baseline MRI (**A**: Sagittal T1, **B**: Axial FLAIR, **C**: Coronal FLAIR) from a 15-year-old female with fulminant MS (Marburg variant, EDSS 8.0). After initial aggressive treatment in 2012, including myeloablation with cyclophosphamide, the patient remained asymptomatic without disease modifying treatment, until a second supratentorial motor relapse in 2015, confirming her MS diagnosis and beginning fingolimod. Since then, no relapses or new T2/enhancing lesions have appeared, and she had an EDSS 1.0 by the time of the second MRI in 2018 (**D**: Sagittal T1, **E**: Axial FLAIR, **F**: Coronal FLAIR). Her Mini-Mental State Examination was 30 (normal), Beck Depression Inventory 4 (without depression), and her fatigue severity score was 4 (significative fatigue). She had below normal performance ($\leq$1.5 standard deviation) in verbal and visual episodic memory, and in information processing speed tests, with the diagnosis of cognitive impairment according to the MACFIMS battery. Note the widespread brain volume loss including cortical grey matter, ventricular width, and corpus callosum atrophy. The patient gave her written informed consent to present this data.

Structural imaging comprise of measurements of brain volume loss (atrophy), which can include global measurements, such as cross-sectional or longitudinal volumetric or 3D whole brain volume loss using semi-automated software (e.g., brain parenchymal fraction (BPF) [68], structural image evaluation using normalization of atrophy SIENAX—SIENA [69,70]), regional measurements of different tissues (e.g., grey matter or white matter volume, also measured by SIENAX), or specific grey or white matter structures (e.g., using voxel-based morphometry or Free Surfer for regional tissue volume loss or cortical thickness, respectively [71]), as well as manual/linear or 2D assessments such as the Corpus Callosum Index [72–74], or the third ventricle width, the frontal horn width, and the intercaudate distance [75].

From a functional point of view, although positron emission tomography (PET) and single photon emission computed tomography (SPECT) have shown correlations between cerebral blood flow and oxygen use with cognitive impairment in MS patients [76,77], functional MRI (fMRI) has gained its place among cognitive researchers in assessing the neural correlates of disability in MS, with an special emphasis on early changes, with a potential role for treatment monitoring (e.g., during cognitive rehabilitation) [78].

Also, recent interest has developed in the study of water diffusivity in normal-appearing white matter (regions of the white matter where no lesion is seen in conventional MRI studies), using diffusion tensor imaging (DTI), that can be related both with structural and functional disconnection between different regions of the brain [79]. Other non-conventional and advanced MRI techniques are also in study, including magnetization transfer imaging (MTI), proton MR spectroscopy (^{1}H-MRS), and iron imaging [80].

Cognitive impairment has been associated with linear measure changes [75], the extent of white matter lesions and lesion load [29,33,37], focal cortical lesions [81], whole brain atrophy [82], diffuse cortical atrophy [81,83,84], regional grey matter structures such as thalamus, caudate, putamen, hippocampus, and amygdala, cerebellum and corpus callosum [67,85], as well as with widespread subtle pathological changes in normal-appearing white matter [83,86], among others.

Neuroanatomical correlates of memory deficits seem to differ across disease stages [87]. Early brain volume loss is a very precise predictor for the presence of cognitive impairment years later [82,83], and although hippocampal atrophy was not significantly seen in patients with CIS suggestive of MS compared with healthy controls in a study using DTI, hippocampal fractional anisotropy was significantly decreased in CIS patients, and mean diffusivity was correlated with verbal episodic memory performance [88]. An interesting study showed that a predictive model of cognitive performance in MS should include bilateral posterior cingulate cortex and bilateral temporal pole cortical thickness, overall white matter lesion load, normal-appearing white matter integrity, and age, reaffirming the multifactorial etiology of MS cognitive impairment [84].

Episodic memory has been correlated with total grey matter and regional cortical structures (e.g., left precuneus [89]); visuospatial memory has been associated with brain MRI total lesion area, T1 lesion, and FLAIR lesion volume, BPF, third ventricular width, and right superior frontal atrophy, among others [90,91]; verbal episodic memory has been associated with total and regional hippocampal atrophy, total lesion load and BPF [90–93]; information processing speed has been correlated with thalamus, whole grey matter atrophy, and third ventricle width [94], cerebellum atrophy [95,96], as well as with less white matter integrity, and increases in functional connectivity [79]; executive disfunction has been associated with frontal lobe structural and functional damage [97,98] and with dorsolateral prefrontal, orbitofrontal, anterior cingulate, and insular areas [99], as well as with thalamic structural and functional changes [100]; PASAT-3" scores have been correlated with cortical and subcortical structures such as bilateral precuneus, posterior cingulate, caudate putamen, and cerebellum [101], and acute changes in PASAT score with no physical changes (EDSS) have been associated with presence of acute gadolinium enhancing lesions [102], with similar results observe with transient SDMT changes [103], proposing that patients could also experience "cognitive relapses".

Concerning social cognition, when assessing regional gray matter atrophy in a cohort of progressive MS patients with social cognitive impairment, significant loss was seen within bilateral cortical regions of orbitofrontal, insula and cerebellum, and right regions of fusiform gyrus, and precuneus [37], while functional MRI studies have shown increased activation in the posterior cingulate cortex and precuneus for the identification of anger and disgust faces, and greater activity in the occipital fusiform gyri, the anterior cingulate, and the inferior frontal cortex for the recognition of neutral faces [104]. Also, increased lesion volume has been correlated with lower success in face emotion recognition [105]. When assessing theory of the mind tasks, it seems that a disconnection syndrome, caused by white matter lesions, could also be one of the possible mechanisms underlying this specific impairment [105–109].

Other regions of interest associated with cognitive performance in multiple cognitive domains include the thalamus, as a relay station or cortico-subcortical and cortico-cortical networks [85] (e.g., global cognitive disfunction, information processing speed, attention, verbal memory, spatial memory, verbal fluency, executive function) [91,110–112]; the cerebellum, as a historically understudied region for cognitive performance (attention, working memory, information processing speed, etc.) [37,95,96]; and the corpus callosum, the main white matter tract of the brain (e.g., information processing speed, working memory, verbal fluency, etc.) [73,74].

Finally, we would like to highlight advances of fMRI and cognitive research in MS [78], although there has been some controversies about the real meaning of fMRI results, it seems that early changes can be seen, even in cognitively preserved patients, including higher recruitment of non-related areas, such as supplementary motor cortex during working memory tasks [113] or by changes in activity properties of regions highly related to cognitive functions, as centrality measures of the default mode network [114], changes that may be used as a biomarker for neurocognitive rehabilitation [115] especially, resting state fMRI [116–118].

6. Treatment of Cognitive Impairment in MS

6.1. Pharmacological Interventions

6.1.1. MS Disease Modifying Therapies

MS specific disease modifying therapies such as the injectables interferon beta, glatiramer acetate; oral agents such as fingolimod, teriflunomide, or dimethyl fumarate; and monoclonal antibodies such as natalizumab, alemtuzumab, and ocrelizumab, have shown significant benefits in reducing the annualized relapse rate and MRI activity (new T2 or gadolinium enhancing lesions), with a more discrete efficacy over reducing disability progression or the brain atrophy rate [2]. However, their specific impact on cognitive impairment remains unclear, mainly because most phase III clinical trials established cognitive impairment as a secondary or tertiary outcome measure. Comparative efficacy on cognitive outcomes across trials is even more difficult, because of the different neuropsychological batteries used, the varied methods for evaluation and outcome analysis, and the differences between populations included in the trials.

Pivotal interferons and glatiramer acetate clinical trials did not include cognitive evaluation as primary endpoints. Intramuscular interferon beta 1a versus placebo included neuropsychological evaluation as a secondary outcome measure and showed 52.7% improvement compared with 29% in the placebo group [119], including processing speed and episodic memory outcomes. In the COGIMUS (Cognitive Impairment in Multiple Sclerosis) study, subcutaneous interferon 1a protected RRMS patients from general cognitive decline when reevaluated at 3 [120] and 5 years [121] after therapy onset. Regarding interferon beta 1b, Pishkin reported only improvement of delayed visual reproduction performance [122], and the Betaferon/Betaseron in Newly Emerging Multiple Sclerosis for Initial Treatment (BENEFIT) trial revealed that in patients with CIS interferon beta 1b had beneficial effects on working memory, and the effects remained over 8 years [123]. Glatiramer Acetate trials, while included BRB-N evaluation, did not show significant differences versus placebo [62].

The GOLDEN Study using once-daily oral fingolimod was compared with interferon beta 1b using a trial design that included cognitive impairment as the primary outcome. This study showed improvement in cognitive function (BRB-N and DKEFS) in both treatment arms, favoring fingolimod on MRI parameters [69], although some baseline imbalances may have favored the interferon beta 1b arm, according to the authors. In a patient-reported outcomes study, evaluating global satisfaction in switching treatment from several disease modifying drugs to teriflunomide and using SDMT to measure cognitive impairment, results showed that patients and physicians reported stability of cognition in a 48-week period [124].

Natalizumab pivotal studies showed that it can reduce the risk of progressive working memory impairment by 43% compared with placebo [125]. In a long-term observational study by Jacques et al., natalizumab was reported to preserve cognition over 7 years of continuous therapy using a computed test and the SDMT. No patient showed evidence of sustained cognitive deterioration over a 24-month period [126]. In a study including 21 patients during a 15-month follow-up period, alemtuzumab showed stable cognitive function using an extensive neuropsychological battery [127]. Ocrelizumab has shown improvement in MS Functional Composite score (a composite measure of walking speed, upper-limb movements, and cognition assessed by PASAT) compared with interferon beta 1a [128].

6.1.2. Cognitive Impairment-Specific Treatment

The use of acetylcholinesterase inhibitors (AChEI) in multiple sclerosis patients remains controversial. Few studies in a small number of MS patient populations reported contradictory results. While Krupp in 2004 reported the positive impact of donepezil in verbal learning and memory in a cohort of 69 patients [129], the same investigator reported no significant effect in 2011, which included 120 MS patients [130]. It is important to stress that long term treatments with AChEI compels one to be aware of the side effects. Regarding memantine, similar contradictory findings were reported in a small number of studies prevailing negative outcomes for this drug [131].

Amphetamines significantly improved visuospatial memory and verbal memory [132], fampridine has shown to be able to improve cognitive fatigue, alertness, psychomotor speed, and verbal fluency [133,134], while no benefit on learning were found using modafinil [135].

6.2. Non-Pharmacological Interventions

6.2.1. Neuropsychological Rehabilitation

Only recently, neuropsychological rehabilitation has been established as a useful therapeutic tool. Multidisciplinary and cognitive-behavioral interventions, computer-assisted training and combinations of the above, have been showing consistently better results [13,136], especially when tailored to individual needs. Evidence-based conclusions have only recently become stronger in regards to which interventions may have real benefits for MS patients. In a recent review article and meta-analysis including literature from 2007 to 2016, only one intervention received support for a practice standard in verbal learning and memory (modified Story Memory Technique—mSMT [137]), two computer programs received support as a practice guideline for attention and multicognitive domains (Attention Process Training—APT [138] and RehaCom [139]), and several studies provided support for the practice option in attention, learning, and memory [140].

6.2.2. Exercise

To date, numerous publications have shown the positive impact of physical exercise on different clinical parameters, but evidence remains to be demonstrated, as clinical trials have shown equivocal results [141,142]. A systematic review by Sandroff et al. showed that a few comparable studies did not yield a significant positive impact of physical exercise on cognitive impairment outcomes [143]. Another systematic review of the impact of yoga also failed to show the effect of this discipline in cognitive impairment [144]. This maybe the result of collectively insufficient well–designed research, and again, the fact that cognitive impairment is maintained as a secondary outcome. The cognitive effects of physical exercise in MS is gaining hype among cognitive researchers, as one relevant intervention both in preventing and improving cognitive outcomes, although clear results, as well as doses and regimens (e.g., aerobic versus weight training), are still missing [13].

7. Conclusions

In the last three decades, increasing knowledge in the field of cognitive impairment in MS has arisen. From defining the most sensitive neuropsychological tests and compound batteries for clinical practice and research, to better understanding the neural correlates in specific populations with assistance from conventional-structural and non-conventional/functional neuroimaging, better and more effective treatment, rehabilitation, and prevention strategies are being proposed.

Cognitive function assessment should be included in the standard clinical evaluation and clinical trials involving MS patients, and treatment strategies should be implemented as supported by current evidence. Limitations are still present, especially due to the validation and standardization of both diagnostic and therapeutic tools.

Due to the devastating impact over the working status, social interaction, and self-care of MS patients, improvement in all the aforementioned areas, as well as education to patients, families, and the community should be stated as a priority, and an unmet need.

References

1. Cree, B.A.; Gourraud, P.A.; Oksenberg, J.R.; Bevan, C.; Crabtree-Hartman, E.; Gelfand, J.M.; Goodin, D.S.; Graves, J.; Green, A.J.; Mowry, E.; et al. Long-term evolution of multiple sclerosis disability in the treatment era. *Ann. Neurol.* **2016**, *80*, 499–510. [PubMed]
2. Thompson, A.J.; Baranzini, S.E.; Geurts, J.; Hemmer, B.; Ciccarelli, O. Multiple sclerosis. *Lancet* **2018**, *391*, 1622–1636. [CrossRef]
3. Miller, D.H.; Leary, S.M. Primary-progressive multiple sclerosis. *Lancet Neurol.* **2007**, *6*, 903–912. [CrossRef]
4. Kakalacheva, K.; L€unemann, J.D. Enviromental triggers of multiple sclerosis. *FEBS Lett.* **2011**, *585*, 3724–3729. [CrossRef] [PubMed]
5. Chitnis, T. Role of puberty in multiple sclerosis risk and course. *Clin. Immunol.* **2013**, *149*, 192–200. [CrossRef]
6. Franciotta, D.; Salvetti, M.; Lolli, F.; Serafini, B.; Aloisi, F. B cells and multiple sclerosis. *Lancet Neurol.* **2008**, *7*, 852–858. [CrossRef]
7. Fletcher, J.M.; Lalor, S.J.; Sweeney, C.M.; Tubridy, N.; Mills, K.H.G.; Lalor, S. T cells in multiple sclerosis and experimental autoimmune encephalomyelitis. *Clin. Exp. Immunol.* **2010**, *162*, 1–11. [CrossRef]
8. Lublin, F.D.; Reingold, S.C.; Cohen, J.A.; Cutter, G.R.; Sørensen, P.S.; Thompson, A.J.; Wolinsky, J.S.; Balcer, L.J.; Banwell, B.; Barkhof, F.; et al. Defining the clinical course of multiple sclerosis: The 2013 revisions. *Neurology* **2014**, *83*, 278–286. [CrossRef]
9. Kurtzke, J.F. Rating neurologic impairment in multiple sclerosis: An expanded disability status scale (EDSS). *Neurology* **1983**, *33*, 1444–1452. [CrossRef]
10. Clemens, L.; Langdon, D. How does cognition relate to employment in multiple sclerosis? A systematic review. *Mult. Scler. Relat. Disord.* **2018**, *26*, 183–191. [CrossRef]
11. Murray, J. Terminology and disease description. In *Multiple Sclerosis the History of a Disease*; DEMOS Medical: New York, NY, USA, 2005; Volume 2, pp. 21–26.
12. Rao, S.; Leo, G.; Bernardin, I.; Unverzagt, F. Cognitive dysfunction in multiple sclerosis: Frequency, patterns, and predictions. *Neurology* **1991**, *41*, 94–97. [CrossRef]
13. Sokolov, A.A.; Grivaz, P.; Bove, R. Cognitive Deficits in Multiple Sclerosis: Recent Advances in Treatment and Neurorehabilitation. *Curr. Treat. Options Neurol.* **2018**, *20*, 53. [CrossRef] [PubMed]
14. American Psychiatric Association. *Diagnostic and Statistical Manual of Mental Disorders*, 5th ed.; American Psychiatric Publishing: Arlington, VA, USA, 2013; pp. 5–25, ISBN 978-0-89042-555-8.
15. Wooddruff, B.K. Disorders of cognition. *Semin. Neurol.* **2011**, *31*, 18–28. [CrossRef] [PubMed]

16. Amato, P.; Langdon, D.; Montalvan, X.; Benedict, R.; DeLuca, J.; Krupp, L.B.; Thompson, A.J.; Comi, G. Treatment of cognitive impairment in multiple sclerosis: Position paper. *J. Neurol.* **2013**, *260*, 1452–1468. [CrossRef] [PubMed]
17. Chiaravaloti, N.D.; DeLuca, J. Cognitive impairment in multiple sclerosis. *Lancet* **2008**, *7*, 1139–1151. [CrossRef]
18. Sumowski, J.F.; Benedict, R.; Enzinger, C.; Filippi, M.; Geurts, J.J.; Hamalainen, P.; Hulst, H.; Inglese, M.; Leavitt, V.M.; Rocca, M.A.; et al. Cognition in multiple sclerosis, State of the field and priorities for the future. *Neurology* **2018**, *90*, 278–288. [CrossRef] [PubMed]
19. DiGiuseppe, G.; Blair, M.; Morrow, S.A. Prevalence of cognitive impairment in newly diagnosed relapsing-remitting multiple sclerosis. *Int. J. MS Care* **2018**, *20*, 153–157. [CrossRef]
20. Vanotti, S.; Caceres, F.J. Cognitive and neuropsychiatric disorders among MS patients from Latin America. *MSJ Exp. Trans. Clin.* **2017**, *3*. [CrossRef]
21. Schiavolin, S.; Leonardi, M.; Giovannetti, A.M.; Antozzi, C.; Brambilla, L.; Confalonieri, P.; Mantegazza, R.; Raggi, A. Factors related to difficulties with employment in patients with multiple sclerosis: A review of 2002–2011 literature. *Int. J. Rehabil. Res.* **2013**, *36*, 105–111. [CrossRef]
22. Raggi, A.; Covelli, V.; Schiavolin, S.; Scaratti, C.; Leonardi, M.; Willems, M. Work-related problems in multiple sclerosis: A literature review on its associates and determinants. *Disabil. Rehabil.* **2016**, *38*, 936–944. [CrossRef]
23. Yamout, B.; Issa, Z.; Herlopian, A.; El Bejjani, M.; Khalifa, A.; Ghadieh, A.S.; Habib, R.H. Predictors of quality of life among multiple sclerosis patients: A comprehensive analysis. *Eur. J. Neurol.* **2013**, *20*, 756–764. [CrossRef] [PubMed]
24. Labbé, T.; Ciampi, E.; Carcamo Rodríguez, C. Social cognition: Concepts, neural basis and its role in multiple sclerosis. *Neurol. Clin. Neurosci.* **2018**, *6*, 3–8. [CrossRef]
25. Dulau, C.; Deloire, M.; Diaz, H.; El Bejjani, M.; Khalifa, A.; Ghadieh, A.S.; Habib, R.H. Social cognition according to cognitive impairment in different clinical phenotypes of multiple sclerosis. *J. Neurol.* **2017**, *264*, 740–748. [CrossRef] [PubMed]
26. Raimo, S.; Trojano, L.; Pappacena, S.; Alaia, R.; Spitaleri, D.; Grossi, D.; Santangelo, G. Neuropsychological Correlates of Theory of Mind Deficits in Patients with Multiple Sclerosis. *Neuropsychology* **2017**. [CrossRef] [PubMed]
27. Carotenuto, A.; Arcara, G.; Orefice, G.; Cerillo, I.; Giannino, V.; Rasulo, M.; Iodice, R.; Bambini, V. Communication in Multiple Sclerosis: Pragmatic Deficit and its Relation with Cognition and Social Cognition. *Arch. Clin. Neuropsychol.* **2017**, *33*, 194–205. [CrossRef] [PubMed]
28. Henry, A.; Tourbah, A.; Chaunu, M.P.; Bakchine, S.; Montreuil, M. Social Cognition Abilities in Patients with Different Multiple Sclerosis Subtypes. *J. Int. Neuropsychol. Soc.* **2017**, *23*, 653–664. [CrossRef]
29. Patil, I.; Young, L.; Sinay, V.; Gleichgerrcht, E. Elevated moral condemnation of third-PARTY violations in multiple sclerosis patients. *Soc. Neurosci.* **2017**, *12*, 308–329. [CrossRef]
30. Mickens, M.N.; Perrin, P.B.; Aguayo, A.; Rabago, B.; Macias-Islas, M.; Arango-Lasprilla, J. Mediational Model of Multiple Sclerosis Impairments, Family Needs, and Caregiver Mental Health in Guadalajara, Mexico. *Behav. Neurol.* **2018**. [CrossRef]
31. Langdon, D.W. Cognition in multiple sclerosis. *Curr. Opin. Neurol.* **2011**, *24*, 244–249. [CrossRef]
32. Benedict, R.H.; Cookfair, D.; Gavett, R.; Gunther, M.; Munschauer, F.; Garg, N.; Weinstock-Guttman, B. Validity of the Minimal Assessment of Cognitive Function in Multiple Sclerosis (MACFIMS). *J. Int. Neuropsychol. Soc.* **2006**, *12*, 549–558. [CrossRef]
33. Deloire, M.S.; Ruet, A.; Hamel, D.; Bonnet, M.; Dousset, V.; Brochet, B. MRI predictors of cognitive outcome in early multiple sclerosis. *Neurology* **2011**, *76*, 1161–1167. [CrossRef] [PubMed]
34. Cotter, J.; Firth, J.; Enzinger, C.; Kontopantelis, E.; Yung, A.R.; Elliott, R.; Drake, R.J. Social cognition in multiple sclerosis: A systematic review and meta-analysis. *Neurology* **2016**, *87*, 1727–1736. [CrossRef] [PubMed]
35. Ruano, L.; Portaccio, E.; Goretti, B.; Niccolai, C.; Severo, M.; Patti, F.; Cilia, S.; Gallo, P.; Grossi, P.; Ghezzi, A.; et al. Age and disability drive cognitive impairment in multiple sclerosis across disease subtypes. *Mult. Scler.* **2017**, *23*, 1258–1267. [CrossRef]

36. Trenova, A.G.; Slavov, G.S.; Manova, M.G.; Aksentieva, J.B.; Miteva, L.D.; Stanilova, S.A. Cognitive impairment in multiple sclerosis. *Folia Med.* **2016**, *58*, 157–163. [CrossRef] [PubMed]
37. Ciampi, E.; Uribe-San-Martin, R.; Vásquez, M.; Ruiz-Tagle, A.; Labbe, T.; Cruz, J.P.; Lillo, P.; Slachevsky, A.; Reyes, D.; Reyes, A.; et al. Relationship between Social Cognition and traditional cognitive impairment in Progressive Multiple Sclerosis and possible implicated neuroanatomical regions. *Mult. Scler. Relat. Disord.* **2018**, *20*, 122–128. [CrossRef] [PubMed]
38. Ntoskou, K.; Messinis, L.; Nasios, G.; Martzoukou, M.; Makris, G.; Panagiotopoulos, E.; Papathanasopoulos, P. Cognitive and Language Deficits in Multiple Sclerosis: Comparison of Relapsing Remitting and Secondary Progressive Subtypes. *Open Neurol. J.* **2018**, *12*, 19–30. [CrossRef] [PubMed]
39. Lezak, M.D.; Howieson, D.B.; Bigler, E.D.; Tranel, D. *Neuropsychological Assessment*, 5th ed.; Oxford University Press: New York, NY, USA, 2012.
40. Thornton, A.E.; Raz, N.; Tucke, K.A. Memory in multiple sclerosis: Contextual encoding defi cits. *J. Int. Neuropsychol. Soc.* **2002**, *8*, 395–409. [CrossRef] [PubMed]
41. Renell, P.G.; Jensen, F.; Henry, J.D. Prospective memory in multiple sclerosis. *J. Int. Neuropsychol. Soc.* **2007**, *13*, 410–416.
42. Sachdev, P.S.; Blacker, D.; Blazer, D.G.; Ganguli, M.; Jeste, D.V.; Paulsen, J.S.; Petersen, R.C. Classifying neurocognitive disorders: The DSM-5 approach. *Nat. Rev. Neurol.* **2014**, *10*, 634–642. [CrossRef] [PubMed]
43. Silva, P.H.R.; Spedo, C.T.; Baldassarini, C.R.; Benini, C.D.; Ferreira, D.A.; Barreira, A.A.; Leoni, R.F. Brain functional and effective connectivity underlying the information processing speed assessed by the Symbol Digit Modalities Test. *Neuroimage* **2019**, *184*, 761–770. [CrossRef]
44. Costa, S.L.; Genova, H.M.; DeLuca, J.; Chiaravalloti, N.D. Information processing speed in multiple sclerosis: Past, present, and future. *Mult. Scler. J.* **2016**, *23*, 772–789. [CrossRef] [PubMed]
45. Grzegorski, T.; Losy, J. Cognitive impairment in multiple sclerosis. *Rev. Neurosci.* **2017**, *7*, 1139–1151.
46. Van Schependom, J.; D'hooghe, M.B.; Cleynhens, K.; D'hooge, M.; Haelewyck, M.C.; De Keyser, J.; Nagels, G. Reduced information processing speed as primum movens for cognitive decline in MS. *Mult. Scler.* **2015**, *21*, 83. [CrossRef] [PubMed]
47. Leavitt, V.M.; Wylie, G.; Krch, D.; Chiaravalloti, N.; DeLuca, J.; Sumowski, J.F. Does slowed processing speed account for executive deficits in multiple sclerosis Evidence from neuropsychological performance and structural neuroimaging. *Rehabil. Psychol.* **2014**, *59*, 422–428. [CrossRef]
48. Prakash, R.S.; Snook, E.M.; Lewis, J.M.; Motl, R.W.; Kramer, A.F. Cognitive impairments in relapsing-remitting multiple sclerosis: A meta-analysis. *Mult. Scler.* **2008**, *14*, 1250–1261. [CrossRef]
49. Frith, C.D.; Frith, U. Social cognition in humans. *Curr. Biol.* **2007**, *17*, R724–R732. [CrossRef]
50. De Bruin, L.; Strijbos, D. Direct social perception, mindreading and Bayesian predictive coding. *Conscious Cogn.* **2015**, *36*, 565–570. [CrossRef]
51. Singer, T.; Lamm, C. The social neuroscience of empathy. *Ann. N. Y. Acad. Sci.* **2009**, *1156*, 81–96. [CrossRef]
52. Ruggieri, V.L. Empathy, social cognition and autism spectrum disorders. *Rev. Neurol.* **2013**, *56*, S13–S21.
53. Baron-Cohen, S. Without a theory of mind one cannot participate in a conversation. *Cognition* **1988**, *29*, 83–84. [CrossRef]
54. Rovira, À.; Wattjes, M.P.; Tintoré, M.; Tur, C.; Yousry, T.A.; Sormani, M.P.; De Stefano, N.; Filippi, M.; Auger, C.; Rocca, M.A.; et al. Evidence-based guidelines: MAGNIMS consensus guidelines on the use of MRI in multiple sclerosis-clinical implementation in the diagnostic process. *Nat. Rev. Neurol.* **2015**, *11*, 471–482. [CrossRef] [PubMed]
55. Wattjes, M.P.; Rovira, À.; Miller, D.; Yousry, T.A.; Sormani, M.P.; de Stefano, M.P.; Tintoré, M.; Auger, C.; Tur, C.; Filippi, M.; et al. Evidence-based guidelines: MAGNIMS consensus guidelines on the use of MRI in multiple sclerosis—Establishing disease prognosis and monitoring patients. *Nat. Rev. Neurol.* **2015**, *11*, 597–606.
56. Beatty, W.W.; Goodkin, D.E. Screening for cognitive impairment in multiple sclerosis. An evaluation of the Mini-Mental State Examination. *Arch. Neurol.* **1990**, *47*, 297–301. [CrossRef] [PubMed]
57. Rao, S.M. *Neuropsychological Screening Battery for Multiple Sclerosis*; National Multiple Sclerosis Society: New York, NY, USA, 1991.
58. Langdon, D.W.; Amato, M.P.; Boringa, J.; Brochet, B.; Foley, F.; Fredrikson, S.; Hämäläinen, P.; Hartung, H.-P.; Krupp, L.; Penner, I.K.; et al. Recommendations for a Brief International Cognitive Assessment for Multiple Sclerosis (BICAMS). *MSJ* **2012**, *18*, 891–898. [CrossRef]

59. Benedict, R.; DeLuca, J.; Phillips, G.; LaRocca, N.; Hudson, L.D.; Rudick, R.; Multiple Sclerosis Outcome Assessments Consortium. Validity of the Symbol Digit Modalities Test as a cognition performance outcome measure formultiple sclerosis. *Mult. Scler. J.* **2017**, *23*, 721–733. [CrossRef] [PubMed]
60. Delis, D.C.; Kramer, J.H.; Kaplan, E.; Ober, B.A. *California Verbal Learning Test*, 2nd ed.; Psychological Corporation: San Antonio, TX, USA, 2000.
61. Gronwall, D. Paced auditory serial addition task: A measure of recovery from concussion. *Percept. Motor Skills* **1977**, *44*, 363–373. [CrossRef]
62. Cutter, G.R.; Baier, M.S.; Rudick, R.A.; Cookfair, D.L.; Fischer, J.S.; Petkau, J.; Syndulko, K.; Weinshenker, B.G.; Antel, J.P.; Confavreux, C.; et al. Development of a Multiple Sclerosis Functional Composite as a clinical trial outcome measure. *Brain* **1999**, *122*, 101–112. [CrossRef]
63. Fischer, J.S.; Rudick, R.A.; Cutter, G.R.; Reingold, S.C. The Multiple Sclerosis Functional Composite Measure (MSFC): An integrated approach to MS clinical outcome assessment. National MS Society Clinical Outcomes Assessment Task Force. *Mult. Scler.* **1999**, *5*, 244–250. [CrossRef]
64. Friesen, W.V.; Ekman, P. *Friesen Pictures of Facial Affect*; Consulting Psychologists Press: Palo Alto, CA, USA, 1976.
65. Funkiewiez, A.; Bertoux, M.; de Souza, L.C.; Lévy, R.; Dubois, B. The sea (social cognition and emotional assessment): A clinical neuropsychological tool for early diagnosis of frontal variant of frontotemporal lobar degeneration. *Neuropsychology* **2012**, *1*, 81–90. [CrossRef]
66. Bertoux, M.; Volle, E.; de Souza, L.C.; Funkiewiez, A.; Dubois, B.; Habert, M.O. Neural correlates of the mini-SEA (Social cognition and Emotional Assessment) in behavioral variant frontotemporal dementia. *Brain Imaging Behav.* **2014**, *1*, 1–6. [CrossRef]
67. Di Filippo, M.; Portaccio, E.; Mancini, A.; Calabresi, P. Multiple sclerosis and cognition: Synaptic failure and network dysfunction. *Nat. Rev. Neurosci.* **2018**, *19*, 599–609. [CrossRef]
68. Zivadinov, R.; Sepcic, J.; Nasuelli, D.; De Masi, R.; Bragadin, L.M.; Tommasi, M.; Zambito-Marsala, S.; Moretti, R.; Bratina, A.; Ukmar, M.; et al. A longitudinal study of brain atrophy and cognitive disturbances in the early phase of relapsing-remitting multiple sclerosis. *J. Neurol. Neurosurg. Psychiatry* **2001**, *70*, 773–780. [CrossRef] [PubMed]
69. Smith, S.M.; Zhang, Y.; Jenkinson, M.; Chen, J.; Matthews, P.M.; Federico, A.; de Stefano, N. Accurate, robust and automated longitudinal and cross-sectional brain change analysis. *NeuroImage* **2002**, *17*, 479–489. [CrossRef] [PubMed]
70. Smith, S.M.; Jenkinson, M.; Woolrich, M.W.; Beckmann, C.F.; Behrens, T.E.J.; Johansen-Berg, H.; Bannister, P.R.; de Luca, M.; Drobnjak, I.; Flitney, D.E.; et al. Advances in functional and structural MR image analysis and implementation as FSL. *NeuroImage* **2004**, *23*, 208–219. [CrossRef] [PubMed]
71. Geurts, J.G.; Calabrese, M.; Fisher, E.; Rudick, R.A. Measurement and clinical effect of grey matter pathology in multiple sclerosis. *Lancet Neurol.* **2012**, *11*, 1082–1092. [CrossRef]
72. Figueira, F.F.; Santos, V.S.; Figueira, G.M.A.; Da Silva, Â.C.M. Corpus callosum index: A practical method for long-term follow-up in multiple sclerosis. *Arq. Neuropsiquiatr.* **2007**, *65*, 931–935. [CrossRef]
73. Yaldizli, Ö.; Penner, I.K.; Frontzek, K.; Naegelin, Y.; Amann, M.; Papadopoulou, A.; Sprenger, T.; Kuhle, J.; Calabrese, P.; Radü, E.W.; et al. The relationship between total and regional corpus callosum atrophy, cognitive impairment and fatigue in multiple sclerosis patients. *Mult. Scler.* **2014**, *3*, 356–364. [CrossRef] [PubMed]
74. Uribe-San-Martín, R.; Ciampi, E.; Di Giacomo, R.; Vásquez, M.; Cárcamo, C.; Godoy, J.; Lo Russo, G.; Tassi, L. Corpus callosum atrophy and post-surgical seizures in temporal lobe epilepsy associated with hippocampal sclerosis. *Epilepsy Res.* **2018**, *142*, 29–35. [CrossRef] [PubMed]
75. Butzkueven, H.; Kolbe, S.C.; Jolley, D.J.; Brown, J.Y.; Cook, M.J.; van der Mei, I.A.; Groom, P.S.; Carey, J.; Eckholdt, J.; Rubio, J.P.; et al. Validation of linear cerebral atrophy markers in multiple sclerosis. *J. Clin. Neurosci.* **2008**, *15*, 130–137. [CrossRef]
76. Lycke, J.; Wikkelso, C.; Bergh, A.C.; Jacobsson, L.; Andersen, O. Regional cerebral blood flow in multiple sclerosis masured by single photon emission tomography with technetium-99m hexamethylpropyleneamine oxime. *Eur. Neurol.* **1993**, *33*, 163–167. [CrossRef] [PubMed]

77. Roelcke, U.; Kappos, L.; Lechner-Scott, J.; Brunnschweiler, H.; Huber, S.; Ammann, W.; Plohmann, A.; Dellas, S.; Maguire, R.P.; Missimer, J.; et al. Reduced glucose metabolism in the frontal cortex and basal ganglia of multiple sclerosis patients with fatigue a 18F-fl uorodeoxyglucose positron emission tomography study. *Neurology* **1997**, *48*, 1566–1571. [CrossRef]
78. Labbé, T.; Ciampi, E.; Cruz, J.P.; Zurita, M.; Uribe, S.; Cárcamo, C. Functional magnetic resonance imaging in the study of multiple sclerosis. *Rev. Neurol.* **2018**, *67*, 91–98.
79. Meijer, K.A.; Muhlert, N.; Cercignani, M.; Sethi, V.; Ron, M.A.; Thompson, A.J.; Miller, D.H.; Chard, D.; Geurts, J.J.; Ciccarelli, O. White matter tract abnormalities are associated with cognitive dysfunction in secondary progressive multiple sclerosis. *Mult. Scler.* **2016**, *22*, 1429–1437. [CrossRef]
80. Giorgio, A.; De Stefano, N. Advanced Structural and Functional Brain MRI in Multiple Sclerosis. *Semin. Neurol.* **2016**, *36*, 163–176. [CrossRef]
81. Calabrese, M.; Agosta, F.; Rinaldi, F.; Mattisi, I.; Grossi, P.; Favaretto, A.; Atzori, M.; Bernardi, V.; Barachino, L.; Rinaldi, L.; et al. Cortical lesions and atrophy associated with cognitive impairment in relapsing-remitting multiple sclerosis. *Arch. Neurol.* **2009**, *66*, 1144–1150. [CrossRef] [PubMed]
82. Summers, M.M.; Fisniku, L.K.; Anderson, V.M.; Miller, D.H.; Cipolotti, I.; Ron, M. Cognitive impairment in relapsing remitting multiple sclerosis can be predicted by imaging performed several years earlier. *Mult. Scler.* **2008**, *14*, 197–204. [CrossRef] [PubMed]
83. Tekok-Kilic, A.; Benedict, R.H.; Weinstock-Gutman, B.; Dwyer, M.G.; Carone, D.; Srinivasaraghavan, B.; Yella, V.; Abdelrahman, N.; Munschauer, F.; Bakshi, R.; et al. Independent contributions of cortical grey matter atrophy and ventricle enlargement for predicting neuropsychological impairment in multiple sclerosis. *Neurology* **2007**, *36*, 1294–1300.
84. Steenwijk, M.D.; Geurts, J.J.G.; Daams, M.; Tijms, B.M.; Wink, A.M.; Balk, L.J.; Tewarie, P.K.; Uitdehaag, B.M.J.; Barkhof, F.; Vrenken, H.; et al. Cortical atrophy patterns in multiple sclerosis are non-random and clinically relevant. *Brain* **2016**, *139*, 115–126. [CrossRef]
85. Kern, K.C.; Gold, S.M.; Lee, B.; Montag, M.; Horsfall, J.; O'Connor, M.F.; Sicotte, N.L. Thalamic-hippocampal-prefrontal disruption in relapsing-remitting multiple sclerosis. *Neuroimage Clin.* **2014**, *8*, 440–447. [CrossRef]
86. Zivadinov, R.; de, M.R.; Nasuelli, D.; Bragadin, L.M.; Ukmar, M.; Pozzi-Mucelli, R.S.; Grop, A.; Cazzato, G.; Zorzon, M. MRI techniques and cognitive impairment in the early phase of relapsing-remitting multiple sclerosis. *Neuroradiology* **2001**, *43*, 272–278. [CrossRef]
87. Sumowski, J.F.; Leavitt, V.M.; Rocca, M.A.; Inglese, M.; Riccitelli, G.; Buyukturkoglu, K.; Meani, A.; Filippi, M. Mesial temporal lobe and subcortical grey matter volumes differentially predict memory across stages of multiple sclerosis. *Mult. Scler.* **2018**, *24*, 675–678. [CrossRef] [PubMed]
88. Planche, V.; Ruet, A.; Coupé, P.; Lamargue-Hamel, D.; Deloire, M.; Pereira, B.; Manjon, J.V.; Munsch, F.; Moscufo, N.; Meier, D.S.; et al. Hippocampal microstructural damage correlates with memory impairment in clinically isolated syndrome suggestive of multiple sclerosis. *Mult. Scler.* **2017**, *23*, 1214–1224. [CrossRef] [PubMed]
89. Aladro, Y.; López-Alvarez, L.; Sánchez-Reyes, J.M.; Hernández-Tamames, J.A.; Melero, H.; Rubio-Fernández, S.; Thuissard, I.; Cerezo-García, M. Relationship between episodic memory and volume of the brain regions of two functional cortical memory systems in multiple sclerosis. *J. Neurol.* **2018**, *265*, 2182–2189. [CrossRef] [PubMed]
90. Benedict, R.H.; Bakshi, R.; Simon, J.H.; Priore, R.; Miller, C.; Munschauer, F. Frontal cortex atrophy predicts cognitive impairment in multiple sclerosis. *J. Neuropsych. Clin. Neurosci.* **2002**, *14*, 44–51. [CrossRef]
91. Houtchens, M.K.; Benedict, R.H.; Kiliiany, R.; Sharma, J.; Jaisani, Z.; Singh, B.; Weinstock-Guttman, B.; Guttmann, C.R.; Bakshi, R. Thalamic atrophy and cognition in multiple sclerosis. *Neurology* **2007**, *69*, 1213–1223. [CrossRef]
92. Sicotte, N.L.; Kern, K.C.; Giesser, B.S.; Arshanapalli, A.; Schultz, A.; Montag, M.; Wang, H.; Bookheimer, S.Y. Regional hippocampal atrophy in multiple sclerosis. *Brain* **2008**, *131*, 1134–1141. [CrossRef]
93. González Torre, J.A.; Cruz Gómez, Á.J.; Belenguer, A.; Sanchis-Segura, C.; Ávila, C.; Forn, C. Hippocampal dysfunction is associated with memory impairment in multiple sclerosis: A volumetric and functional connectivity study. *Mult. Scler.* **2017**, *23*, 1854–1863. [CrossRef]

94. Minagar, A.; Barnett, M.H.; Benedict, R.H.B.; Pelletier, D.; Pirko, I.; Sahraian, M.A.; Frohman, E.; Zivadinov, R. The thalamus and multiple sclerosis: Modern views on pathologic, imaging, and clinical aspects. *Neurology* **2013**, *80*, 210–219. [CrossRef]
95. Ruet, A.; Hamel, D.; Deloire, M.S.; Charré-Morin, J.; Saubusse, A.; Brochet, B. Information processing speed impairment and cerebellar dysfunction in relapsing-remitting multiple sclerosis. *J. Neurol. Sci.* **2014**, *347*, 246–250. [CrossRef]
96. Moroso, A.; Ruet, A.; Lamargue-Hamel, D.; Munsch, F.; Deloire, M.; Coup, P.; Ouallet, J.C.; Planche, V.; Moscufo, N.; Meier, D.S.; et al. Posterior lobules of the cerebellum and information processing speed at various stages of multiple sclerosis. *J. Neurol. Neurosurg. Psychiatry* **2017**, *88*, 146–151.
97. Foong, J.; Rozewicz, L.; Quaghebeur, G.; Davie, C.A.; Kartsounis, L.D.; Thompson, A.J.; Miller, D.H.; Ron, M.A. Executive function in multiple sclerosis. The role of frontal lobe pathology. *Brain* **1997**, *120*, 15–26. [CrossRef]
98. Muhlert, N.; Sethi, V.; Schneider, T.; Daga, P.; Cipolotti, L.; Haroon, H.A.; Parker, G.J.M.; Ourselin, S.; Wheeler-Kingshott, C.A.M.; Miller, D.H.; et al. Diffusion MRI-based cortical complexity alterations associated with executive function in multiple sclerosis. *J. Magn. Reson. Imaging* **2013**, *38*, 54–63.
99. Weygandt, M.; Wakonig, K.; Behrens, J.; Meyer-Arndt, L.; Söder, E.; Brandt, A.U.; Bellmann-Strobl, J.; Ruprecht, K.; Gold, S.M.; Haynes, J.-D.; et al. Brain activity, regional gray matter loss, and decision-making in multiple sclerosis. *Mult. Scler.* **2017**, *24*, 1163–1173. [CrossRef]
100. Koini, M.; Filippi, M.; Rocca, M.A.; Yousry, T.; Ciccarelli, O.; Tedeschi, G.; Gallo, A.; Ropele, S.; Valsasina, P.; Riccitelli, G.; et al. Correlates of Executive Functions in Multiple Sclerosis Based on Structural and Functional MR Imaging: Insights from a Multicenter Study. *Radiology* **2016**, *280*, 869–879. [CrossRef] [PubMed]
101. Matias-Guiu, J.A.; Cortés-Martínez, A.; Montero, P.; Pytel, V.; Moreno-Ramos, T.; Jorquera, M.; Yus, M.; Arrazola, J.; Matías-Guiu, J. Structural MRI correlates of PASAT performance in multiple sclerosis. *BMC Neurol.* **2018**, *20*, 214. [CrossRef] [PubMed]
102. Bellmann-Strobl, J.; Wuerfel, J.; Aktas, O.; Dorr, J.; Wernecke, K.D.; Zipp, F.; Paul, F. Poor PASAT performance correlates with MRI contrast enhancement in multiple sclerosis. *Neurology* **2009**, *73*, 1624–1627. [CrossRef]
103. Pardini, M.; Uccelli, A.; Grafman, J.H.; Yaldizli, O.; Mancardi, G.L.; Roccatagliata, L. Isolated cognitive relapses in multiple sclerosis. *J. Neurol. Neurosurg. Psychiatry* **2014**, *85*, 1035–1037. [CrossRef] [PubMed]
104. Jehna, M.; Langkammer, C.; Wallner-Blazek, M.; Neuper, C.; Loitfelder, M.; Ropele, S.; Fuchs, S.; Khalil, M.; Pluta-Fuerst, A.; Fazekas, F.; et al. Cognitively preserved MS patients demonstrate functional differences in processing neutral and emotional faces. *Brain Imaging Behav.* **2011**, *5*, 241–251. [CrossRef]
105. Mike, A.; Strammer, E.; Aradi, M.; Orsi, G.; Perlaki, G.; Hajnal, A.; Sandor, J.; Banati, M.; Illes, E.; Zaitsev, A.; et al. Disconnection mechanism and regional cortical atrophy contribute to impaired processing of facial expressions and theory of mind in multiple sclerosis: A structural MRI study. *PLoS ONE* **2013**, *8*, e82422. [CrossRef]
106. Calabrese, P.; Penner, I.K. Cognitive dysfunctions in multiple sclerosis "a multiple disconnection syndrome". *J. Neurol.* **2007**, *254*, 18–21. [CrossRef]
107. Henry, A.; Tourbah, A.; Chaunu, M.; Rumbach, L.; Montreuil, M.; Bakchine, S. Social cognition impairments in relapsing-remitting multiple sclerosis. *J. Int. Neuropsychol. Soc.* **2011**, *17*, 1122–1131. [CrossRef] [PubMed]
108. Batista, S.; d'Almeida, O.C.; Afonso, A.; Freitas, S.; Macário, C.; Sousa, L.; Castelo-Branco, M.; Santana, I.; Cunha, L. Impairment of social cognition in multiple sclerosis: Amygdala atrophy is the main predictor. *Mult. Scler.* **2017**, *23*, 1358–1366. [CrossRef] [PubMed]
109. Chalah, M.A.; Ayache, S.S. Deficits in Social Cognition: An Unveiled Signature of Multiple Sclerosis. *J. Int. Neuropsychol. Soc.* **2017**, *23*, 266–286. [CrossRef] [PubMed]
110. Benedict, R.H.; Hulst, H.E.; Bergsland, N.; Schoonheim, M.M.; Dwyer, M.G.; Weinstock-Guttman, B.; Geurts, J.J.; Zivadinov, R. Clinical significance of atrophy and white matter mean diffusivity within the thalamus of multiple sclerosis patients. *Mult. Scler.* **2013**, *19*, 1478–1484. [CrossRef] [PubMed]
111. Schoonheim, M.M.; Hulst, H.E.; Brandt, R.B.; Strik, M.; Wink, A.M.; Uitdehaag, B.M.J.; Barkhof, F.; Geurts, J.J.G. Thalamus structure and function determine severity of cognitive impairment in multiple sclerosis. *Neurology* **2015**, *84*, 776–783. [CrossRef] [PubMed]

112. Bisecco, A.; Rocca, M.A.; Pagani, E.; Mancini, L.; Enzinger, C.; Gallo, A.; Vrenken, H.; Stromillo, M.L.; Copetti, M.; Thomas, D.L.; et al. Connectivity-based parcellation of the thalamus in multiple sclerosis and its implications for cognitive impairment: A multicenter study. *Hum. Brain Mapp.* **2015**, *36*, 2809–2825. [CrossRef]
113. Nelson, F.; Akhtar, M.A.; Zúñiga, E.; Perez, C.A.; Hasan, K.M.; Wilken, J.; Wolinsky, J.S.; Narayana, P.A.; Steinberg, J.L. Novel fMRI working memory paradigm accurately detects cognitive impairment in multiple sclerosis. *Mult. Scler.* **2016**, *23*, 836–847. [CrossRef]
114. Eijlers, A.J.; Meijer, K.A.; Wassenaar, T.M.; Steenwijk, M.D.; Uitdehaag, B.M.; Barkhof, F.; Wink, A.M.; Geurts, J.J.; Schoonheim, M.M. Increased default-mode network centrality in cognitively impaired multiple sclerosis patients. *Neurology* **2017**, *88*, 952–960. [CrossRef]
115. Campbell, J.; Langdon, D.; Cercignani, M.; Rashid, W. A randomised controlled trial of efficacy of cognitive rehabilitation in multiple sclerosis: A cognitive, behavioural, and MRI study. *Neural Plast.* **2016**, *2016*, 4292585. [CrossRef]
116. Pinter, D.; Beckmann, C.; Koini, M.; Pirker, E.; Filippini, N.; Pichler, A.; Fuchs, S.; Fazekas, F.; Enzinger, C. Reproducibility of resting state connectivity in patients with stable multiple sclerosis. *PLoS ONE* **2016**, *11*, e0152158. [CrossRef]
117. Boutiere, C.; Rey, C.; Zaaraoui, W.; Le Troter, A.; Rico, A.; Crespy, L.; Achard, S.; Reuter, F.; Pariollaud, F.; Wirsich, J.; et al. Improvement of spasticity following intermittent theta burst stimulation in multiple sclerosis is associated with modulation of resting-state functional connectivity of the primary motor cortices. *Mult. Scler.* **2017**, *23*, 855–863. [CrossRef] [PubMed]
118. Pareto, D.; Sastre-Garriga, J.; Alonso, J.; Galán, I.; Arévalo, M.J.; Renom, M.; Montalban, X.; Rovira, À. Classic Block Design "Pseudo"-Resting-State fMRI Changes After a Neurorehabilitation Program in Patients with Multiple Sclerosis. *J. Neuroimaging* **2018**, *28*, 313–319. [CrossRef]
119. Fisher, R.L.; Priore, R.L.; Jacobs, L.D.; Cookfair, D.L.; Rudick, R.A.; Herndon, R.M.; Richert, J.R.; Salazar, A.M. Neuropsychological effects of interferón beta 1 a in relapsing multiple sclerosis. *Ann. Neurol.* **2000**, *48*, 885–892. [CrossRef]
120. Patti, F.; Amato, M.P.; Bastianello, S.; Caniatti, L.; Di Monte, E.; Ferrazza, P.; Goretti, B.; Gallo, P.; Brescia Morra, V.; Lo Fermo, S.; et al. Effects of immunomodulatory treatment with subcutaneous interferon beta-1a on cognitive decline in mildly disabled patients with relapsing-remitting multiple sclerosis. *Mult. Scler.* **2010**, *16*, 68–77. [CrossRef] [PubMed]
121. Patti, F.; Morra, V.B.; Amato, M.P.; Trojano, M.; Bastianello, S.; Tola, M.R.; Cottone, S.; Plant, A.; Picconi, O. Subcutaneous interferon β-1a may protect against cognitive impairment in patients with relapsing-remitting multiple sclerosis: 5-year follow-up of the COGIMUS study. *PLoS ONE* **2013**, *8*, e74111. [CrossRef] [PubMed]
122. Pliskin, N.H.; Hamer, D.P.; Goldstein, D.S.; Towle, V.L.; Reder, A.T.; Noronha, A.; Arnason, B.G. Improved delayed visual reproduction test performance in multiple sclerosis patients receiving interferon beta-1b. *Neurology* **1996**, *47*, 1463–1468. [CrossRef] [PubMed]
123. Edan, G.; Kappos, L.; Montalbán, X.; Polman, C.H.; Freedman, M.S.; Hartung, H.-P.; Miller, D.; Barkhof, F.; Herrmann, J.; Lanius, V.; et al. Longterm impact of interferon beta-1b in patients with CIS: 8-year follow-up of BENEFIT. *J. Neurol. Neurosurg. Psychiatry* **2014**, *85*, 1183–1189. [CrossRef]
124. Weinstein, A.; Schwid, S.I.; Schiffer, R.B.; McDermott, M.P.; Giang, D.W.; Goodman, A.D. Neuropsychologic status in multiple sclerosis after treatment with glatiramer. *Arch. Neurol.* **1999**, *56*, 319–324. [CrossRef]
125. Weinstock-Guttman, B.; Galetta, S.L.; Giovannoni, G.; Havrdova, E.; Hutchinson, M.; Kappos, L.; O'Connor, P.W.; Phillips, J.T.; Polman, C.; Stuart, W.H.; et al. Additional efficacy endpoints from pivotal natalizumab trials in relapsing-remitting MS. *J. Neurol.* **2012**, *259*, 898–905. [CrossRef]
126. Jacques, F.H.; Harel, B.T.; Schembri, A.J.; Paquette, C.; Bilodeau, B.; Kalinowski, P.; Roy, R. Cognitive evolution in natalizumab-treated multiple sclerosis patients. *MSJ* **2016**, *2*. [CrossRef]
127. Riepl, E.; Pfeuffer, S.; Ruck, T.; Lohmannt, H.; Wiendl, H.; Meuth, S.G.; Johnen, A. Alemtuzumab improves cognitive proccesing speed in active multiple sclerosis—A longitudinal observational study. *Front. Neurol.* **2018**, *8*, 730. [CrossRef] [PubMed]
128. Hauser, S.L.; Bar-Or, A.; Comi, G.; Giovannoni, G.; Hartung, H.-P.; Hemmer, B.; Lublin, F.; Montalban, X.; Rammohan, K.W.; Selmaj, K.; et al. Ocrelizumab versus Interferon Beta-1a in Relapsing Multiple Sclerosis. *N. Engl. J. Med.* **2017**, *376*, 221–234. [CrossRef] [PubMed]

129. Krupp, L.B.; Christodoulou, C.; Melville, P.; Scherl, W.F.; MacAllister, W.S.; Elkins, L.E. Donepezil improved memory in multiple sclerosis in a randomized clinical trial. *Neurology* **2004**, *63*, 1579–1585. [CrossRef] [PubMed]
130. Krupp, L.B.; Christodoulou, C.; Melville, P.; Scherl, W.F.; Pai, L.Y.; Muenz, L.R.; He, D.; Benedict, R.H.; Goodman, A.; Rizvi, S.; et al. Multicenter randomized clinical trial of donepezil for memory impairment in multiple sclerosis. *Neurology* **2011**, *76*, 1500–1507. [CrossRef] [PubMed]
131. Lovera, J.F.; Frohman, E.; Brown, T.; Bandari, D.; Nguyen, L.; Yadav, V.; Stuve, O.; Karman, J.; Bogardus, K.; Heimburger, G.; et al. Memantine for cognitive impairment in multiple sclerosis: A randomized placebo-controlled trial. *Mult. Scler.* **2010**, *16*, 715–723. [CrossRef] [PubMed]
132. Sumowski, J.F.; Chiaravalloti, N.; Erlanger, D.; Kaushik, T.; Benedict, R.H.B.; DeLuca, J. L-amphetamine improves memory in MS patients with objective memory impairment. *Mult. Scler.* **2011**, *17*, 1141–1145. [CrossRef] [PubMed]
133. Broicher, S.D.; Filli, L.; Geisseler, O.; Germann, N.; Zörner, B.; Brugger, P.; Linnebank, M. Positive effects of fampridine on cognition, fatigue and depression in patients with multiple sclerosis over 2 years. *J. Neurol.* **2018**, *265*, 1016–1025. [CrossRef] [PubMed]
134. Pavsic, K.; Pelicon, K.; Ledinek, A.H.; Sega, S. Short-term impact of fampridine on motor and cognitive functions, mood and quality of life among multiple sclerosis patients. *Clin. Neurol. Neurosurg.* **2015**, *139*, 35–40. [CrossRef] [PubMed]
135. Ford-Johnson, L.; DeLuca, J.; Zhang, J.; Elovic, E.; Lengenfelder, J.; Chiaravalloti, N.D. Cognitive effects of modafinil in patients with multiple sclerosis: A clinical trial. *Rehabil. Psychol.* **2016**, *61*, 82–91. [CrossRef]
136. Millera, E.; Morelc, A.; Redlickaa, J.; Millera, I.; Salukc, J. Pharmacological and Non-pharmacological Therapies of Cognitive Impairment in Multiple Sclerosis. *Curr. Neuropharmacol.* **2018**, *16*, 475–483. [CrossRef]
137. Chiaravalloti, N.D.; Moore, N.B.; Nikelshpur, O.M.; DeLuca, J. An RCT to treat learning impairment in multiple sclerosis: The MEMREHAB trial. *Neurology* **2013**, *81*, 2066–2072. [CrossRef] [PubMed]
138. Amato, M.P.; Goretti, B.; Viterbo, R.G.; Portaccio, E.; Niccolai, C.; Hakiki, B.; Iaffaldano, P.; Trojano, M. Computer-assisted rehabilitation of attention in patients with multiple sclerosis: Results of a randomized, double-blind trial. *Mult. Scler. J.* **2014**, *20*, 91–98. [CrossRef] [PubMed]
139. De Giglio, L.; De Luca, F.; Prosperini, L.; Borriello, G.; Bianchi, V.; Pantano, P.; Pozzilli, C. A low-cost cognitive rehabilitation with a commercial video game improves sustained attention and executive functions in multiple sclerosis: A pilot study. *Neurorehabil. Neural Repair.* **2015**, *29*, 453–461. [CrossRef] [PubMed]
140. Goverover, Y.; Chiaravalloti, N.D.; O'Brien, A.R.; DeLuca, J. Evidenced-Based Cognitive Rehabilitation for Persons with Multiple Sclerosis: An Updated Review of the Literature From 2007 to 2016. *Arch. Phys. Med. Rehabil.* **2018**, *99*, 390–407. [CrossRef]
141. Carter, A.; Daley, A.; Humphreys, L.; Snowdon, N.; Woodroofe, N.; Petty, J.; Roalfet, Al.; Tosh, J.; Sharrack, B.; Saxton, J. Pragmatic intervention for increasing self-directed exercise behaviour and improving important health outcomes in people with multiple sclerosis: A randomised controlled trial. *Mult. Scler.* **2014**, *20*, 1112–1122. [CrossRef]
142. Briken, S.; Gold, S.M.; Patra, S.; Vettorazzi, E.; Harbs, D.; Tallner, A.; Ketels, G.; Schulz, K.H.; Heesen, C. Effects of exercise on fitness and cognition in progressive MS: A randomized, controlled pilot trial. *Mult. Scler.* **2014**, *20*, 382–390. [CrossRef] [PubMed]
143. Sandroff, B.M.; Motl, R.W.; Scudder, M.R.; DeLuca, J. Systematic, Evidence-Based Review of Exercise, Physical Activity, and Physical Fitness Effects on Cognition in Persons with Multiple Sclerosis. *Neuropsychol. Rev.* **2016**, *26*, 271–294. [CrossRef]
144. Cramer, H.; Lauche, R.; Azizi, H.; Dobos, G. ; Langhorst J Yoga for Multiple Sclerosis: A Systematic Review and Meta-Analysis. *PLoS ONE* **2014**, *9*, e112414. [CrossRef]

4

Comprehensive Analysis of the Immune and Stromal Compartments of the CNS in EAE Mice Reveal Pathways by Which Chloroquine Suppresses Neuroinflammation

Rodolfo Thome, Alexandra Boehm, Larissa Lumi Watanabe Ishikawa, Giacomo Casella, Jaqueline Munhoz, Bogoljub Ciric, Guang-Xian Zhang and Abdolmohamad Rostami *

Department of Neurology, Thomas Jefferson University, Philadelphia, PA 19107, USA; rodolfo.thome@jefferson.edu (R.T.); alexandra.boehm@jefferson.edu (A.B.); larissa.ishikawa@jefferson.edu (L.L.W.I.); giacomo.casella@jefferson.edu (G.C.); jlima.munhoz@gmail.com (J.M.); bogoljub.ciric@jefferson.edu (B.C.); guang-xian.zhang@jefferson.edu (G.-X.Z.)

* Correspondence: a.m.rostami@jefferson.edu

Abstract: Multiple sclerosis (MS) and experimental autoimmune encephalomyelitis (EAE) are neuroinflammatory diseases of the central nervous system (CNS), where leukocytes and CNS resident cells play important roles in disease development and pathogenesis. The antimalarial drug chloroquine (CQ) has been shown to suppress EAE by modulating dendritic cells (DCs) and Th17 cells. However, the mechanism of action by which CQ modulates EAE is far from being elucidated. Here, we comprehensively analyzed the CNS of CQ and PBS-treated EAE mice to identify and characterize the cells that are affected by CQ. Our results show that leukocytes are largely modulated by CQ and have a reduction in the expression of inflammatory markers. Intriguingly, CQ vastly modulated the CNS resident cells astrocytes, oligodendrocytes (OLs) and microglia (MG), with the latter producing IL-10 and IL-12p70. Overall, our results show a panoramic view of the cellular components that are affect by CQ and provide further evidence that drug repurposing of CQ will be beneficial to MS patients.

Keywords: chloroquine; EAE; dendritic cells; microglia; astrocytes; oligodendrocytes

1. Introduction

MS and EAE are inflammatory diseases of the CNS. Although the mechanisms that trigger MS are not fully elucidated, studies in EAE have uncovered the major role played by T cells in disease development, severity, and recovery [1]. Inflammatory $CD4^+$ T cells differentiate into IFN-γ^+ Th1 cells and IL-17^+ Th17 cells and migrate to the CNS where they induce inflammation and the chemoattraction of myeloid cells [2–5]. We and others have shown that the cytokine GM-CSF is an essential mediator of pathogenic Th17 cells [6–8]. Moreover, GM-CSF is induced in Th17 cells by IL-23R stimulation [7,9]. Conversely, Foxp3-expressing regulatory T (Treg) cells suppress Th1/Th17 cells and overall inflammation through contact-dependent and independent mechanisms [10]. Additionally, Treg cells were shown to promote remyelination [11,12]. In this context, antigen-presenting cells, such as dendritic cells (DCs), may direct T cell differentiation to Th17/Th1 and Treg cell phenotypes [13–15].

CNS resident cells are affected by local inflammation and may contribute to neurodegeneration in EAE. At early stages of EAE, microglia (MG) acquire an inflammatory M1 profile with the production of IL-1β, IL-6 and nitric oxide (NO), which shifts towards a tissue repair-associated M2 phenotype at later stages [16–18]. MG-derived IL-1β promote neuroinflammation and MG proliferation in an autocrine manner [19]. Moreover, MG-astrocyte crosstalk greatly influences the outcome of neuroinflammation in EAE [20,21]. Inflammatory A1 astrocytes actively induce damage to oligodendrocytes (OLs) and neurons, promote leukocyte infiltration and aid neuroinflammatory processes [22,23]. These observations illustrate the complex network and interactions among peripherally-derived leukocytes and CNS resident cells in EAE and MS. Thus, drugs that target multiple cell types while inducing tissue repair are of great importance in MS therapy.

Chloroquine (CQ) is a known antimalarial drug with anti-inflammatory properties [24]. CQ modulates monocyte activation and TNF-α production [25,26]. CQ also inhibits lysosomal maturation and antigen-processing [27–29]. By modulating DCs and Th17 cells, CQ has been shown to suppress EAE [27,30,31]. However, the mechanisms by which CQ suppresses EAE are far from being elucidated. CQ induces tolerogenic DCs in a STAT1-dependent manner [32]. Interestingly, CQ inhibited Th17 cell differentiation in a STAT-1-independent and T-bet-dependent fashion [31]. These observations suggest that CQ interferes with multiple cell types and influences diverse signaling pathways to suppress inflammation. The identification of such cell types and pathways may provide a better understanding of the mechanisms by which CQ suppresses EAE and may shed light on new therapeutic targets in MS.

In this study, we comprehensively characterized the phenotype and activity of peripherally derived leukocytes and CNS resident cells in CQ-treated EAE mice. We observed that CQ suppressed inflammatory leukocytes while also modulating MG and astrocytes. Further analyses revealed that CQ reduced IL-23R expression in $CD4^+$ T cells and IL-23 production by MG. Moreover, CQ stimulated MG to produce IL-10 and IL-12p70, which stimulated IL-10 production in T cells and refrained astrocyte activation. Together, our results show that CQ has a broad action by modulating leukocytes and CNS resident cells to suppress EAE and provide further evidence that drug repurposing of CQ is beneficial to patients with MS.

2. Methods

2.1. *Animals*

We used 8–12 week old male and female C57BL/6 and B6SJLF1 mice from the Jackson Laboratory (Bar Harbor, ME, USA). Mice were acclimated in clean cages in a controlled environment with food and water ad libitum. Experiments detailed in this study were approved by Thomas Jefferson University's IACUC under protocol numbers 01970 and 02034.

2.2. *EAE Induction and Evaluation*

To induce and evaluate EAE, we followed previously described protocols [33,34]. Mice were subcutaneously immunized with 200 μg of MOG_{35-55} peptide (Genscript) and equal volume of Complete Freund's adjuvant supplemented with 10 mg/mL of heat-killed *Mycobacterium tuberculosis* H37Ra. Additionally, mice were intraperitoneally injected with 240 ng of Pertussis toxin at 0 and 2 days after immunization. EAE development was analyzed daily and scored on a 0–5 scale, where: 0—no clinical sign, 1—limp tail, 2—hind paw weakness, 3—hind paw paralysis, 4—hind paw paralysis and front paw weakness, 5—full paralysis/death.

2.3. *CQ Treatment*

The dosage for CQ treatment has been assessed before [35]. Mice were treated with CQ (chloroquine diphosphate salt, Sigma-Aldrich) at a 5 mg/kg concentration via i.p. injections. The pH in CQ solution was 7.2. Control mice were injected with diluent solution (phosphate-buffered saline 0.02 M pH 7.2).

2.4. *Isolation of Mononuclear Cells in the CNS of Mice with EAE*

Mononuclear cells from the CNS of EAE mice were isolated by Percol gradient centrifugation following published reports [32–34]. In brief, euthanized mice were perfused with ice-cold PBS and the CNS tissue was collected and incubated with 700 μg/mL Liberase TL (Sigma-Aldrich, St. Louis, MO,

USA) at 37 °C for 30 min. To remove myelin debris, the digested tissue was centrifuged in a 30% Percol solution. MNCs were recovered from the bottom of the tube and used for flow cytometry analyses.

2.5. Flow Cytometry

For detection of intracellular cytokines by flow cytometry, cells were stimulated with PMA (50 ng/mL), ionomycin (500 ng/mL) and GolgiPlug (1 μg/mL) in IMDM complete medium for 3 h at 37 °C. Cells were washed in FACS buffer (PBS/2% FBS) and stained with fluorochrome labeled Abs to surface molecules for 20 min at 4 °C. Cells were then fixed and permeabilized (Invitrogen/ThermoFisher, Waltham, MA, USA) and incubated with antibodies against intracellular antigens for 18 h at 4 °C. Immediately before acquisition, cells were washed and resuspended in PBS. We utilized a FACSAria Fusion (BD Biosciences) flow cytometer for acquisition and FlowJo VX (Tristar Inc., Ashland, OR, USA) for analyses. Antibodies used in this study were anti-mouse: CD45 (30-F11), TCR-β (H57-597), CD4 (GK1.5), CD8 (53-6.7), GFAP (2E1.E9), CD11b (M1/70), Ly6C (HK1.4), CD11c (N418), MHC-II (M5/114.15.2), CD80 (16-10A1), CD86 (GL-1), pSTAT1 (A15158B), pSTAT3 (13A3-1), mTOR (O21-404, from BD Biosciences), IL-1β (NJTEN3, from eBioscience/ThermoFisher), IL-6 (MP5-20F3), IL-10 (JES5-16E3), IL-12p70 (C15.6, from BD Biosciences), IL-17A (TC11-18H10.1), IL-23 (N71-1183, from BD Biosciences), GM-CSF (MP1-22E9), Foxp3 (FJK-16s, from eBioscience/ThermoFisher, Waltham, MA, USA), IL-23R (12B2B64), IL-10R (1B1.3a), Granzyme B (GB11), and IRF8 (V3GYWCH, from eBioscience/ThermoFisher). All antibodies used in this study were purchased from Biolegend, San Diego, CA, USA, except where mentioned otherwise.

2.6. Isolation of Primary MG and CQ Treatment

$CD11b^+$ MG were isolated from MNCs obtained from the CNS of P0–P3 pups using magnetic beads (Miltenyi Biotec., Auburn, CA, USA). This isolation procedure yielded a consistent purity of 95% of $CD11b^+$ cells assessed by flow cytometry. MG were activated with LPS (100 ng/mL) with or without CQ (50 μM) for 18 h at 37 °C. The optimal CQ concentration for in vitro treatment of myeloid cells has been determined before [27]. At the end of culture time, MG cells were processed for flow cytometry, RNA extraction and co-culture.

2.7. PCRArray and Gene Ontology Analysis

RNA was extracted and reverse-transcribed from primary MG utilizing commercially available kits (RNAeasy extraction kit and high capacity RNA-to-cDNA kit, respectively, both from ThermoFisher). The cDNA was tested for quality and purity in a nanodrop equipment before being subjected to PCRArray (ThermoFisher). Gene ontology analysis was performed with CytoScape v3.8 (CytoScape.org).

2.8. Co-Culture of MG and T Cells

Primary MG were treated as above and extensively washed with Iscove's Modified Dulbecco Medium (IMDM) to remove LPS and CQ from the cells. In total, 50,000 MG were seeded into each well of a 96 U-bottom well plate. Then, $CD4^+$ T cells were isolated from spleens of naïve mice using magnetic beads (Miltenyi Biotec) and 100,000 cells were seeded on each well on top of MG. As controls, T cells were cultured without MG. As stimulus, cells were incubated with agonistic anti-CD3 antibody at a concentration of 0.5 μg/mL. For these analyses, co-stimulation was provided by MG without the need for anti-CD28 antibodies. Cells were incubated for 72 h at 37 °C as described [32], and then, analyzed by flow cytometry.

2.9. Co-Culture of MG and Astrocytes

Primary MG were treated as above and extensively washed with Iscove's Modified Dulbecco Medium (IMDM) to remove LPS and CQ from the cells. In total, 50,000 MG were seeded into each well of a 96 U-bottom well plate. Then, 50,000 C8D30 astrocytes (ATCC-CRL-2534) were seeded on each well on top of MG. As controls, astrocytes were cultured without MG. Cells were incubated for 48 h at 37 °C before being collected and analyzed by flow cytometry.

2.10. Statistical Analyses

Daily clinical scores among experimental groups in EAE were compared by two-way ANOVA and post-tested with Sidak. Comparisons between two groups were carried out with unpaired Student's *t* test and Welch's correction. Values of $p < 0.05$ were defined as significant.

3. Results

3.1. CQ Reduces Ongoing Inflammation in Relapsing EAE

CQ has been shown to prevent EAE development when given prophylactic and to reduced EAE severity when given at disease onset [31,35]. However, if CQ is able to suppress ongoing relapsing EAE is unknown. B6SJLF1 mice, the offspring of C57BL/6 and SJL mice, develop relapsing EAE when immunized with MOG_{35-55} [36,37]. We immunized mice to develop EAE and CQ treatment started at the onset of clinical signs of EAE. Mice treated with PBS fully developed disease clinical signs and the characteristic relapsing feature of this model (Figure 1A). However, mice treated with CQ developed a significantly less severe EAE compared with PBS-treated mice (Figure 1A). These results are on par with those observed in chronic EAE in C57BL/6 mice (Figure 1B). B6SJLF1 mice treated with CQ had a significant decrease in the infiltration of leukocytes to the CNS compared with those treated with PBS (Figure 1C). A similar trend was observed in treated C57BL/6 mice (Figure 1C). These results show that CQ is a potent agent in suppressing the clinical development of two models of EAE.

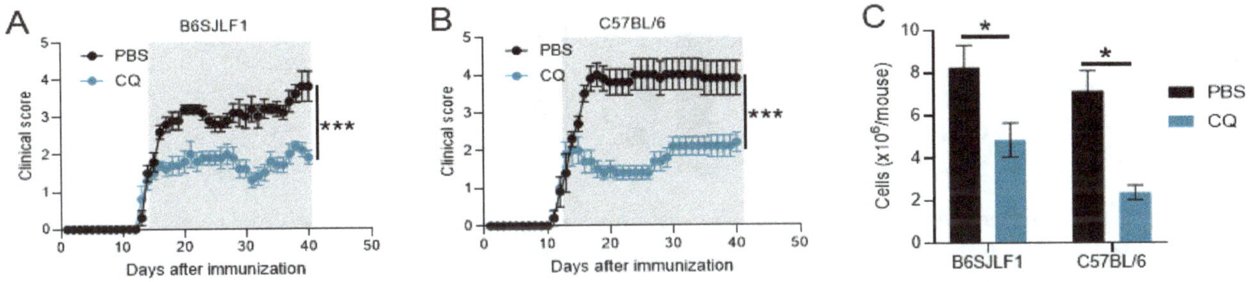

Figure 1. Chloroquie (CQ) suppresses neuroinflammation in two models of experimental autoimmune encephalomyelitis (EAE). C57BL/6 and B6SJLF1 mice ($n = 5$/group) were immunized to induce EAE. At the onset and until the end of experimentation, mice were treated with CQ (5 mg/kg) via i.p. everyday. (**A**) Disease development in B6SJLF1 mice and in (**B**) C57BL/6 mice. (**C**) CNS cells were analyzed at day 21 post-immunization. Values of $p < 0.05$ (*) and < 0.001 (***) were considered statistically significative. Results are from three independent experiments.

3.2. Peripherally-Derived Leukocytes Are Modulated in CQ-Treated Mice

We analyzed the phenotype of leukocytes in the CNS of CQ-treated EAE B6SJLF1 mice. We observed a significant reduction in numbers of $CD45^{high}$ leukocyte in mice treated with CQ compared with those treated with PBS (Figure 1C). Furthermore, DCs and macrophages from CQ-treated mice presented a reduced expression of the molecules involved in antigen-presentation and activation: class II MHC, CD80, CD86 in comparison with controls (Figure 2A). Analyses of the signaling mediators pSTAT1, pSTAT3, and mTOR in peripherally derived myeloid cells from CQ-treated mice revealed a decrease in the expression of pSTAT3 and mTOR in DCs and macrophages, but not in neutrophils in comparison with those from PBS-treated mice (Figure 2C). pSTAT1 was significantly upregulated in DCs and macrophages while pSTAT3 was upregulated in neutrophils (Figure 2C). There was no significant difference in mTOR expression in neutrophils between the two groups of mice (Figure 2C).

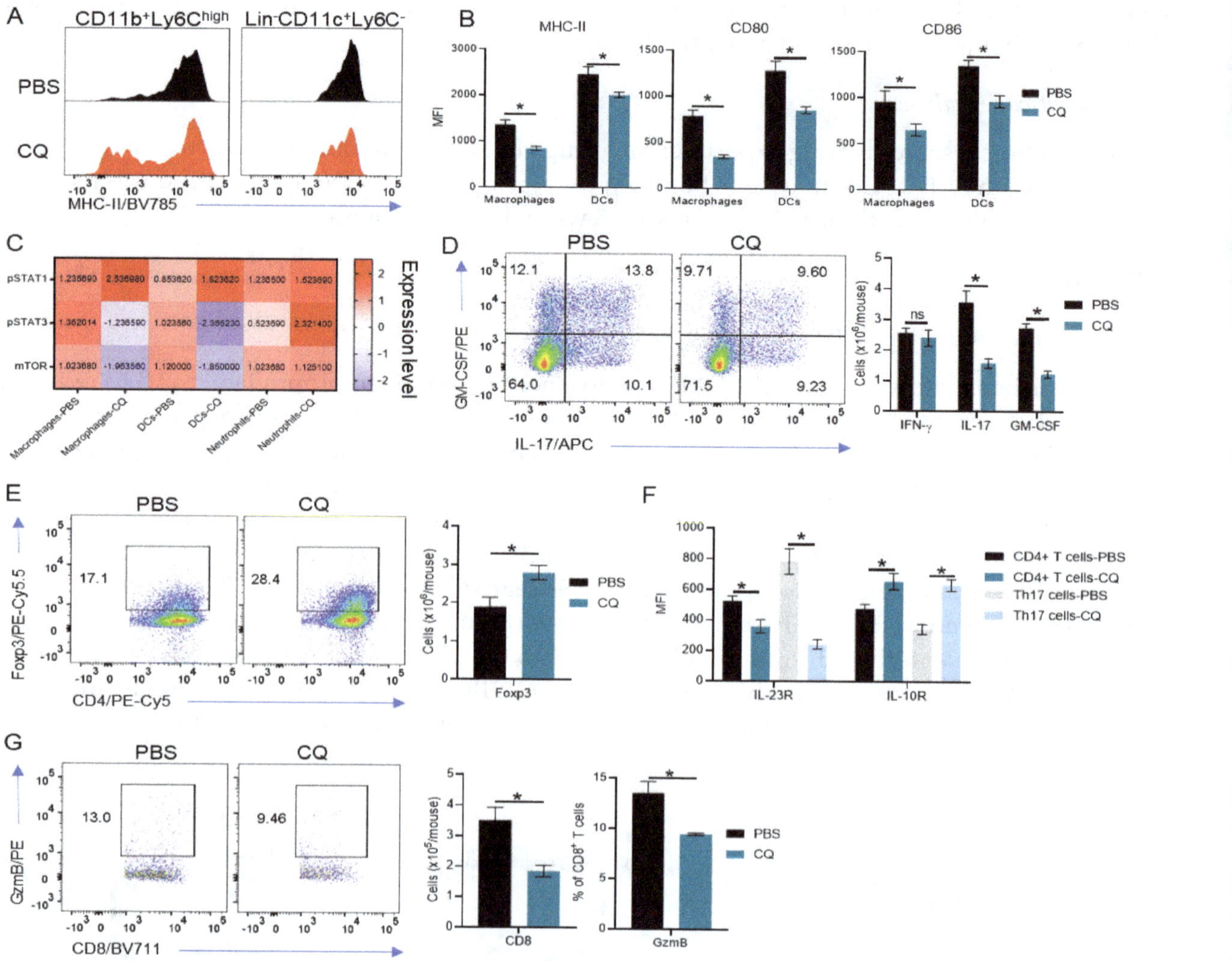

Figure 2. Comprehensive analysis of the immune compartment in the central nervous system (CNS) of CQ-treated mice. CNS cells from EAE B6SJLF1 mice ($n = 5$/group) at day 21 post-immunization were analyzed by flow cytometry. (**A**) Representative histogram for MHC-II expression in CD11b$^+$Ly6C^{high} macrophages and in Lin$^-$CD11c$^+$Ly6C$^-$ DCs. (**B**) MHC-II, CD80 and CD86 expression in macrophages and dendritic cells (DCs). (**C**) Mean fluorescent values for pSTAT1, pSTAT3 and mTOR in macrophages, DCs and Ly6G$^+$ neutrophils were measured by flow cytometry. (**D**) Infiltrating GM-CSF-, IFN-γ and IL-17-producing CD4$^+$ T cells in the CNS of EAE mice. (**E**) Numbers of Foxp3$^+$ Treg cells. (**F**) Analysis of IL-23R and IL-10R in total CD4$^+$ T cells and in Th17 cells in the CNS of EAE mice. (**G**) Analysis of total CD8$^+$ T cell GzmB-producing CD8$^+$ T cell infiltration in the CNS of EAE mice. Values of $p < 0.05$ (*) were considered statistically significative. Ns: not significative. Results are from three independent experiments.

We also observed a significant decrease in IL-17$^+$ and GM-CSF$^+$CD4$^+$ T cells in the CNS of CQ-treated mice compared with PBS-treated ones (Figure 2D). No significant differences were observed in Th1 cells (Figure 2D). Foxp3$^+$ Treg cells were upregulated in CQ-treated mice compared with controls (Figure 2E). Interestingly, we observed a significant decrease in the expression of IL-23R and an increase in the expression of IL-10R in total CD4$^+$ T cells and more drastically in Th17 cells (Figure 2F). CD8$^+$ T cells numbers were reduced and had lower expression of Granzyme B in CQ-treated mice compared with PBS-treated mice (Figure 2G). B cells did not show significant differences in numbers, MHC-II expression and in cytokine production (not shown). Combined, these results show that CQ modulates both myeloid and lymphoid leukocyte populations in the CNS of EAE mice.

3.3. MG and Astrocytes Are Modulated by CQ

We then analyzed the effect of CQ treatment on CNS resident cells of EAE mice. We observed that GFAP$^+$ astrocytes presented as two populations GFAP$^+$ and GFAP^{high} (Figure 3A), which reflect their activation profile. GFAP^{high} are reactive astrocytes that are involved in scar formation and oligodendrocyte death [38,39]. We observed a significant decrease in GFAP^{high} astrocytes in CQ-treated mice compared with PBS-treated controls (Figure 3A). Moreover, astrocytes from CQ-treated mice showed an increase in IL-10 production and a decrease in IL-6 and IL-1β production in comparison with cells from PBS-treated mice (Figure 3B).

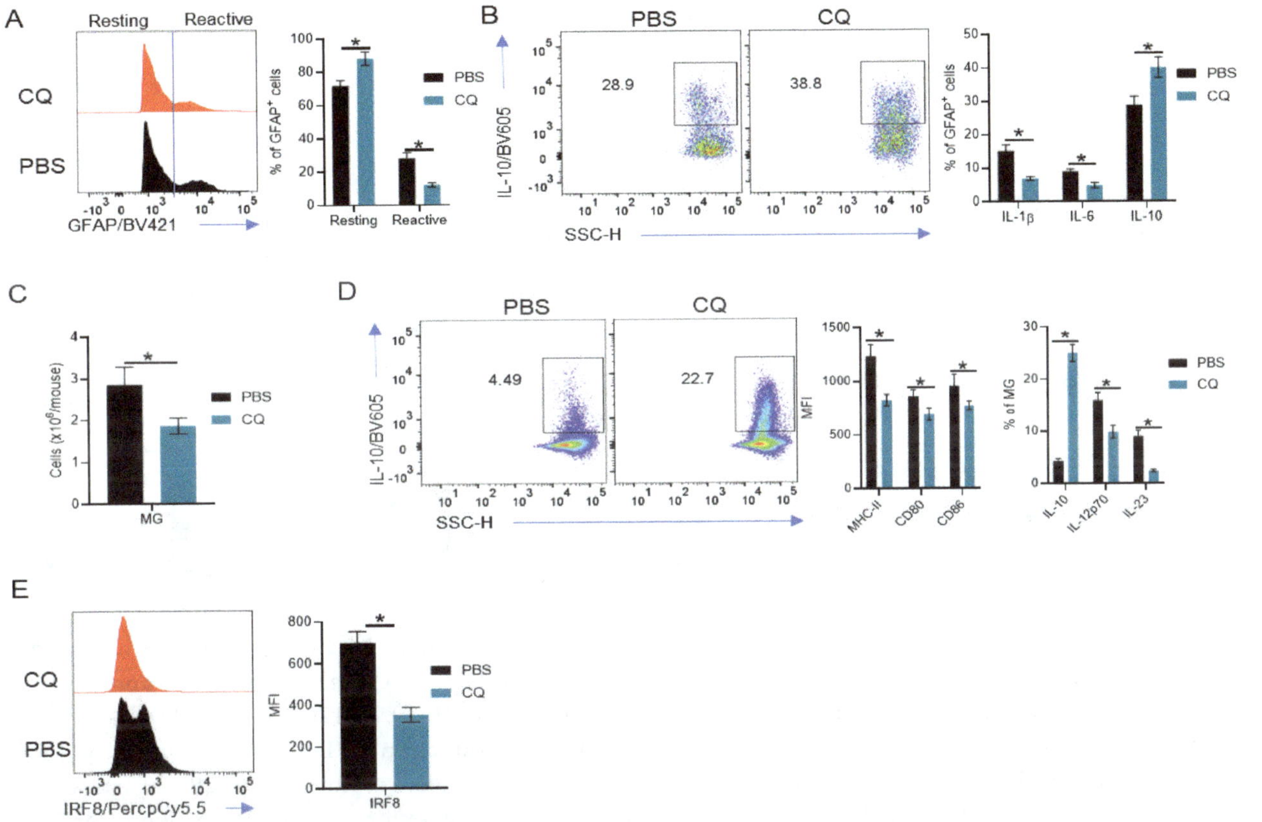

Figure 3. Comprehensive analysis of the stromal compartment in the CNS of CQ-treated mice. CNS cells from EAE B6SJLF1 mice (n = 5/group) at day 21 post-immunization were analyzed by flow cytometry. (**A**) Analysis of resting (GFAP$^{+/low}$) and reactive (GFAP^{high}) astrocytes. (**B**) Analysis of IL-1β, IL-6 and IL-10 production by astrocytes. (**C**) Absolute numbers of MG (CD45$^{+/low}$CD11b$^+$Ly6C$^-$) in the CNS of CQ- and PBS-treated mice. (**D**) Analysis of the expression of the antigen-presenting molecules MHC-II, CD80 and CD86 and of the cytokine profile of MG. (**E**) IRF8 expression in MG from CQ- and PBS-treated mice. Values of $p < 0.05$ (*) were considered statistically significative. Results are from three independent experiments.

Furthermore, MG greatly influences astrocyte activation [40,41] and provides additional antigen stimulation to T cells in the CNS [42–44]. Thus, we investigated the phenotype of MG in mice treated with CQ. Our results showed that the numbers of MG were reduced in the CNS of CQ-treated mice compared with those from PBS-treated mice (Figure 3C). Interestingly, MG from CQ-treated mice had an increase in IL-10 and IL-12p70 cytokine production while MHC-II, CD80 and CD86 levels were decreased in comparison with MG from PBS-treated mice (Figure 3D). Moreover, we observed a significant decrease in IL-23 production in MG from CQ-treated mice compared with controls (Figure 3D). The transcriptional factor IRF8, which promotes MG differentiation and aids in IL-1β production by MG [45–48], was significantly reduced in MG from CQ-treated mice (Figure 3E). Together, these results reveal a portrait of CNS resident cells in EAE mice treated with CQ, where astrocytes and MG acquire an immunomodulatory phenotype.

3.4. CQ Induces IL-10 and IL-12p70 in MG Which Enhances IL-10 Production by T Cells and Reduces Astrocyte Activation

Finally, we investigated whether CQ modulates MG directly. We isolated primary MG and activated the cells with LPS for 18 h in the presence or absence of CQ. Then, the RNA from MG was analyzed by PCRArray. We observed that CQ reduced the expression of genes associated with inflammation (Cd40, H2-eb, Il1b, Il6, Tnfa, Il23a), while increasing those related to immune modulation (Il10, Lag3, Entpd1, Cd274) (Figure 4A). Moreover, CQ-treated MG produced significantly more IL-10 and IL-12p70 and less IL-23 than PBS-treated MG (Figure 4B).

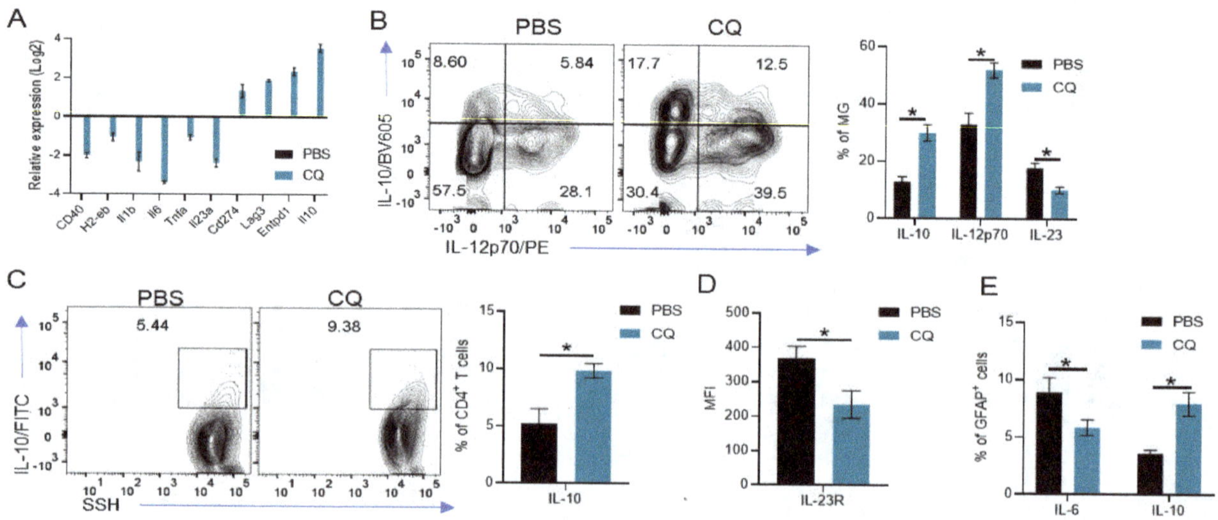

Figure 4. CQ-treated MG modulates T cells and astrocytes. Primary MG were activated with LPS (100 ng/mL) in the presence or absence of CQ (50 μM) for 18 h. (**A**) Gene expression analysis in CQ-treated MG compared with PBS-treated ones. (**B**) Analysis of IL-10, IL-12p70 and IL-23 production by MG. (**C**) MG were co-cultured with $CD4^+$ T cells and the production of IL-10 was analyzed by flow cytometry. (**D**) IL-23R in $CD4^+$ T cells cultured with MG. (**E**) MG were cultured with C8D30 astrocytic cells and the production of IL-6 and IL-10 was analyzed by flow cytometry. Cultures were carried out in triplicate. Values of $p < 0.05$ (*) were considered statistically significative. Results from three independent experiments.

To test their effect on $CD4^+$ T cell activation, we co-cultured CQ-treated MG with $CD4^+$ T cells isolated from naïve WT mice. We observed that CQ-treated MG induced significantly more IL-10 production in T cells than PBS-treated MG (Figure 4C). Moreover, IL-23R in T cells cultured with CQ-treated MG was downregulated when compared with T cells cultured with PBS-treated MG (Figure 4D).

To test the effect of CQ-treated MG on astrocyte activation, we co-cultured MG with the astrocytic cell line C8D30. We observed that CQ-treated MG induced a significant increase in IL-10 production by astrocytes, while PBS-treated MG induced higher IL-6 production (Figure 4E). Collectively, our results show a pivotal role of CNS resident cells, especially MG, on CQ-induced immunosuppression in EAE.

4. Discussion

In this study, we show that CQ modulates a broad array of cell subtypes to reduce EAE severity. Although the therapeutic effect of CQ in EAE was shown before, its underlying mechanism of action remains to be fully elucidated. Here, our results have uncovered a portrait of the CNS resident and infiltrating cells after CQ treatment. We observed that CQ reduced the numbers and phenotype of inflammatory leukocytes and also upregulated the expression of modulatory mediators in leukocytes and CNS resident cells.

EAE is a T cell-dependent model of MS, where pathogenic Th1 and Th17 cells play a major role in disease severity and development [1]. In addition, GM-CSF production grants pathogenicity of Th17 cells [7]. Thus, we investigated the profile of $CD4^+$ T cells in CQ-treated mice and compared them with those found in PBS-treated mice. Our results showed that CQ inhibited differentiation of Th17 and GM-CSF^+ $CD4^+$ T cells without disturbing the frequencies of Th1 cells. This finding is in line with a recent publication from our group, where we show that Th17 cells are more sensitive to CQ treatment [31]. Moreover, CQ reduces the differentiation of Th17 cells by inducing the expression of T-bet [31]. GM-CSF production in Th17 cells is induced through stimulation of the IL-23 receptor [7,9]. Interestingly, CQ reduced the expression of IL-23R on $CD4^+$ T cells. These results show that CQ modulates T cells through different mechanisms: either by suppressing their differentiation into inflammatory Th17 cells or by reducing their pathogenicity through downregulation of IL-23R.

We also observed a reduction in $CD8^+$ T cells numbers in the CNS of CQ-treated mice. Although EAE is mainly a Th cell model, $CD8^+$ T cells were shown to play an important role shaping the phenotype of $CD4^+$ T cells during EAE through the Qa-1 receptor [49,50]. In fact, pathogenic MOG-reactive $CD8^+$ T cells cooperate with Th cells to promote sustained CNS inflammation in EAE [51], whereas dual modulation of $CD8^+$ and $CD4^+$ T cells proved to be more efficient in suppressing EAE [52]. Our results showed that CQ induced suppression of both $CD8^+$ and $CD4^+$ T cells, which may account for its efficiency in reducing EAE severity.

We have showed previously that CQ induces $Foxp3^+$ Treg cells indirectly by stimulating tolerogenic DCs [35]. Additionally, CQ directly modulates DCs by inducing iNOS and pSTAT1 expression, and the lack of these molecules abrogated the tolerogenic phenotype of CQ-treated DCs [30,32]. A similar increase in $Foxp3^+$ Treg cells in models of inflammatory bowel disease and lupus was observed [53,54]. CQ directly induced Foxp3 expression in T cells in a Nurr1-dependent manner [53]. Thus, the literature data show that CQ induces STAT1 in DCs, T-bet in Th17 cells and Nurr1 in naïve T cells [32,53,54]. In line with this observation, CQ modulates tumor infiltrating macrophages through stimulation of the NF-kB signaling pathway [29]. In the present study, we show that STAT3 and mTOR signaling pathways in myeloid cells were also affected by CQ. Specifically, pSTAT1 was upregulated in DCs and macrophages, while pSTAT3 was upregulated in neutrophils. mTOR was decreased in DCs and macrophages, and unaffected in neutrophils. These results show that CQ induces different signaling cascades in various leukocytes.

MG are CNS resident cells that closely resemble peripheral macrophages [55,56]. MG act as a first line defense in the CNS against infections [16,21,46]. In EAE, MG cooperate with local inflammation and provide antigen-stimulation to infiltrating T cells [40,43]. Thus, we analyzed MG phenotype in CQ-treated mice, and we found that CQ inhibited MG activation. Moreover, we observed a reduced production of IL-23 and an increase in IL-10 and IL-12p70 cytokines in MG from CQ-treated mice. CQ modulated MG directly in in vitro experiments and conferred an anti-inflammatory profile in them. In co-culture experiments with total $CD4^+$ T cells, CQ-treated MG reduced GM-CSF production and increased IL-10 production. These results are in line with our in vivo observations, where $CD4^+$ T cells had a reduced GM-CSF and increased IL-10 production while IL-23R expression was also reduced.

In prophylactical treatment with CQ, it is possible that EAE amelioration relied on the modulation of antigen-presenting cells, such as DCs and macrophages [27,35]. However, during ongoing EAE, there is a possibility that CQ acts directly on Th17 cells in the CNS and on MG to refrain further T cell activation and promote an immunosuppressive microenvironment [31,57,58]. In line with this, MG modulated T cells and astrocytes. Astrocytes cultured with CQ-treated MG showed a reduced production of IL-6 and IL-1β and an increase in IL-10 production. Ultimately, paralysis and weakness are a result of the loss of neuronal transmission, and OL play an important role in maintaining neuronal growth and providing the myelin sheaths [59–61]. We observed that CQ-treated mice had more MBP^+ OLs than PBS-treated mice (not shown). We did not investigate whether CQ induces myelination directly or if this finding is a by-stander result of reduced inflammation in the CNS, which warrant further investigations.

Overall, results presented in this study clearly show that CQ suppresses ongoing neuroinflammation by acting in both leukocytes and CNS resident cells. This finding places CQ as a promising therapeutic agent due to its modulation of both inflammation and neurodegeneration, and strengthen the basis for the use of CQ in patients with MS. The majority of FDA-approved drugs to treat MS target leukocytes and inflammation with limited effect on CNS resident cells [62–64]. Moreover, CQ has high bioavailability when taken orally [65,66], which increases acceptability among patients. Thus, we believe that CQ would be as efficient as, if not better than, current FDA-approved drugs in the treatment of MS.

5. Conclusions

Our results show that CQ is a potent modulator of the immune system and CNS resident cells. Moreover, CQ suppressed EAE progression and interfered with the activation of leukocytes and MG. CQ-treated MG-derived cytokines modulated T cells and astrocytes towards an anti-inflammatory phenotype that likely influenced the inflammation in the CNS. Overall, our data reveal a novel pathway by which CQ suppresses neuroinflammation that can be harnessed to develop novel strategies to treat MS.

Author Contributions: R.T., A.B., L.L.W.I., and J.M. performed the experiments. R.T., G.C., B.C. and G.-X.Z. analyzed the data. R.T. and A.R. wrote the manuscript. A.R. supervised the study. All authors have read and agreed to the published version of the manuscript.

Acknowledgments: We would like to thank Katherine Regan for help editing this manuscript.

References

1. Glatigny, S.; Bettelli, E. Experimental Autoimmune Encephalomyelitis (EAE) as Animal Models of Multiple Sclerosis (MS). *Cold Spring Harb. Perspect. Med.* **2018**, *8*, a028977. [CrossRef]
2. Baron, J.L.; Madri, J.A.; Ruddle, N.H.; Hashim, G.; Janeway, C.A. Surface expression of alpha 4 integrin by CD4 T cells is required for their entry into brain parenchyma. *J. Exp. Med.* **1993**, *177*, 57–68. [CrossRef] [PubMed]
3. Voskuhl, R.R.; Martin, R.; Bergman, C.; Dalal, M.; Ruddle, N.H.; McFarland, H.F. T helper 1 (Th1) functional phenotype of human myelin basic protein-specific T lymphocytes. *Autoimmunity* **1993**, *15*, 137–143. [CrossRef] [PubMed]
4. Veldhoen, M.; Hocking, R.J.; Flavell, R.A.; Stockinger, B. Signals mediated by transforming growth factor-beta initiate autoimmune encephalomyelitis, but chronic inflammation is needed to sustain disease. *Nat. Immunol.* **2006**, *7*, 1151–1156. [CrossRef] [PubMed]
5. Zhang, Z.; Zhenyi, X.; Ying, L.; Hongkun, L.; Xiangdong, G.; Yan, L.; Hongwei, Y.; Lijuan, Z.; Yurong, D.; Zhi, Y. MicroRNA-181c promotes Th17 cell differentiation and mediates experimental autoimmune encephalomyelitis. *Brain Behav. Immun.* **2018**, *70*, 305–314. [CrossRef]
6. Pare, A.; Mailhot, B.; Lévesque, S.A.; Juzwik, C.; Doss, P.M.I.A.; Lécuyer, M.; Prat, A.; Rangachari, M.; Fournier, A.; Lacroix, S. IL-1beta enables CNS access to CCR2(hi) monocytes and the generation of pathogenic cells through GM-CSF released by CNS endothelial cells. *Proc. Natl. Acad. Sci. USA* **2018**, *115*, E1194–E1203. [CrossRef]
7. El-Behi, M.; Ciric, B.; Hong, D.; Yaping, Y.; Cullimore, M.; Safavi, F.; Guang-Xian, Z.; Dittel, B.N.; Rostami, A. The encephalitogenicity of T(H)17 cells is dependent on IL-1- and IL-23-induced production of the cytokine GM-CSF. *Nat. Immunol.* **2011**, *12*, 568–575. [CrossRef]
8. Codarri, L.; Gyülvészi, G.; Tosevski, V.; Hesske, L.; Fontana, A.; Magnenat, L.; Suter, T.; Bechere, B. RORgammat drives production of the cytokine GM-CSF in helper T cells, which is essential for the effector phase of autoimmune neuroinflammation. *Nat. Immunol.* **2011**, *12*, 560–567. [CrossRef]

9. Komuczki, J.; Tuzlak, S.; Friebel, E.; Hartwig, T.; Spath, S.; Rosenstiel, P.; Waisman, A.; Opitz, L.; Oukka, M.; Schreiner, B.; et al. Fate-Mapping of GM-CSF Expression Identifies a Discrete Subset of Inflammation-Driving T Helper Cells Regulated by Cytokines IL-23 and IL-1beta. *Immunity* **2019**, *50*, 1289–1304. [CrossRef]
10. Dominguez-Villar, M.; Hafler, D.A. Regulatory T cells in autoimmune disease. *Nat. Immunol.* **2018**, *19*, 665–673. [CrossRef]
11. McIntyre, L.L.; Greilach, S.A.; Othy, S.; Sears-Kraxberger, I.; Wi, B.; Ayala-Angulo, J.; Vu, E.; Pham, Q.; Silva, J.; Dang, K.; et al. Regulatory T cells promote remyelination in the murine experimental autoimmune encephalomyelitis model of multiple sclerosis following human neural stem cell transplant. *Neurobiol. Dis.* **2020**, *140*, 104868. [CrossRef] [PubMed]
12. Dombrowski, Y.; O'Hagan, T.; Dittmer, M.; Penalva, R.; Mayoral, S.R.; Bankhead, P.; Fleville, S.; Eleftheriadis, G.; Chao, Z.; Naughton, M.; et al. Regulatory T cells promote myelin regeneration in the central nervous system. *Nat. Neurosci.* **2017**, *20*, 674–680. [CrossRef] [PubMed]
13. Bailey, S.L.; Schreiner, B.; McMahon, E.J.; Miller, S.D. CNS myeloid DCs presenting endogenous myelin peptides 'preferentially' polarize CD4+ T(H)-17 cells in relapsing EAE. *Nat. Immunol.* **2007**, *8*, 172–180. [CrossRef] [PubMed]
14. Louveau, A.; Herz, J.; Alme, M.N.; Salvador, A.F.; Dong, M.Q.; Viar, K.E.; Herod, S.G.; Knopp, J.; Setliff, J.C.; Lupi, A.L.; et al. CNS lymphatic drainage and neuroinflammation are regulated by meningeal lymphatic vasculature. *Nat. Neurosci.* **2018**, *21*, 1380–1391. [CrossRef] [PubMed]
15. Mundt, S.; Mrdjen, D.; Utz, S.G.; Greter, M.; Schreiner, B.; Becher, B. Conventional DCs sample and present myelin antigens in the healthy CNS and allow parenchymal T cell entry to initiate neuroinflammation. *Sci. Immunol.* **2019**, *4*, eaau8380. [CrossRef]
16. Chu, F.; Shi, M.; Zheng, C.; Shen, D.; Zhu, J.; Zheng, X.; Cui, L. The roles of macrophages and microglia in multiple sclerosis and experimental autoimmune encephalomyelitis. *J. Neuroimmunol.* **2018**, *318*, 1–7. [CrossRef]
17. Tanabe, S.; Saitoh, S.; Miyajima, H.; Itokazu, T.; Yamashita, T. Microglia suppress the secondary progression of autoimmune encephalomyelitis. *Glia* **2019**, *67*, 1694–1704. [CrossRef]
18. Zabala, A.; Vazquez-Villoldo, N.; Rissiek, B.; Gejo, J.; Martin, A.; Palomino, A.; Perez-Samartín, A.; Pulagam, K.R.; Lukowiak, M.; Capetillo-Zarate, E.; et al. P2X4 receptor controls microglia activation and favors remyelination in autoimmune encephalitis. *EMBO Mol. Med.* **2018**, *10*, e8743. [CrossRef]
19. Zhang, C.J.; Jiang, M.; Zhou, H.; Liu, W.; Wang, C.; Kang, Z.; Han, B.; Zhang, Q.; Chen, X.; Xiao, J.; et al. TLR-stimulated IRAKM activates caspase-8 inflammasome in microglia and promotes neuroinflammation. *J. Clin. Investig.* **2018**, *128*, 5399–5412. [CrossRef]
20. Rothhammer, V.; Borucki, D.M.; Tjon, E.M.; Takenaka, M.C.; Chao, C.C.; Ardura-Fabregat, A.; Alves de Lima, K.; Gutiérrez-Vázquez, C.; Hewson, P.; Staszewski, O.; et al. Microglial control of astrocytes in response to microbial metabolites. *Nature* **2018**, *557*, 724–728. [CrossRef]
21. Domingues, H.S.; Portugal, C.C.; Socodato, R.; Relvas, J.B. Oligodendrocyte, Astrocyte, and Microglia Crosstalk in Myelin Development, Damage, and Repair. *Front. Cell Dev. Biol.* **2016**, *4*, 71. [PubMed]
22. Chrzanowski, U.; Bhattarai, S.; Scheld, M.; Clarner, T.; Fallier-Becker, P.; Beyer, C.; Rohr, S.O.; Schmitz, C.; Hochstrasser, T.; Schweiger, F.; et al. Oligodendrocyte degeneration and concomitant microglia activation directs peripheral immune cells into the forebrain. *Neurochem. Int.* **2019**, *126*, 139–153. [CrossRef] [PubMed]
23. Liddelow, S.A.; Guttenplan, K.A.; Clarke, L.E.; Bennett, F.C.; Bohlen, C.J.; Schirmer, L.; Bennett, M.L.; Münch, A.E.; Chung, W.; Peterson, T.C.; et al. Neurotoxic reactive astrocytes are induced by activated microglia. *Nature* **2017**, *541*, 481–487. [CrossRef] [PubMed]
24. Thome, R.; Lopes, S.C.P.; Costa, F.T.M.; Verinaud, L. Chloroquine: Modes of action of an undervalued drug. *Immunol. Lett.* **2013**, *153*, 50–57. [CrossRef] [PubMed]
25. Jang, C.H.; Choi, J.H.; Byun, M.S.; Jue, D.M. Chloroquine inhibits production of TNF-alpha, IL-1beta and IL-6 from lipopolysaccharide-stimulated human monocytes/macrophages by different modes. *Rheumatology* **2006**, *45*, 703–710. [CrossRef] [PubMed]
26. Long, Y.; Liu, X.; Wang, N.; Zhou, H.; Zheng, J. Chloroquine attenuates LPS-mediated macrophage activation through miR-669n-regulated SENP6 protein translation. *Am. J. Transl. Res.* **2015**, *7*, 2335–2345.

27. Thome, R.; Issayama, L.K.; DiGangi, R.; Bombeiro, A.L.; da Costa, T.A.; Ferreira, I.T.; de Oliveira, A.L.R.; Verinaud, L. Dendritic cells treated with chloroquine modulate experimental autoimmune encephalomyelitis. *Immunol. Cell Biol.* **2014**, *92*, 124–132. [CrossRef]
28. Mauthe, M.; Orhon, I.; Rocchi, C.; Zhou, X.R.; Luhr, M.; Hijlkema, K.-J.; Coppes, R.P.; Engedal, N.; Mari, M.; Reggiori, F. Chloroquine inhibits autophagic flux by decreasing autophagosome-lysosome fusion. *Autophagy* **2018**, *14*, 1435–1455. [CrossRef]
29. Chen, D.; Xie, J.; Fiskesund, R.; Dong, W.Q.; Liang, X.Y.; Lv, J.D.; Jin, X.; Liu, J.Y.; Mo, S.Q.; Zhang, T.Z.; et al. Chloroquine modulates antitumor immune response by resetting tumor-associated macrophages toward M1 phenotype. *Nat. Commun.* **2018**, *9*, 873. [CrossRef]
30. Verinaud, L.; Issayama, L.K.; Zanucoli, F.; de Carvalho, A.C.; da Costa, T.A.; Di Gangi, R.; Bonfanti, A.P.; Ferreira, I.T.; de Oliveira, A.L.R.; Machado, D.R.S.; et al. Nitric oxide plays a key role in the suppressive activity of tolerogenic dendritic cells. *Cell Mol. Immunol.* **2015**, *12*, 384–386. [CrossRef]
31. Thome, R.; Boehm, A.; Ishikawa, L.L.W.; Casella, G.; Munhoz, J.; Ciric, B.; Zhang, G.X.; Rostami, A. Chloroquine reduces Th17 cell differentiation by stimulating T-bet expression in T cells. *Cell Mol. Immunol.* **2020**.
32. Thome, R.; Bonfanti, A.P.; Rasouli, J.; Mari, E.R.; Zhang, G.X.; Rostami, A.; Verinaud, L. Chloroquine-treated dendritic cells require STAT1 signaling for their tolerogenic activity. *Eur. J. Immunol.* **2018**, *48*, 1228–1234. [CrossRef] [PubMed]
33. Thome, R.; Moore, J.N.; Mari, E.R.; Rasouli, J.; Hwang, D.; Yoshimura, S.; Ciric, B.; Zhang, G.X.; Rostami, A.M. Induction of Peripheral Tolerance in Ongoing Autoimmune Inflammation Requires Interleukin 27 Signaling in Dendritic Cells. *Front. Immunol.* **2017**, *8*, 1392. [CrossRef] [PubMed]
34. Yoshimura, S.; Thome, R.; Konno, S.; Mari, E.R.; Rasouli, J.; Hwang, D.; Boehm, A.; Li, Y.; Zhang, G.X.; Ciric, B.; et al. IL-9 Controls Central Nervous System Autoimmunity by Suppressing GM-CSF Production. *J. Immunol.* **2020**, *204*, 531–539. [CrossRef] [PubMed]
35. Thome, R.; Moraes, A.S.; Bombeiro, A.L.; Farias Ados, S.; Francelin, C.; da Costa, T.A.; Di Gangi, R.; dos Santos, L.M.; de Oliveira, A.L.; Verinaud, L. Chloroquine treatment enhances regulatory T cells and reduces the severity of experimental autoimmune encephalomyelitis. *PLoS ONE* **2013**, *8*, e65913. [CrossRef]
36. Skundric, D.S.; Dai, R.; Zakarian, V.L.; Zhou, W. Autoimmune-induced preferential depletion of myelin-associated glycoprotein (MAG) is genetically regulated in relapsing EAE (B6 x SJL) F1 mice. *Mol. Neurodegener.* **2008**, *3*, 7. [CrossRef]
37. Zhang, G.X.; Yu, S.; Gran, B.; Li, J.; Calida, D.; Ventura, E.; Chen, X.; Rostami, A. T cell and antibody responses in remitting-relapsing experimental autoimmune encephalomyelitis in (C57BL/6 x SJL) F1 mice. *J. Neuroimmunol.* **2004**, *148*, 1–10. [CrossRef]
38. Frik, J.; Merl-Pham, J.; Plesnila, N.; Mattugini, N.; Kjell, J.; Kraska, J.; Gómez, R.M.; Hauck, S.M.; Sirko, S.; Götz, M. Cross-talk between monocyte invasion and astrocyte proliferation regulates scarring in brain injury. *EMBO Rep.* **2018**, *19*, e45294. [CrossRef]
39. Anderson, M.A.; Ao, Y.; Sofroniew, M.V. Heterogeneity of reactive astrocytes. *Neurosci. Lett.* **2014**, *565*, 23–29. [CrossRef]
40. Norden, D.M.; Trojanowski, P.J.; Villanueva, E.; Navarro, E.; Godbout, J.P. Sequential activation of microglia and astrocyte cytokine expression precedes increased Iba-1 or GFAP immunoreactivity following systemic immune challenge. *Glia* **2016**, *64*, 300–316. [CrossRef]
41. Shinozaki, Y.; Shibata, K.; Yoshida, K.; Shigetomi, E.; Gachet, C.; Ikenaka, K.; Tanaka, K.F.; Koizumi, S. Transformation of Astrocytes to a Neuroprotective Phenotype by Microglia via P2Y1 Receptor Downregulation. *Cell Rep.* **2017**, *19*, 1151–1164. [CrossRef] [PubMed]
42. Wlodarczyk, A.; Løbner, M.; Cédile, O.; Owens, T. Comparison of microglia and infiltrating CD11c(+) cells as antigen presenting cells for T cell proliferation and cytokine response. *J. Neuroinflamm.* **2014**, *11*, 57. [CrossRef] [PubMed]
43. Matsumoto, Y.; Ohmori, K.; Fujiwara, M. Immune regulation by brain cells in the central nervous system: Microglia but not astrocytes present myelin basic protein to encephalitogenic T cells under in vivo-mimicking conditions. *Immunology* **1992**, *76*, 209–216. [PubMed]
44. Hu, J.; He, H.; Yang, Z.; Zhu, G.; Kang, L.; Jing, X.; Lu, H.; Song, W.; Bai, B.; Tang, H. Programmed Death Ligand-1 on Microglia Regulates Th1 Differentiation via Nitric Oxide in Experimental Autoimmune Encephalomyelitis. *Neurosci. Bull.* **2016**, *32*, 70–82. [CrossRef]

45. Zhou, N.; Liu, K.; Sun, Y.; Cao, Y.; Yang, J. Transcriptional mechanism of IRF8 and PU.1 governs microglial activation in neurodegenerative condition. *Protein Cell* **2019**, *10*, 87–103. [CrossRef]
46. Kierdorf, K.; Erny, D.; Goldmann, T.; Sander, V.; Schulz, C.; Perdiguero, E.G.; Wieghofer, P.; Heinrich, A.; Riemke, P.; Hölscher, C.; et al. Microglia emerge from erythromyeloid precursors via Pu.1- and Irf8-dependent pathways. *Nat. Neurosci.* **2013**, *16*, 273–280. [CrossRef]
47. Masuda, T.; Iwamoto, S.; Mikuriya, S.; Tozaki-Saitoh, H.; Tamura, T.; Tsuda, M.; Inoue, K. Transcription factor IRF1 is responsible for IRF8-mediated IL-1beta expression in reactive microglia. *J. Pharmacol. Sci.* **2015**, *128*, 216–220. [CrossRef]
48. Masuda, T.; Tsuda, M.; Yoshinaga, R.; Tozaki-Saitoh, H.; Ozato, K.; Tamura, T.; Inoue, K. IRF8 is a critical transcription factor for transforming microglia into a reactive phenotype. *Cell Rep.* **2012**, *1*, 334–340. [CrossRef]
49. Jiang, H.; Braunstein, N.S.; Yu, B.; Winchester, R.; Chess, L. CD8+ T cells control the TH phenotype of MBP-reactive CD4+ T cells in EAE mice. *Proc. Natl. Acad. Sci. USA* **2001**, *98*, 6301–6306. [CrossRef]
50. Leuenberger, T.; Paterka, M.; Reuter, E.; Herz, J.; Niesner, R.A.; Radbruch, H.; Bopp, T.; Zipp, F.; Siffrin, V. The role of CD8+ T cells and their local interaction with CD4+ T cells in myelin oligodendrocyte glycoprotein35-55-induced experimental autoimmune encephalomyelitis. *J. Immunol.* **2013**, *191*, 4960–4968. [CrossRef]
51. Bettini, M.; Rosenthal, K.; Evavold, B.D. Pathogenic MOG-reactive CD8+ T cells require MOG-reactive CD4+ T cells for sustained CNS inflammation during chronic EAE. *J. Neuroimmunol.* **2009**, *213*, 60–68. [CrossRef] [PubMed]
52. Pei, W.; Wan, X.; Shahzad, K.A.; Zhang, L.; Song, S.; Jin, X.; Wang, L.; Zhao, C.; Shen, C. Direct modulation of myelin-autoreactive CD4(+) and CD8(+) T cells in EAE mice by a tolerogenic nanoparticle co-carrying myelin peptide-loaded major histocompatibility complexes, CD47 and multiple regulatory molecules. *Int. J. Nanomed.* **2018**, *13*, 3731–3750. [CrossRef] [PubMed]
53. Park, T.Y.; Jang, Y.; Kim, W.; Shin, J.; Toh, H.T.; Kim, C.H.; Yoon, H.S.; Leblanc, P.; Kim, K.S. Chloroquine modulates inflammatory autoimmune responses through Nurr1 in autoimmune diseases. *Sci. Rep.* **2019**, *9*, 15559. [CrossRef] [PubMed]
54. An, N.; Chen, Y.; Wang, C.; Yang, C.; Wu, Z.H.; Xue, J.; Ye, L.; Wang, S.; Liu, H.F.; Pan, Q. Chloroquine Autophagic Inhibition Rebalances Th17/Treg-Mediated Immunity and Ameliorates Systemic Lupus Erythematosus. *Cell Physiol. Biochem.* **2017**, *44*, 412–422. [CrossRef] [PubMed]
55. Prinz, M.; Erny, D.; Hagemeyer, N. Ontogeny and homeostasis of CNS myeloid cells. *Nat. Immunol.* **2017**, *18*, 385–392. [CrossRef]
56. Bennett, M.L.; Bennett, F.C.; Liddelow, S.A.; Ajami, B.; Zamanian, J.L.; Fernhoff, N.B.; Mulinyawe, S.B.; Bohlen, C.J.; Adil, A.; Tucker, A.; et al. New tools for studying microglia in the mouse and human CNS. *Proc. Natl. Acad. Sci. USA* **2016**, *113*, E1738–E1746. [CrossRef]
57. Chu, T.; Tran, T.; Yang, F.; Beech, W.; Cole, G.M.; Frautschy, S.A. Effect of chloroquine and leupeptin on intracellular accumulation of amyloid-beta (A beta) 1-42 peptide in a murine N9 microglial cell line. *FEBS Lett.* **1998**, *436*, 439–444. [CrossRef]
58. Koch, M.W.; Zabad, R.; Giuliani, F.; Hader, W., Jr.; Lewkonia, R.; Metz, L.; Wee Yong, V. Hydroxychloroquine reduces microglial activity and attenuates experimental autoimmune encephalomyelitis. *J. Neurol. Sci.* **2015**, *358*, 131–137. [CrossRef]
59. Barateiro, A.; Brites, D.; Fernandes, A. Oligodendrocyte Development and Myelination in Neurodevelopment: Molecular Mechanisms in Health and Disease. *Curr. Pharm. Des.* **2016**, *22*, 656–679. [CrossRef]
60. Domingues, H.S.; Cruz, A.; Chan, J.R.; Relvas, J.B.; Rubinstein, B.; Pinto, I.M. Mechanical plasticity during oligodendrocyte differentiation and myelination. *Glia* **2018**, *66*, 5–14. [CrossRef]
61. Foster, A.Y.; Bujalka, H.; Emery, B. Axoglial interactions in myelin plasticity: Evaluating the relationship between neuronal activity and oligodendrocyte dynamics. *Glia* **2019**, *67*, 2038–2049. [CrossRef]
62. Aharoni, R.; Eilam, R.; Domev, H.; Labunskay, G.; Sela, M.; Arnon, R. The immunomodulator glatiramer acetate augments the expression of neurotrophic factors in brains of experimental autoimmune encephalomyelitis mice. *Proc. Natl. Acad. Sci. USA* **2005**, *102*, 19045–19050. [CrossRef] [PubMed]
63. Maarouf, A.; Boutière, C.; Rico, A.; Audoin, B.; Pelletier, J. How much progress has there been in the second-line treatment of multiple sclerosis: A 2017 update. *Rev. Neurol.* **2018**, *174*, 429–440. [CrossRef] [PubMed]

64. Vargas, D.L.; Tyor, W.R. Update on disease-modifying therapies for multiple sclerosis. *J. Investig. Med.* **2017**, *65*, 883–891. [CrossRef] [PubMed]

65. Krishna, S.; White, N.J. Pharmacokinetics of quinine, chloroquine and amodiaquine. *Clin. Pharmacokinet.* **1996**, *30*, 263–299. [CrossRef]

66. Gustafsson, L.L.; Walker, O.; Alván, G.; Beermann, B.; Estevez, F.; Gleisner, L.; Lindström, B.; Sjöqvist, F. Disposition of chloroquine in man after single intravenous and oral doses. *Br. J. Clin. Pharmacol.* **1983**, *15*, 471–479. [CrossRef]

5

A Multiple *N*-Glucosylated Peptide Epitope Efficiently Detecting Antibodies in Multiple Sclerosis

Francesca Nuti [1], Feliciana Real Fernandez [1], Giuseppina Sabatino [1,2], Elisa Peroni [1,3], Barbara Mulinacci [1,†], Ilaria Paolini [1,‡], Margherita Di Pisa [1,§], Caterina Tiberi [1,||], Francesco Lolli [4], Martina Petruzzo [5], Roberta Lanzillo [5], Vincenzo Brescia Morra [5], Paolo Rovero [2,6] and Anna Maria Papini [1,2,3,*]

1 Interdepartmental Research Unit of Peptide and Protein Chemistry and Biology, Department of Chemistry "Ugo Schiff", University of Florence, Via della Lastruccia 13, 50019 Sesto Fiorentino, Italy; francesca.nuti@unifi.it (F.N.); feliciana.realfernandez@unifi.it (F.R.F.); giuseppina.sabatino@cnr.it (G.S.); elisa.peroni@cyu.fr (E.P.); barbaramulinacci@gmail.com (B.M.); ilariapao@gmail.com (I.P.); marghedipi@gmail.com (M.D.P.); caterina.tiberi@gmail.com (C.T.)

2 CNR-IC Istituto di Cristallografia, Via Paolo Gaifami 18, 95126 Catania, Italy; paolo.rovero@unifi.it

3 UMR 8076 CNRS-BioCIS Team of Chemical Biology and PeptLab@UCP Platform of Peptide and Protein Chemistry and Biology, Neuville Campus, CY Cergy Paris Université, 5 mail Gay-Lussac, 95031 Cergy-Pontoise CEDEX, France

4 Department of Clinical and Experimental Biomedical Sciences "Mario Serio" and Careggi University Hospital, University of Florence, Largo Brambilla 3, 50134 Florence, Italy; lolli@unifi.it

5 Multiple Sclerosis Clinical Care and Research Centre, Department of Neurosciences, Reproductive Sciences and Odontostomatology, Federico II University, Via Sergio Pansini 5, 80131 Naples, Italy; martinapetruzzo@gmail.com (M.P.); roberta.lanzillo@unina.it (R.L.); vincenzo.bresciamorra2@unina.it (V.B.M.)

6 Interdepartmental Research Unit of Peptide and Protein Chemistry and Biology, Department of Neurosciences, Psychology, Drug Research and Child Health–Section of Pharmaceutical Sciences and Nutraceutics, University of Florence, Via Ugo Schiff 6, 50019 Sesto Fiorentino, Italy

* Correspondence: annamaria.papini@unifi.it

† Current address: Crelux GmbH, am Klopferspitz 19a, 82152 Martinsried, Germany.

‡ Current address: Isvea srl, Via Basilicata 1/3, Località Fosci, 53036 Poggibonsi, Siena, Italy.

§ Current address: Flamma SpA, Via Bedeschi 22, 24040 Chignolo d'Isola, Bergamo, Italy.

|| Current address: "Stabilimento Chimico Farmaceutico Militare", Via Reginaldo Giuliani 201, 50141 Firenze, Italy.

Abstract: Diagnostics of Multiple Sclerosis (MS) are essentially based on the gold standard magnetic resonance imaging. Few alternative simple assays are available to follow up disease activity. Considering that the disease can remain elusive for years, identification of antibodies fluctuating in biological fluids as relevant biomarkers of immune response is a challenge. In previous studies, we reported that anti-*N*-glucosylated (*N*-Glc) peptide antibodies that can be easily detected in Solid-Phase Enzyme-Linked ImmunoSorbent Assays (SP-ELISA) on MS patients' sera preferentially recognize hyperglucosylated adhesin of non-typeable *Haemophilus Influenzae*. Since multivalency can be useful for diagnostic purposes to allow an efficient coating in ELISA, we report herein the development of a collection of Multiple *N*-glucosylated Peptide Epitopes (*N*-Glc MEPs) to detect anti-*N*-Glc antibodies in MS. To this aim, a series of *N*-Glc peptide antigens to be represented in the *N*-GlcMEPs were tested in competitive ELISA. We confirmed that the epitope recognized by antibodies shall contain at least 5-mer sequences including the fundamental *N*-Glc moiety. Using a 4-branched dendrimeric lysine scaffold, we selected the *N*-Glc MEP **24**, carrying the minimal epitope Asn(Glc) anchored to a polyethylene glycol-based spacer (PEG) containing a 19-atoms chain, as an efficient multivalent probe to reveal specific and high affinity anti-*N*-Glc antibodies in MS.

Keywords: Multiple Sclerosis; antibody detection; ELISA; multivalency; N-glucosylated peptide epitopes

---

1. Introduction

Multiple Sclerosis (MS) is the most frequent, chronic, inflammatory, demyelinating, disabling disease of the central nervous system, mainly caused by an autoimmune response to self-antigens in genetically susceptible individuals. MS diagnosis and prognosis are mainly supported by magnetic resonance imaging (MRI) that up to now is considered the gold standard diagnostic technique [1]. To the best of our knowledge, there is still no biological marker relevant not only for MS diagnosis but also for its prognosis [2–4]. In the last few years, the role of autoantibodies in MS and their identification have been re-evaluated [5–8]. In particular, a cell-based assay to detect antibodies to myelin oligodendrocyte glycoprotein (MOG), one of the candidate protein autoantigens in MS, has been proposed. However, the real antigen(s) responsible of anti-MOG antibody recognition in the assay remain elusive.

Covid-19, triggering the coronavirus pandemic era we have been living in 2020, marks the return of the old and familiar, but unfortunately misunderstood, enemy killing more human beings than natural disasters: viruses, bacteria, and parasites killers that our modern world tried to fight mainly by social distancing.

Historically, protein antigens isolated from biological material or reproduced by recombinant technologies were used to detect antibodies, but this approach has sometimes turned out as unrealistic. The main limiting factor depends on epitope recognition because of sequence mutations, incorrect folding, lack of post-translational modifications (aberrant versus native), and nonspecific binding.

Peptides mimicking the appropriate epitopes can be valuable tools. In fact, peptides that can be synthetically produced as unique molecules, can increase specificity of antibody recognition, eliminating or minimizing potential cross-reactivity with structurally similar fragments in non-relevant proteins [9–11].

Several Enzyme-Linked ImmunoSorbent Assays (ELISA) based on synthetic peptides have been proposed to detect antibodies in different diseases like Acquired ImmunoDeficiency Syndrome (AIDS), Infectious Bronchitis (IB), Severe Acute Respiratory Syndrome (SARS), and Bluetongue (BT) [12,13]. However, peptide-based ELISA can have some practical limitations, such as the antigen immobilization that can ultimately affects the sensitivity of the assay, particularly when short sequences (7–8 amino acids) are used [14,15]. Surface functionalization and biomolecular interactions can overcome these disadvantages, such as in the streptavidin-biotin system [16].

An interesting strategy to increase surface binding on the ELISA plate, improving sensitivity, is based on multimeric peptide dendrimers. In particular, Multiple Antigen Peptides (MAPs) are an optimal compromise between short peptide epitopes and recombinant or native antigens. It is widely recognized, that surface antibody binding is increased by multivalent presentation of the antigen. In fact, multivalent interactions can be collectively much stronger than the sum of the corresponding monovalent interactions [17,18]. Therefore, MAPs represent a useful chemically unambiguous system to explore antigen-antibody interaction, thanks to their shape and globular physical characteristics [19,20].

Moreover, aberrant Post-Translational Modifications (PTMs) of antigens, can play a fundamental role in triggering antibodies. Particularly, the *N*-glycosylation has been described as possible PTM involved in an antibody-mediated form of MS [21,22].

In previous studies, by a structure-based design, we developed a collection of synthetic glycopeptides, characterized by β-turn structures optimally exposing the sugars as minimal epitopes. We demonstrated that the β-D-glucopyranosyl moiety (Glc) linked to an Asn residue (*N*-Glc) on the tip of the turn is fundamental for antibody recognition in an MS patients' population. *N*-Glc is a prokaryote-specific modification that is found in selected Gram-negative bacteria, where it is most commonly found on cell-surface proteins such as (autotransporter) adhesins, biosynthesized as part of the three-protein HMW cluster including the *N*-glucosyl transferase HMW1C. We demonstrated that anti-*N*-Glc peptide antibodies, easily detected by a Solid-Phase (SP)-ELISA [22,23], preferentially recognize hyperglucosylated adhesin of non-typeable *Haemophilus influenzae* (NTHi) particularly the C-terminal portion HMW1(1205-1526) termed HMW1ct. This was the first example of an N-glucosylated native antigen that can be considered a relevant candidate for triggering pathogenic antibodies in MS [24]. The protein HMW1ct is expressed as a mixture of three *N*-Glc variants containing 7, 8, and 9 Glc moieties on Asn residues inside the consensus sequence NX(S/T) in a 1:1:1 ratio. Since the NTHi cell-surface adhesins are widely glucosylated, the *N*-Glc residues are likely to be exposed conceptually in vivo in a multivalent shape, thus potentially favoring the emergence of a rough immunological response.

In the present study, we aimed to reproduce multivalent exposure of *N*-Glc epitopes to increase coating efficiency on the ELISA microplate for the detection of anti-*N*-Glc antibodies in MS, reminiscent of an early infection. First of all, by ELISA experiments, both competitive and in solid-phase, we defined the *N*-Glc epitopes (assuring the specificity and selectivity of autoantibody recognition), decreasing the length of the originally developed *N*-glucosylated β-turn synthetic antigenic probes. Then, the best efficiency of coating to the polystyrene ELISA plate was guaranteed, considering the concept of the multivalency to increase the antibody binding affinity. In particular, the selected short epitopes were conjugated to 4-branched dendrimeric lysine scaffolds creating Multiple *N*-Glucosylated Peptide Epitopes (*N*-Glc MEPs). Therefore, the novel *N*-Glc MEPs were developed with the aim not only to enhance the diagnostic performance of the assay but also the coating efficiency of the minimal epitopes to the polystyrene ELISA plate.

2. Materials and Methods

2.1. Synthesis of the N-Glc Peptides

N-Glc peptide epitopes **2–22** (Tables 1 and 2) were synthesized following the Fmoc/tBu manual strategy. Experimental details and analytical data of the synthetic molecules are reported in the Supplementary Materials (Tables S1 and S2).

Table 1. Shortened *N*-glucosylated (*N*-Glc) sequences of CSF114(Glc).

Peptide Name Number	*N*-Glucosylated Peptide Sequence
CSF114(Glc) (**1**)	TPRVERN(Glc)GHSVFLAPYGWMVK
[Asn^7(Glc)] CSF114(1–18) (**2**)	Ac-TPRVERN(Glc)GHSVFLAPYGW-NH_2
[Asn^7(Glc)] CSF114(1–16) (**3**)	Ac-TPRVERN(Glc)GHSVFLAPY-NH_2
[Asn^7(Glc)] CSF114(1–14) (**4**)	Ac-TPRVERN(Glc)GHSVFLA-NH_2
[Asn^7(Glc)] CSF114(2–13) (**5**)	Ac-PRVERN(Glc)GHSVFL-NH_2
[Asn^7(Glc)] CSF114(4–11) (**6**)	Ac-VERN(Glc)GHSV-NH_2
[Asn^7(Glc)] CSF114(5–10) (**7**)	Ac-ERN(Glc)GHS-NH_2
[Asn^7(Glc)] CSF114(6–9) (**8**)	Ac-RN(Glc)GH-NH_2

Table 2. *N*-Glc tri- and pentapeptides as synthetic antigens.

Glucosylated Core Peptide	Glucosylated Tripeptides	Glucosylated Pentapeptides
Selected NXT/S sequences	Ac-N(Glc)GS-NH_2 (**9**);	Ac-ERN(Glc)GS-NH_2 (**16**);
	Ac-N(Glc)GT-NH_2 (**10**);	Ac-ERN(Glc)GT-NH_2 (**17**);
	Ac-N(Glc)KS-NH_2 (**11**);	Ac-ERN(Glc)KS-NH_2 (**18**);
	Ac-N(Glc)KT-NH_2 (**12**).	Ac-ERN(Glc)KT-NH_2 (**19**)
CSF114(Glc)	Ac-N(Glc)GH-NH_2 (**13**);	Ac-ERN(Glc)GH-NH_2 (**20**);
	Ac-N(Glc)KH-NH_2 (**14**)	Ac-ERN(Glc)KH-NH_2 (**21**)
[Asn^{31}(Glc)]hMOG(30–50)	Ac-N(Glc)AT-NH_2 (**15**)	Ac-KGN(Glc)AT-NH_2 (**22**)

2.2. *Synthesis of N-Glc Multiple Epitope Peptides (N-Glc MEPs)*

N-Glc MEPs **23–26** (see Section 3.4) were synthesized following the protocol described in the Supplementary Materials. Analytical data are reported in Table S3.

2.3. *Immunological Assays*

Multiple Sclerosis (MS) patients' sera samples were collected in the Multiple Sclerosis Clinical Care and Research Centre, Department of Neurosciences, Reproductive Sciences and Odontostomatology, Federico II University (Naples, Italy). Sera samples were obtained for diagnostic purposes, from patients and healthy blood donors who had given their informed consent, and stored at −20 °C until use. The present study was conducted in accordance with the Declaration of Helsinki. All experimental protocols performed were approved by the Ethics Committee 2006 and 2017 (protocol n. 120/06 and 160/17, respectively). The MS group consisted of relapsing-remitting MS (RR-MS) patients after a diagnostic lumbar puncture, cerebrospinal fluid analysis, and MRI examination and fulfilled established international diagnostic criteria [25,26]. Blood samplings in the patients' group were performed during the routine follow-up study, while the healthy control samples were carried out during routine health checks or blood donations.

2.3.1. Inhibition ELISA

Ninety-six-well activated polystyrene ELISA plates (NUNC Maxisorb, Sigma Aldrich, Milano, Italy) were coated with 1 µg per 100 µL of the type I′ beta turn glucosylated peptide CSF114(Glc) or MEPs per well, in pure carbonate buffer 0.05 M (pH 9.6) and incubated at 4 °C overnight. Washing steps were executed with an automatic Hydroflex microplate washer (Tecan Italia, Milano, Italy). After five washes with washing buffer containing 0.9% NaCl and 0.05% Tween 20, nonspecific binding sites were blocked with 100 µL per well fetal calf serum (FCS) buffer solution (10% in washing buffer) at room temperature for 60 min.

Antibody affinity was measured following the inhibition methods reported elsewhere [27,28]. Semi-saturating sera dilution was calculated in preliminary titration curves (absorbance 0.7). Six different concentrations of each synthetic antigenic peptide probe were used as inhibitors. Then, sera samples at the selected dilution were incubated in parallel with increasing concentrations of the synthetic shortened peptide sequences (range 1×10^{-10} to 1×10^{-4}) for 60 min at room temperature. All inhibition experiments were performed in duplicate or triplicate for each single MS patient's serum positive to CSF114(Glc) separately. All experiments were repeated at least twice on two different working days.

After three washes, uninhibited antibodies were identified by adding 100 µL/well of alkaline phosphatase-conjugated anti-human immunoglobulin G (IgG, Sigma-Aldrich, Milano, Italy) diluted 1:8000 in washing buffer containing 10% FCS. The microplates were then incubated 3 h at room temperature and, after three washes, 100 µL of substrate solution consisting of 1 mg/mL *p*-nitrophenyl phosphate (Sigma-Aldrich, Milano, Italy) in 10% diethanolamine buffer (pH 9.8) were added. After approximately 30 min, the reaction was stopped with 1M NaOH solution (50 µL/well), and the absorbance was read in a multichannel ELISA reader (Tecan Sunrise, Männedorf, Switzerland) at 405 nm. The selected ELISA microplates, coating conditions, reagent dilutions, buffers, and incubation times were previously tested [24,29]. The relationship between peptide concentrations and the absorbance values was represented graphically in absorbance inhibition percentage, and half-maximal response concentration values (IC50) were calculated.

2.3.2. Solid-Phase ELISA (SP-ELISA)

Immunoassays, to detect IgM or IgG antibodies in sera, were performed by SP-ELISA coating the synthetic peptides on 96-well plates (Nunc Maxisorp, Sigma−Aldrich, Milano, Italy).

Polystyrene 96-well ELISA plates were coated with a 10 µg/mL solution of diluted synthetic peptides, independently, in pure carbonate buffer 0.05 M (pH 9.6). After overnight incubation at

4 °C, plates were washed three times using washing buffer. Nonspecific binding sites were blocked with 100 μL/well of fetal calf serum buffer (10% FCS in washing buffer) at room temperature for 1 h. FCS buffer was removed and plates were incubated overnight with sera (diluted 1:100 in FCS buffer, 100 μL/well) at 4 °C. After three washes, plates were treated with 100 μL/well of anti-human IgG or IgM alkaline phosphatase-conjugated specific antibodies diluted in FBS buffer (1:8000 and 1:200, respectively). After 3 h of incubation at room temperature and three washes, 100 μL of substrate buffer was added to each well. After 15–30 min incubation at room temperature, the absorbance of each plate was read in a multichannel ELISA reader at 405 nm. The antibody levels are expressed as absorbance in arbitrary units at 405 nm.

2.4. Statistical Analysis

Data are expressed as measured absorbance values at 405 nm calculated as the mean ± SD. Statistical analysis was performed using the software GraphPad Prism version 6.01 (Graphpad Software Inc., La Jolla, CA, USA). Descriptive statistics was used to calculate mean and standard deviation for continuous variables and percentage for categorical variables. Mann–Whitney U tests were used to compare antibody response distributions. Differences were deemed statistically significant when p value < 0.05 (two-tailed test). Non-parametric Spearman's rho and related 95% confidence intervals were used to assess correlation between pair of tests. A p value < 0.05 (two-tailed test) was considered as significant. Receiver Operating Characteristic (ROC) curve analysis was employed to calculate cut-off values, establishing sensitivities and sensibilities.

3. Results

In previous studies, we reported the cross-reactivity between the *N*-glucosylated adhesin antigen HMW1ct-Glc and anti-CSF114(*N*-Glc) IgG antibodies in MS patients' sera by competitive ELISA [25]. The HMW1C from NTHi is one of the first examples of soluble bacterial protein glycosyltransferases capable of performing *N*-glycosylation with simple hexoses (i.e., glucose) on asparagine residues in conserved Asn-Xaa-Ser/Thr motifs [29,30]. On the other hand, CSF114(Glc) is a structure-based designed 21-mer peptide (TPRVERN(Glc)GHSVFLAPYGWMVK) that was optimized as a type I′ beta-turn structure because of its ability to expose at the best, at position 7, the minimal, but fundamental moiety Asn(*N*-Glc), in the epitope for autoantibody recognition in the solid-phase conditions of the immunoenzymatic assay [31].

Starting from this assumption, preliminary experiments were performed to select the shortest peptide sequences corresponding to the epitope(s) to be presented in multiple copies in fully characterized multivalent Multiple Epitope Peptides (MEPs) to detect antibodies in MS patients' sera by SP-ELISA. The use of MEPs for specific antibody detection can pave the way for the development of a simple tool to identify immune responses to aberrant glycosylations, such as *N*-glucosylation in MS possibly linked to an early non-typeable *Haemophilus influenzae* bacterial infection.

3.1. Antibody Detection in Solid-Phase ELISA (SP-ELISA) Is Affected by the Length of the Peptide Antigen

First of all, we investigated the influence of the length of shortened peptide sequences of the synthetic antigenic probe CSF114(Glc) on the efficiency both in antibody recognition and on the coating in the SP-ELISA. At this purpose, the glucopeptide sequence was tightened down step-by-step and the shortened peptides **2–5** (Table 1) derived from CSF114(Glc) were synthesized (as described in the Supplementary Materials) and characterized using analytical Reverse-Phase High Performance Liquid Chromatography (RP-HPLC) and ElectroSpray Ionisation Mass Spectrometry (ESI-MS) (Table S1). The shortened peptide sequences were acetylated at the *N*-terminus and amides at the *C*-terminus, in order to dislodge free terminal charges, which are not present in the native protein sequence and might hamper the antibody recognition [32].

SP-ELISA, against pools of positive MS sera and healthy controls (Figure 1), clearly showed a progressive decrease in antibody titre in parallel with the decrease in peptide length. In fact, the 12-mer glucopeptide **5** completely lost its ability to identify antibodies in SP-ELISA, possibly because of an inefficient coating. Therefore 14 residues appeared to be the minimum length necessary for antibody identification in SP-ELISA, probably because shorter immobilized glucopeptide sequences (<14) are only partially prone to expose the epitope for antibody binding.

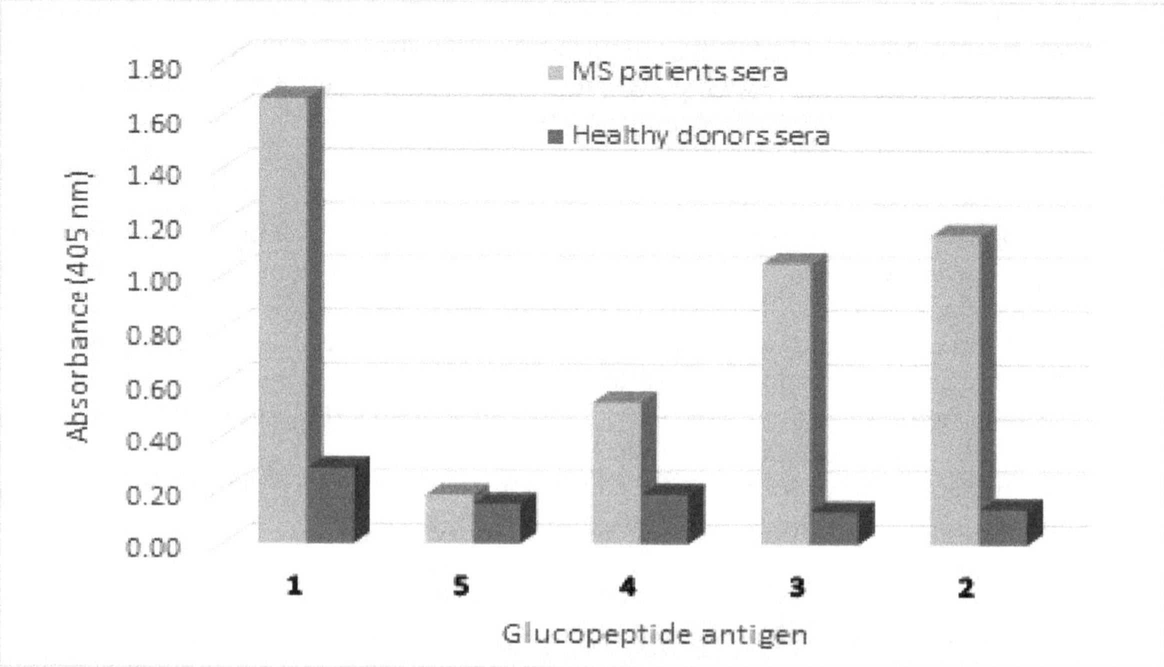

Figure 1. Antibody titres (expressed as Absorbance values) in Multiple Sclerosis (MS) patients' and healthy blood donors' sera against the glucopeptide antigens CSF114(Glc) (**1**), [Asn^7(Glc)]CSF114(1–18) (**2**), [Asn^7(Glc)]CSF114(1–16) (**3**), [Asn^7(Glc)]CSF114(1–14) (**4**), and [Asn^6(Glc)]CSF114(2–13) (**5**).

3.2. Antibody Affinity of Shortened CSF114(Glc) Glucopeptide Sequences in Competitive ELISA: Shortening CSF114(Glc) Does not Affect Antibody Epitope Recognition

Considering that SP-ELISA allows to evaluate fundamentally the relative antibody affinity that depends on the exposure of the peptide in the solid-phase conditions of the assay, we also investigated the absolute antibody affinity against the CSF114(Glc) shortened sequences by a competitive ELISA. For this purpose, the *N*-glucosylated β-turn peptide structure CSF114(Glc) was tightened down again step-by-step with the aim to identify the critical epitope displaying optimal antibody binding reactivity in the competitive in vitro assay.

Further, we investigated the role of the amino acids surrounding the previously identified minimal epitope Asn(*N*-Glc) [24]. In particular, we developed the synthetic shorter sequences **6–8** that were tested in competitive ELISA in parallel to **2–5** (Table 1).

All the synthetic glucopeptides were used as inhibitors in competitive ELISA using anti-CSF114(Glc) antibodies in one representative positive MS patient's serum. The IC50 s were calculated applying the non-linear regression least squares (ordinary) fit to the experimental data for each peptide, and values are summarized in the Supplementary Materials (Table S4). As shown in Figure 2, the full length CSF114(Glc) showed the highest degree of binding affinity (IC50 = 0.009 μM, Table S4 in the Supplementary Materials). Despite 14 residues are the minimum for antibody recognition in SP-ELISA, the inhibitory activity is still optimal when the epitope region is included in ca. 11 amino acid residues as **5** and **4** display (IC50 = 0.035 μM and 0.014 μM, respectively). On the other hand, the 4-mer glucopeptide **8** and the 6-mer glucopeptide **7** displayed the lowest inhibitory potency (IC50 = 2.2 μM and 3.5 μM, respectively), but, in any case, all are able to inhibit antibodies.

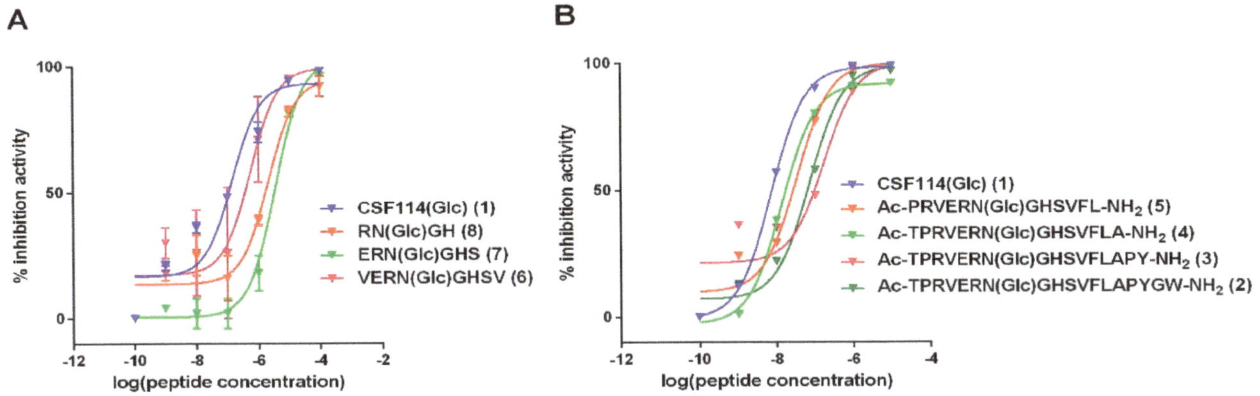

Figure 2. Inhibition curves: (**A**) Inhibition curve of anti-CSF114(Glc) IgG antibodies from a representative MS serum with *N*-glucosylated peptides, [Asn^7(Glc)]CSF114(4–11) (**6**), [Asn^7(Glc)]CSF114(5–10) (**7**), and [Asn^7(Glc)]CSF114(6–9) (**8**) in comparison with the *N*-glucosylated peptide CSF114(Glc) (**1**) in a competitive Enzyme-Linked ImmunoSorbent Assay (ELISA). (**B**) Inhibition curve of anti-CSF114(Glc) IgG antibodies from a representative MS serum with glucopeptides: [Asn^7(Glc)]CSF114 (1–18) (**2**), [Asn^7(Glc)]CSF114 (1–16) (**3**), [Asn^7(Glc)]CSF114 (1–14) (**4**), [Asn^7(Glc)]CSF114 (2–13) (**5**) in comparison with the glucopeptide CSF114(Glc) in a competitive ELISA. The results are expressed as percentage of inhibition activity of representative MS serum (ordinate axis) versus the peptide concentrations (M) in logarithmical scale.

3.3. Study of the Possible Role of a Consensus Sequence Surrounding N(Glc) in Antibody Recognition

Taking into consideration that shorter glucopeptides **6** and **8** displayed antibody affinity in competitive ELISA, we decided to investigate a series of *N*-Glc tri- and pentapeptides as synthetic antigens, undertaking a deductive approach to rule out *N*-glycosylation consensus sequences (sequons).

As a proof of concept, among the possible combinations of tripeptide sequons NX(T/S), we selected the ones containing X = Gly or Lys. In particular, we synthesized *N*(Glc)GS (**9**), *N*(Glc)GT (**10**), *N*(Glc)KS (**11**), and *N*(Glc)KT (**12**). Moreover, we synthesized *N*(Glc)GH (**13**) and *N*(Glc)KH (**14**), derived from the original glucosylated core of CSF114(Glc), that did not correspond to a consensus sequence. Then, we included the sequon *N*(Glc)AT (**15**), present both in the human myelin oligodendrocyte glycoprotein (MOG) sequence [Asn^{31}(Glc)]hMOG(30–50) (an antigenic immunodominant epitope recognizing also antibodies in MS) [33], but also highly represented (3 out of 12 positions) in the C-terminal portion HMW1(1205–1526), i.e., HMW1ct hyperglucosylated adhesin of non-typeable *Haemophilus influenzae* (NTHi) (N at positions 3, 7, and 9) [25] together with *N*(Glc)GS (**9**). Moreover, considering that a tripeptide sequence is probably not long enough for a good antigen-antibody interaction, the following step in the identification of the epitope was to test the pentapeptides **16–22**, including the sequons. At this purpose the two amino acids placed in positions –B2 and –B1 in the CSF114(Glc) sequence were added to allow the spatial hint in the shape of a β-turn, with Asn(Glc) on the tip. The same idea was applied to the sequon *N*(Glc)AT (**15**), inserting amino acids in positions 29 and 30 of hMOG(30–50) sequence, originally containing Asn(Glc) at position 31 [33].

Therefore, glucosylated tri- and pentapeptides **9–22** (Table 2) were synthesized, purified, and characterized as described in detail in the Supplementary Materials.

The antibody affinity of tripeptides **9–15** and pentapeptides **16–22** was evaluated by competitive ELISA compared to the original *N*-glucosylated β-turn peptide sequence (Figure 3). CSF114(Glc) was coated onto the ELISA microplate and patients' sera were incubated with different shortened peptide concentrations. IC50 values were reported in the Supplementary Materials (Table S5).

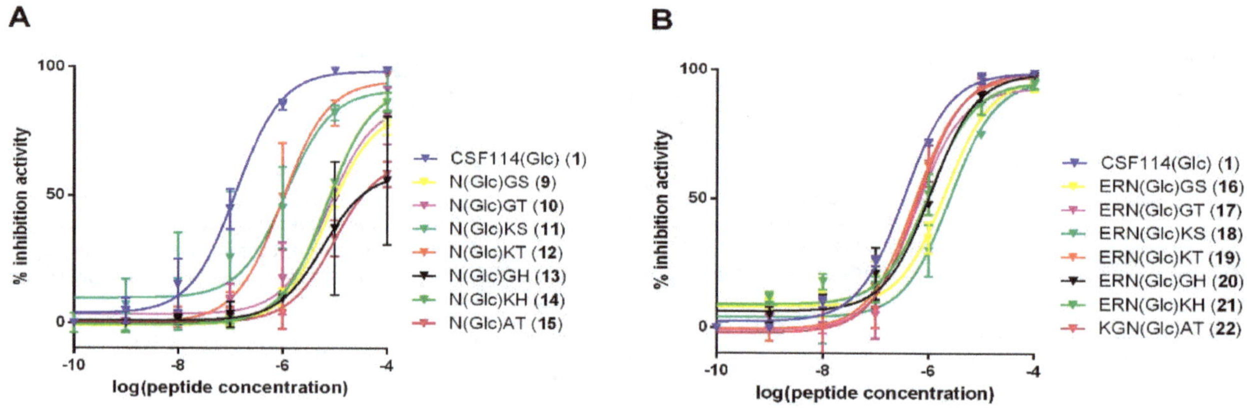

Figure 3. Inhibition curves: (**A**) Inhibition curve of anti-CSF114(Glc) IgG antibodies from a representative MS serum with the tripeptides **9–15**: Ac-N(Glc)GS-NH_2 (**9**), Ac-N(Glc)GT-NH_2 (**10**), Ac-N(Glc)KS-NH_2 (**11**), Ac-N(Glc)KT-NH_2 (**12**), Ac-N(Glc)GH-NH_2 (**13**) Ac-N(Glc)KH-NH_2 (**14**), Ac-N(Glc)AT-NH_2 (**15**), in comparison with the glucopeptide CSF114(Glc) (**1**) in a competitive ELISA. (**B**) Inhibition curve of anti-CSF114(Glc) IgG antibodies from a representative MS serum with the pentapeptides **16–22**: Ac-ERN(Glc)GS-NH_2 (**16**), Ac-ERN(Glc)GT-NH_2 (**17**), Ac-ERN(Glc)KS-NH_2 (**18**); Ac-ERN(Glc)KT-NH_2 (**19**), Ac-ERN(Glc)GH-NH_2 (**20**), Ac-ERN(Glc)KH-NH_2 (**21**); Ac-N(Glc)AT-NH_2 (**22**), in comparison with the glucopeptide CSF114(Glc) in a competitive ELISA. The results are expressed as the percentage of inhibition activity of a representative MS serum (ordinate axis) versus the peptide concentrations (M) in logarithmical scale.

Inhibition curves of the tripeptides **9–15** and pentapeptides **16–22** are shown in Figure 3. The original sequence of CSF114(Glc) presented the best inhibitory activity (IC50 = 0.34 μM, Table S5). The shortest tripeptide probes **9–15** recognized anti-CSF114(Glc) antibodies even if with an affinity lower than the synthetic glucosylated 21mer-peptide (Figure 1). Among all the tripeptides tested, the glucopeptides Ac-N(Glc)KS-NH_2 (**11**) and Ac-N(Glc)KT-NH_2 (**12**) showed the best inhibitory activity (IC50 = 1.1 and 0.97 μM, respectively, Table S5).

The longer linear sequences **16–22** exhibited high inhibition efficacy in competitive ELISA, better than their corresponding tripeptide analogs **9–15**. In particular, the pentapeptide Ac-ERN(Glc)KT-NH_2 (**19**) presented the best inhibitory activity (IC50 = 0.54 μM, Table 3) followed by the pentapeptides Ac-ERN(Glc)GT-NH_2 (**17**) (IC50 = 0.58 μM) and Ac-KGN(Glc)AT-NH_2 (**22**) (IC50 = 0.60 μM). This result indicates that the IC50 values for *N*-Glc pentapeptides are closely similar, and no substantial differences were observed among the pentapeptides tested, independently of the sequence.

Table 3. Receiver Operating Characteristic (ROC) analysis. Values obtained from ROC-analysis of *N*-Glc MEPs **23–26** and the glycopeptide CSF114(Glc) (**1**) for the area under the curve, *p* value, established cut-off and the corresponding sensitivity, specificity, and likelihood ratio.

Compound	Area Under Curve (AUC)				Criterion Value and Coordinates			
	AUC	Standard Error (SE)	95% Confidence Interval	*p*-Value	Cut-Off	Sensitivity (%)	Specificity (%)	Likelihood Ratio
N-Glc MEP (**23**)	0.5747	0.1073	0.3643 to 0.7850	0.4899	>1.057	17.65 (3.799 to 43.43)	92.31 (63.97 to 99.81)	2.294
N-Glc MEP (**24**)	0.5249	0.1100	0.3092 to 0.7406	0.8180	>0.6104	35.29 (14.21 to 61.67)	92.31 (63.97 to 99.81)	4.588
N-Glc MEP (**25**)	0.7511	0.09376	0.5673 to 0.9350	0.02023	>1.053	38.46 (13.86 to 68.42)	82.35 (56.57 to 96.20)	2.179
N-Glc MEP (**26**)	0.6380	0.1041	0.4339 to 0.8421	0.2018	>1.029	30.77 (9.092 to 61.43)	82.35 (56.57 to 96.20)	1.744
CSF114(Glc) (**1**)	0.6516	0.1049	0.4458 to 0.8573	0.1610	>0.7575	47.06 (22.98 to 72.19)	92.31 (63.97 to 99.81)	6.118

3.4. N-Glc Multiple Epitope Peptides (N-Glc MEPs) to Mimic Multivalency in SP-ELISA

In order to mimic a multivalent presentation of the minimal but fundamental epitope Asn(*N*-Glc), and increasing at the same time the efficiency in coating to the ELISA polystyrene plate of short linear peptides, we synthesized different *N*-Glc MEPs based on a dendrimeric lysine scaffold, having in common Asn(Glc) [34].

Starting from a lysine tetrameric core, we synthesized five *N*-Glc MEPs **23–26** bearing spacers of different length: β-Alanine and two different polyethylene glycol-based spacers (PEG), containing 9- and 19-atoms chain, respectively. The following antigens were selected: (i) the β-turn *N*-glucosylated pentapeptide ERN(Glc)GH (**12**) and (ii) the simple minimal *N*-glucosylated asparagine epitope Asn(Glc). The spacers were introduced to avoid steric hindrance possibly hampering antibody binding. The *N*-Glc MEP structures are reported in Figure 4.

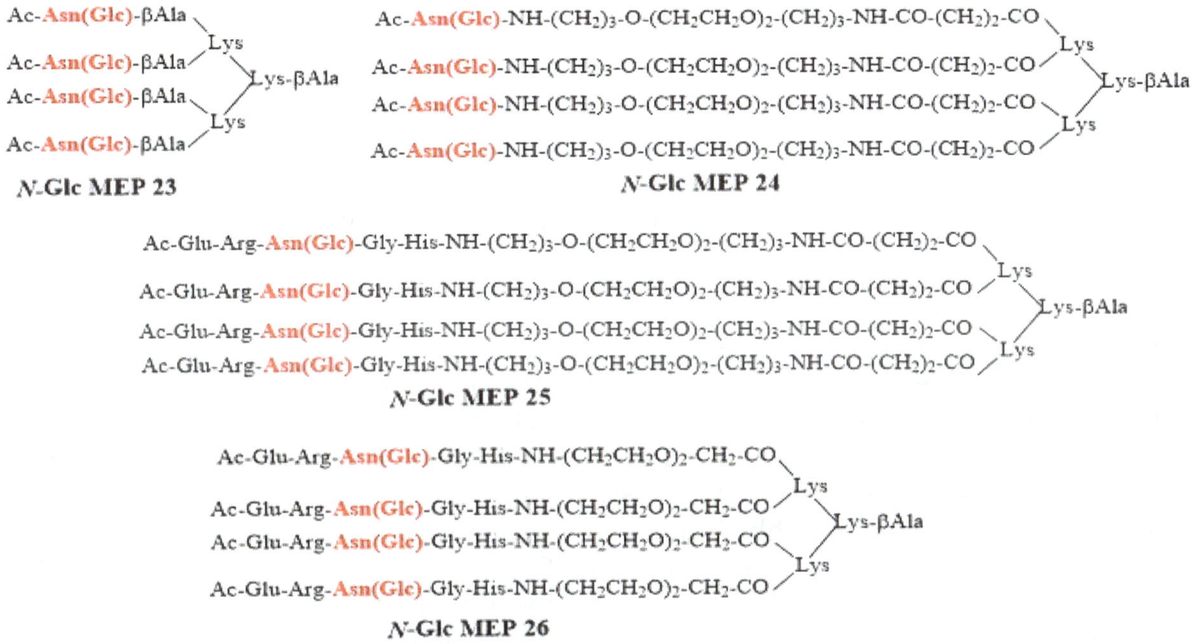

Figure 4. Collection of the synthetic *N*-Glc Multiple Epitope Peptides (MEPs).

The *N*-Glc MEPs were synthesized starting from $Fmoc_4$-Lys_2-Lys-β-Ala-Wang resin, according to the general procedure described in details in the Supplementary Materials. The Fmoc-Asn(β$GlcAc_4$)-OH building block was synthesized according to the method developed by Paolini et al. [35]. *N*-Glc MEPs were acetylated on the *N*-terminal function. All the *N*-Glc MEPs were purified by semi-preparative RP-HPLC, and characterized by RP-HPLC and ESI-MS (Table S3).

We assessed IgG isotype antibodies against *N*-Glc MEPs **23–26** in a cohort of 16 MS patients, previously selected on their reactivity to the original *N*-glucosylated type I′ β-turn peptide structure CSF114(Glc), and compared to 14 healthy blood donors as controls (Figure 5).

The Receiver Operating Characteristic (ROC) analysis was employed to perform an accurate comparative investigation of the performances of the different *N*-Glc MEPs, evaluating their discrimination power at the different cut-off values. Sensitivity, specificity, and likelihood ratios were also calculated [36]. Selected cut-off values, sensitivities, and the rest of the statistical parameters are shown in Table 3 (ROC curves are reported in Figure S1 in the Supplementary Materials). The characteristics of the curves, their shape and steepness, and their underlying area provide evidence that the synthetic *N*-Glc MEPs are able to identify antibodies in MS patients' sera.

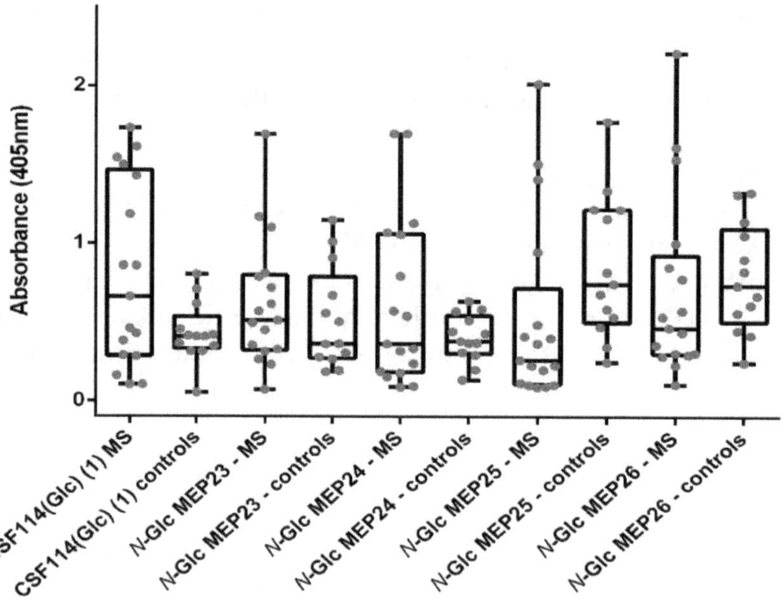

Figure 5. Antibody responses (expressed as Absorbance values) against the synthetic *N*-Glc MEPs. Data distribution of IgG antibodies against the glucopeptide CSF114(Glc) and the synthetic *N*-Glc MEPs **23–26** obtained by SP-ELISA (grey). Box and whiskers (min to max) are plotted for each data group (black).

Despite *N*-Glc MEP **25** and **26** presented the best Area Under the Curve (AUC) values (0.7511 and 0.6380, respectively), observing the data distribution we assume that their ability to identify specific MS antibodies is lower compared with *N*-Glc MEPs **23** and **24**. This is justified with the increased means of the antibody titers in controls compared to MS patients in both *N*-Glc MEP **25** and **26**, which apparently improved AUC and p values, but are due to non-specific interactions. In fact, the specificities calculated for *N*-Glc MEPs **25** and **26** are sensibly decreased compared with CSF114(Glc) (82.35% and 92.31%, respectively). Considering the sensitivity values, once the specificity is fixed in 92.31%, the *N*-Glc MEP **24** presented the best performance identifying as positive the 35.29% of the MS patients.

Consequently, we decided to deepen on *N*-Glc MEP **24** ability (containing only *N*-Glc moieties) to recognize specific MS antibodies in patients' sera. At this purpose, *N*-Glc MEP **24** was tested against an increased number of MS patients' sera (81) and healthy controls' (30) sera, in parallel, to the glucopeptide CSF114(Glc) as reference. Data distribution of IgG and IgM antibody titers identified by SP-ELISA are reported in Figure 6A,B.

The non-parametric Mann–Whitney test was applied to evaluate significant differences between MS patients' and controls' groups. The results showed significant differences (p value < 0.001, two-tailed test) for CSF114(Glc), both for IgM and IgG-type antibodies. Slightly different results were observed in the case of *N*-Glc MEP **24**. In fact, the differences among groups were statistically significant when IgM-isotype antibodies were detected (p value $= 0.0001$, two-tailed test). On the other hand, the IgGs against the multivalent *N*-Glc MEP **24** showed no level of significance (p value $= 0.3611$, Two-tailed test). In our opinion, the IgG antibody response as detected by *N*-Glc MEP **24** appears to be less specific because it detects a "noise" level in the control group, forcing a decreased specificity to maintain sensibility when selecting the corresponding cut-off.

Among the absorbance values of MS patients, the frequencies of the anti-CSF114(Glc) antibodies significantly correlated with the ones against the *N*-Glc MEP **24** (p value < 0.0001, two-tailored); the Spearman's correlation coefficients (rho values) were $r = 0.7507$ and 0.7424 for IgG and IgM, respectively (Figure 6C,D).

Then, we investigated the absolute antibody affinity of *N*-Glc MEP **24** in a competitive ELISA. In a set of three MS positive sera tested in parallel, the multivalent *N*-Glc MEP **24** inhibited the binding of antibodies to the glycopeptide CSF114(Glc), giving rise to contrasting inhibition curves among the different representative sera employed (Figure S2 in the Supplementary Materials). Data of serum MS1 (Figure S2A in the Supplementary Materials) showed that the affinity of *N*-Glc MEP **24** was lower than CSF114(Glc) (IC50 = 2.145×10^{-8} M and 5.200×10^{-7} M, respectively), whereas serum MS2 exhibited superimposable affinity (IC50 = 6.373×10^{-8} M and 6.088×10^{-8} M respectively). Moreover, in MS3 serum IC50 was lower for *N*-Glc MEP **24** compared to CSF114(Glc) (IC50 = 2.145×10^{-8} M and 5.116×10^{-9} M, respectively). This finding indicates that the *N*-Glc MEP **24** shares similar epitopes, all including the Asn(*N*-Glc) residue. In particular, its antibody affinity can be slightly different among the MS patients, probably because of the differential innate and adaptive immune responses typical of each subject.

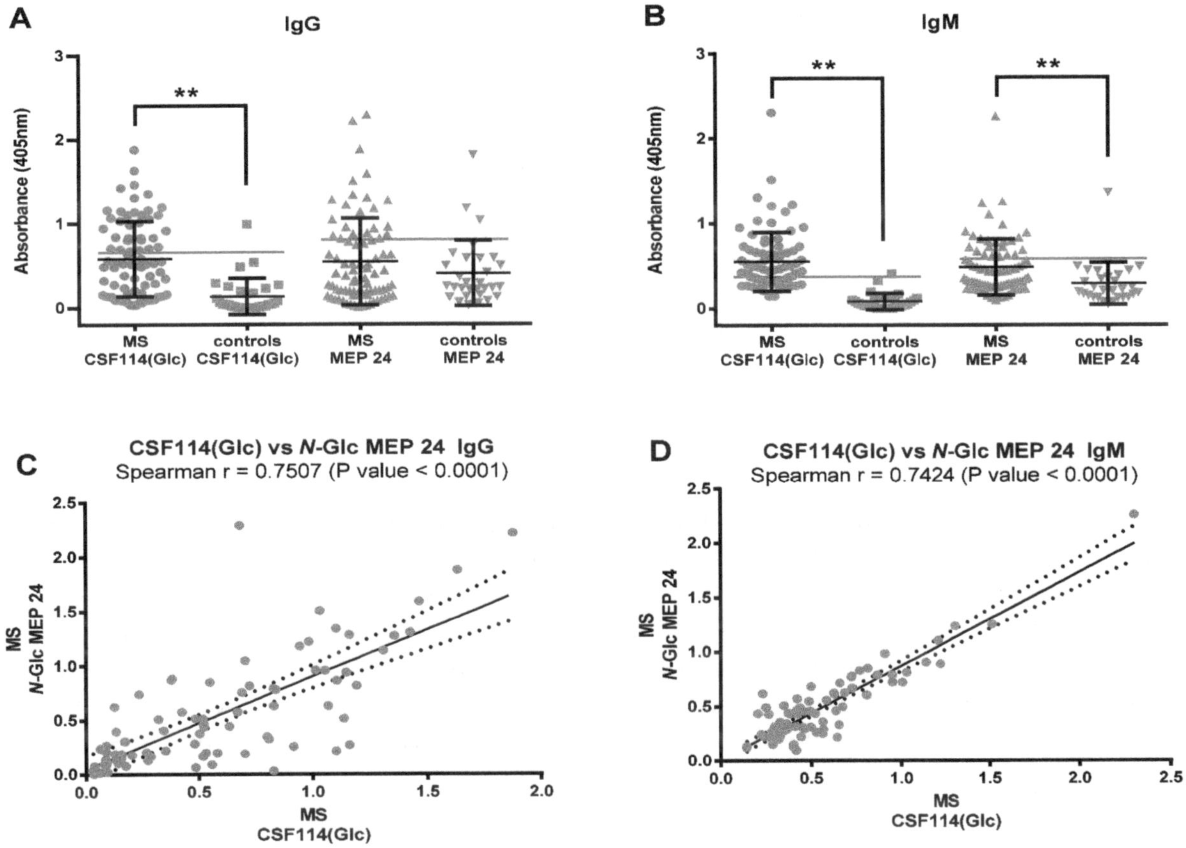

Figure 6. Data of antibody responses against the glucopeptide CSF114(Glc) and *N*-Glc MEP **24**. Data distribution of IgG (**A**) and IgM (**B**) antibody titers in 81 MS patients' sera and 30 controls' sera identified by SP-ELISA against the peptide sequences CSF114(Glc) and the synthetic multivalent *N*-Glc MEP **24**. Data are expressed as mean values ± standard deviation with a significance level ** $p < 0.001$ (two-tailed Mann–Whitney non-parametric test). Selected cut-off values for each compound are plotted in red. Correlation between CSF114(Glc) and *N*-Glc MEP **24** both for IgG (**C**) and for IgM (**D**) are shown. The Spearman's correlation coefficients (rho values) and the corresponding p values are reported in each plot. Regressions lines are plotted in black (dashed lines show the 95% confidence interval of the best-fit line).

4. Discussion

Multiple sclerosis diagnosis is still very challenging, relying on clinical and radiological criteria and in the absence of "better explanations" [37], the development of simple diagnostics detecting specific biomarkers is highly warranted. Moreover, native structures triggering specific antibodies in

Multiple Sclerosis (MS) are still uncharacterized. Consequently, surrogate antigens used to identify antibodies in MS by ELISA are elusive. In spite of the fact that MS is considered mainly a T-cell mediated disease, the role of B-cells is increasingly appreciated. In this scenario, we demonstrated for the first time that an aberrant *N*-glucosylation is part of a relevant epitope that was identified by the structure-based designed β-turn 21-mer glucopeptide CSF114(Glc). This synthetic tool was instrumental for the discovery of antibodies in an MS patients' population preferentially recognizing the hyperglucosylated bacterial adhesin of non-typeable *Haemophilus influenzae*. With the idea in mind that multivalent presentation of glucosylated asparagine residues may occur in a variety of native antigens, as in the case of citrullination in rheumatoid arthritis [38], we focused on the development of a synthetic tool enhancing the role of multiple aberrant modifications versus amino acid sequences. We simplified the antigen to be synthetically produced in a multiple format, taking into consideration that peptide dendrimers are considered protein-like multivalent materials, whose architecture is a key parameter for activity [39,40]. Therefore, we selected the multivalent epitope peptide *N*-Glc MEP **24**, based on a lysine-dendritic scaffold (relatively simple to be produced), carrying four copies of the minimal glucosylated epitope Asn(Glc) anchored to a PEG-based spacer containing a 19-atoms chain [41]. In previous studies, we demonstrated that CSF114(Glc) shortened epitopes lost specificity and sensitivity for IgM antibodies in MS patients' sera by SP-ELISA [29], sensibly decreasing the diagnostic potential of the synthetic antigen. On the contrary, *N*-Glc MEP **24** displays an interesting ability to identify in SP-ELISA both IgG and IgM antibodies in a large number of MS patients' sera (81) compared to controls (30), with a sensitivity of 35% (95% CI: 14.21–61.67) and a specificity of 92.31 (95% CI: 63.97–99.81). This result is particularly relevant, since it offers the possibility to detect with the same tool both IgMs and IgGs in MS, thus increasing the diagnostic and prognostic value of the antigen thanks to multivalent presentation of the minimal epitope [24].

5. Conclusions

The present study reported the development of new *N*-glucosylated Multivalent Epitope Peptides for the detection of anti-*N*(Glc) antibodies in Multiple Sclerosis. After a preliminary screening of several short linear peptide epitopes and multiple epitope peptides, the promising results suggest that multivalent interaction can be useful in designing SP-ELISA to detect antibodies to aberrant *N*-glucosylation in Multiple Sclerosis for both diagnostic and prognostic purposes. Indeed, the multivalent *N*-Glc MEP **24** ligand, carrying the minimal glucosylated epitope Asn (Glc) anchored to the 19-atoms PEG-based spacer, can be an efficient probe to reveal both IgM and IgG autoantibodies as disease biomarkers.

Supplementary Materials:
Details of the synthetic procedures, analytical and immunochemical characterization of the synthetic antigenic probes are reported online. Table S1: Shortened CSF114(Glc)-sequences of peptides **2–8.**, Table S2: Sequences and chemical data for the *N*-glucosylated (*N*-Glc) peptides **9–22**, Table S3: Analytical data of the Multiple *N*-glucosylated Peptide Epitopes (*N*-Glc MEPs) **23–26**, Table S4: Calculated half maximal inhibitory concentration (IC50). Calculated Log 1/IC50 with the Std errors and the IC50 with the Corresponding Confidence Interval (CI) for the shortened peptides versus CSF114(Glc), Table S5: Calculated Log 1/IC50 with the Std errors and the IC50 with the Corresponding Confidence Interval (CI) for the Peptides **9–22** and CSF114(Glc) (**1**), Figure S1: Received Operating Characteristic (ROC) analysis. ROC curve analysis of anti-CSF114(Glc) antibodies and anti-*N*-Glc MEPs **23–26** in Multiple Sclerosis versus controls determined by SP-ELISA, Figure S2: Competitive ELISA experiments with CSF114(Glc) and *N*-Glc MEP 24. Inhibition curves of anti-CSF114(Glc) antibodies with *N*-Glc MEP **24** compared with CSF114(Glc) in a competitive ELISA. The results are expressed as percentage of inhibition (ordinate axis) of three representative MS sera: MS1 (A), MS2 (B) and MS3 (C) versus the peptide concentrations (M) in logarithmical scale.

Author Contributions: F.R.F. and E.P. performed the immunoassays; I.P., B.M., M.D.P., C.T., F.N., F.R.F., G.S. performed the syntheses of the synthetic antigenic probes and glucosylated building blocks; M.P., R.L., and V.B.M. provided sera samples and oversaw the data collection; F.L., F.R.F. and E.P. performed data analyses of immunoassays; A.M.P. and P.R. conceived and designed the research project, supervised the research, reviewed and edited the final manuscript. All authors have read and agreed to the published version of the manuscript.

Acknowledgments: The authors would like to acknowledge Francis Ciolli and Giada Rossi for their technical assistance.

References

1. de Seze, J.; Vermersch, P. Sequential magnetic resonance imaging follow-up of multiple sclerosis before the clinical phase. *Mult. Scler.* **2005**, *11*, 395–397. [CrossRef]
2. Lanzillo, R.; Prinster, A.; Scarano, V.; Liuzzi, R.; Coppola, G.; Florio, C.; Salvatore, E.; Schiavone, V.; Brunetti, A.; Muto, M.; et al. Neuropsychological assessment, quantitative MRI and ApoE gene polymorphisms in a series of MS patients treated with IFN beta-1b. *J. Neurol. Sci.* **2006**, *245*, 141–145. [CrossRef] [PubMed]
3. Freedman, M.S.; Thompson, E.J.; Deisenhammer, F.; Giovannoni, G.; Grimsley, G.; Keir, G.; Ohman, S.; Racke, M.K.; Sharief, M.; Sindic, C.J.M.; et al. Recommended standard of cerebrospinal fluid analysis in the diagnosis of multiple sclerosis: A consensus statement. *Arch. Neurol.* **2005**, *62*, 865–870. [CrossRef] [PubMed]
4. Luque, F.A.; Jaffe, S.L. Cerebrospinal fluid analysis in multiple sclerosis. *Int. Rev. Neurobiol.* **2007**, *79*, 341–356. [PubMed]
5. Reindl, M.; Jarius, S.; Rostasy, K.; Berger, T. Myelin oligodendrocyte glycoprotein antibodies: How clinically useful are they? *Curr. Opin. Neurol.* **2017**, *30*, 295–301. [CrossRef] [PubMed]
6. Waters, P.J.; Komorowski, L.; Woodhall, M.; Lederer, S.; Majed, M.; Fryer, J.; Mills, J.; Flanagan, E.P.; Irani, S.R.; Kunchok, A.C. A multicenter comparison of MOG-IgG cell-based assays. *Neurology* **2019**, *92*, e1250–e1255. [CrossRef]
7. Papp, V.; Langkilde, A.R.; Blinkenberg, M.; Schreiber, K.; Jensen, P.E.H.; Sellebjerg, F. Clinical utility of anti-MOG antibody testing in a Danish cohort. *Mult. Scler. Relat. Disord.* **2018**, *26*, 61–67. [CrossRef]
8. de Seze, J. Myelin oligodendrocyte glycoprotein antibodies in neuromyelitis optica spectrum disorder. *Curr. Opin. Neurol.* **2019**, *32*, 111–114.
9. Meloen, R.H.; Puijk, W.C.; Langeveld, J.P.; Langedijk, J.P.; Timmerman, P. Design of synthetic peptides for diagnostics. *Curr. Protein Pept. Sci.* **2003**, *4*, 253–260. [CrossRef]
10. Papini, A.M. The use of post-translationally modified peptides for detection of biomarkers of immune-mediated diseases. *J. Pept. Sci.* **2009**, *15*, 621–628. [CrossRef]
11. Ballew, J.T.; Murray, J.A.; Collin, P.; Mäki, M.; Kagnoff, M.F.; Kaukinen, K.; Daugherty, P.S. Antibody biomarker discovery through in vitro directed evolution of consensus recognition epitopes. *Proc. Natl. Acad. Sci. USA* **2013**, *110*, 19330–19335. [CrossRef] [PubMed]
12. Gómara, M.J.; Fernández, L.; Pérez, T.; Ercilla, G.; Haro, I. Assessment of synthetic chimeric multiple antigenic peptides for diagnosis of GB virus C infection. *Anal. Biochem.* **2010**, *396*, 51–58. [CrossRef] [PubMed]
13. Tarradas, J.; Monsó, M.; Muñoz, M.; Rosell, R.; Fraile, L.; Frías, M.T.; Domingo, M.; Andreu, D.; Sobrino, F.; Ganges, L. Partial protection against classical swine fever virus elicited by dendrimeric vaccine-candidate peptides in domestic pigs. *Vaccine* **2011**, *29*, 4422–4429. [CrossRef]
14. Buus, S.; Rockberg, J.; Forsström, B.; Nilsson, P.; Uhlen, M.; Schafer-Nielsen, C. High-resolution mapping of linear antibody epitopes using ultrahigh-density peptide microarrays. *Mol. Cell. Proteom.* **2012**, *11*, 1790–1800. [CrossRef] [PubMed]
15. Hebbes, T.R.; Turner, C.H.; Thorne, A.W.; Crane-Robinson, C. A "minimal epitope" anti-protein antibody that recognises a single modified amino acid. *Mol. Immunol.* **1989**, *26*, 865–873. [CrossRef]
16. Waritani, T.; Chang, J.; McKinney, B.; Terato, K. An ELISA protocol to improve the accuracy and reliability of serological antibody assays. *MethodsX* **2017**, *4*, 153–165. [CrossRef]
17. Mammen, M.; Choi, S.K.; Whitesides, G.M. Polyvalent Interactions in Biological Systems: Implications for Design and Use of Multivalent Ligands and Inhibitors. *Angew. Chem. Int. Ed. Engl.* **1998**, *37*, 2754–2794. [CrossRef]
18. Liu, S.P.; Zhou, L.; Lakshminarayanan, R.; Beuerman, R.W. Multivalent Antimicrobial Peptides as Therapeutics: Design Principles and Structural Diversities. *Int. J. Pept. Res. Ther.* **2010**, *16*, 199–213. [CrossRef]
19. Joshi, V.G.; Dighe, V.D.; Thakuria, D.; Malik, Y.S.; Kumar, S. Multiple antigenic peptide (MAP): A synthetic peptide dendrimer for diagnostic, antiviral and vaccine strategies for emerging and re-emerging viral diseases. *Indian J. Virol.* **2013**, *24*, 312–320. [CrossRef] [PubMed]
20. Tam, J.P.; Zavala, F. Multiple antigen peptide. A novel approach to increase detection sensitivity of synthetic peptides in solid-phase immunoassays. *J. Immunol. Methods* **1989**, *124*, 53–61. [CrossRef]

21. Doyle, H.A.; Mamula, M.J. Post-translational protein modifications in antigen recognition and autoimmunity. *Trends Immunol.* **2001**, *22*, 443–449. [CrossRef]
22. Lolli, F.; Mazzanti, B.; Pazzagli, M.; Peroni, E.; Alcaro, M.C.; Sabatino, G.; Lanzillo, R.; Brescia Morra, V.; Santoro, L.; Gasperini, C.; et al. The glycopeptide CSF114(Glc) detects serum antibodies in multiple sclerosis. *J. Neuroimmunol.* **2005**, *167*, 131–137. [CrossRef]
23. Lolli, F.; Mulinacci, B.; Carotenuto, A.; Bonetti, B.; Sabatino, G.; Mazzanti, B.; D'Ursi, A.M.; Novellino, E.; Pazzagli, M.; Lovato, L.; et al. An N-glucosylated peptide detecting disease-specific autoantibodies, biomarkers of multiple sclerosis. *Proc. Natl. Acad. Sci. USA* **2005**, *102*, 10273–10278. [CrossRef]
24. Walvoort, M.T.; Testa, C.; Eilam, R.; Aharoni, R.; Nuti, F.; Rossi, G.; Lanzillo, R.; Papini, A.M.; Imperiali, B.; Rovero, P.; et al. Antibodies from multiple sclerosis patients preferentially recognize hyperglucosylated adhesin of non-typeable *Haemophilus influenzae*. *Sci. Rep.* **2017**, *7*, 44969. [CrossRef]
25. Polman, C.H.; Reingold, S.C.; Banwell, B.; Clanet, M.; Cohen, J.A.; Filippi, M.; Fujihara, K.; Havrdova, E.; Hutchinson, M.; Kappos, L.; et al. Diagnostic criteria for multiple sclerosis: 2010 revisions to the McDonald criteria. *Ann. Neurol.* **2011**, *69*, 292–302. [CrossRef] [PubMed]
26. Thompson, A.J.; Banwell, B.L.; Barkhof, F.; Carroll, W.M.; Coetzee, T.; Comi, G.; Correale, J.; Fazekas, F.; Filippi, M.; Freedman, M.S. Diagnosis of multiple sclerosis: 2017 revisions of the Mc Donald criteria. *Lancet Neurol.* **2018**, *17*, 162–173. [CrossRef]
27. Rath, S.; Stanley, C.M.; Steward, M.W. An inhibition enzyme immunoassay for estimating relative antibody affinity and affinity heterogeneity. *J. Immunol. Methods* **1988**, *106*, 245–249. [CrossRef]
28. Real Fernández, F.; Di Pisa, M.; Rossi, G.; Auberger, N.; Lequin, O.; Larregola, M.; Benchohra, A.; Mansuy, C.; Chessaing, G.; Lolli, F.; et al. Antibody recognition in multiple sclerosis and Rett syndrome using a collection of linear and cyclic N-glucosylated antigenic probes. *Biopolymers* **2015**, *104*, 560–576. [CrossRef]
29. Schwarz, F.; Fan, Y.Y.; Schubert, M.; Aebi, M. Cytoplasmic N-glycosyltransferase of Actinobacillus pleuropneumoniae is an inverting enzyme and recognizes the NX(S/T) consensus sequence. *J. Biol. Chem.* **2011**, *286*, 35267–35274. [CrossRef]
30. Choi, K.J.; Grass, S.; Paek, S.; St Geme, J.W.; Yeo, H.J. The Actinobacillus pleuropneumoniae HMW1C-like glycosyltransferase mediates N-linked glycosylation of the Haemophilus influenzae HMW1 adhesin. *PLoS ONE* **2010**, *5*, e15888. [CrossRef]
31. Carotenuto, A.; D'Ursi, A.M.; Mulinacci, B.; Paolini, I.; Lolli, F.; Papini, A.M.; Novellino, E.; Rovero, P. Conformation-activity relationship of designed glycopeptides as synthetic probes for the detection of autoantibodies, biomarkers of multiple sclerosis. *J. Med. Chem.* **2006**, *49*, 5072–5079. [CrossRef] [PubMed]
32. Van Regenmortel, M.H.V. Antigenicity and Immunogenicity of Synthetic Peptides. *Biologicals* **2001**, *29*, 209–213. [CrossRef] [PubMed]
33. Mazzucco, S.; Matà, S.; Vergelli, M.; Fioresi, R.; Nardi, E.; Mazzanti, B.; Chelli, M.; Lolli, F.; Giannenschi, M.; Pinto, F.; et al. Synthetic glycopeptide of human myelin oligodendrocyte glycoprotein to detect antibody responses in multiple sclerosis and other neurological diseases. *Bioorg. Med. Chem. Lett.* **1999**, *9*, 167–172. [CrossRef]
34. Araújo, P.R.; Ferreira, A.W. High diagnostic efficiency of IgM-ELISA with the use of multiple antigen peptides (MAP1) from T. gondii ESA (SAG-1, GRA-1 and GRA-7), in acute toxoplasmosis. *Rev. Inst. Med. Trop. Sao Paulo* **2010**, *52*, 63–68. [CrossRef] [PubMed]
35. Paolini, I.; Nuti, F.; de la Cruz Pozo-Carrero, M.; Barbetti, F.; Kolesinska, B.; Kaminski, Z.J.; Chelli, M.; Papini, A.M. A convenient microwave-assisted synthesis of N-glycosyl amino acids. *Tetrahedron Lett.* **2007**, *48*, 2901–2904. [CrossRef]
36. Habbema, J.D.; Eijkemans, R.; Krijnen, J.; Knottnerus, J.E. Analysis of data on the accuracy of diagnostic tests. In *The Evidence Base of Clinical Diagnosis*; Knottnerus, J.E., Ed.; BMJ Books: London, UK, 2002; pp. 117–143.
37. Calabrese, M.; Gasperini, C.; Tortorella, C.; Schiavi, G.; Frisullo, G.; Ragonese, P.; Fantozzi, R.; Prosperini, L.; Annovazzi, P.; Cordioli, C.; et al. "Better explanations" in multiple sclerosis diagnostic workup: A 3-year longitudinal study. *Neurology* **2019**, *92*, e2527–e2537. [CrossRef]
38. Migliorini, P.; Pratesi, F.; Tommasi, C.; Anzilotti, C. The immune response to citrullinated antigens in autoimmune diseases. *Autoimmun. Rev.* **2005**, *4*, 561–564. [CrossRef]
39. Gestwicki, J.E.; Cairo, C.W.; Strong, L.E.; Oetjen, K.A.; Kiessling, L.L. Influencing receptor-ligand binding mechanisms with multivalent ligand architecture. *J. Am. Chem. Soc.* **2002**, *124*, 14922–14933. [CrossRef]

40. Sadler, K.; Tam, J.P. Peptide dendrimers: Applications and synthesis. *J. Biotechnol.* **2002**, *90*, 195–229. [CrossRef]
41. Weimer, B.C.; Walsh, M.K.; Wang, X. Influence of a poly-ethylene glycol spacer on antigen capture by immobilized antibodies. *J. Biochem. Biophys. Methods* **2000**, *45*, 211–219. [CrossRef]

6

Whole-Transcriptome Analysis in Peripheral Blood Mononuclear Cells from Patients with Lipid-Specific Oligoclonal IgM Band Characterization Reveals Two Circular RNAs and Two Linear RNAs as Biomarkers of Highly Active Disease

Leire Iparraguirre [1], Danel Olaverri [1,2], Telmo Blasco [1,2], Lucía Sepúlveda [1,3], Tamara Castillo-Triviño [4], Mercedes Espiño [5], Lucienne Costa-Frossard [5], Álvaro Prada [6], Luisa María Villar [3,5], David Otaegui [1,3] and Maider Muñoz-Culla [1,3,*]

1 Multiple Sclerosis Group, Neurosciences Area, Biodonostia Health Research Institute, 20014 San Sebastian, Spain; leire.iparraguirre@biodonostia.org (L.I.); a904612@alumni.unav.es (D.O.); tblasco@tecnun.es (T.B.); lucia.sepulveda@biodonostia.org (L.S.); david.otaegui@biodonostia.org (D.O.)
2 Department of Biomedical Engineering and Sciences, Tecnun-Universidad de Navarra, Manuel de Lardizábal 15, 20018 San Sebastián, Spain
3 Spanish Network of Multiple Sclerosis, 08028 Barcelona, Spain; luisamaria.villar@salud.madrid.org
4 Multiple Sclerosis Group, Neurosciences Area, Biodonostia Health Research Institute, Neurology Department, Basque Health Service, 20014 San Sebastian, Spain; TAMARA.CASTILLOTRIVINO@osakidetza.eus
5 Departments of Immunology and Neurology, Multiple Sclerosis Unit, Hospital Ramon y Cajal, (IRYCIS), 28034 Madrid, Spain; mercedes.espino@salud.madrid.org (M.E.); lucienne.costa@salud.madrid.org (L.C.-F.)
6 Multiple Sclerosis Group, Neurosciences Area, Biodonostia Health Research Institute, Immunology Department, Basque Health Service, 20014 San Sebastian, Spain; ALVAROJOSE.PRADAINURRATEGUI@osakidetza.eus
* Correspondence: maider.munoz@biodonostia.org

Abstract: The presence of anti-myelin lipid-specific oligoclonal IgM bands (LS-OCMBs) has been defined as an accurate predictor of an aggressive evolution of multiple sclerosis. However, the detection of this biomarker is performed in cerebrospinal fluid, a quite invasive liquid biopsy. In the present study we aimed at studying the expression profile of miRNA, snoRNA, circRNA and linearRNA in peripheral blood mononuclear cells (PBMCs) from patients with lipid-specific oligoclonal IgM band characterization. We included a total of 89 MS patients, 47 with negative LS-OCMB status and 42 with positive status. Microarray (miRNA and snoRNA) and RNA-seq (circular and linear RNAs) were used to perform the profiling study in the discovery cohort and candidates were validated by RT-qPCR in the whole cohort. The biomarker potential of the candidates was evaluated by ROC curve analysis. RNA-seq and RT-qPCR validation revealed that two circular (hsa_circ_0000478 and hsa_circ_0116639) and two linear RNAs (*IRF5* and *MTRNR2L8*) are downregulated in PBMCs from patients with positive LS-OCMBs. Finally, those RNAs show a performance of a 70% accuracy in some of the combinations. The expression of hsa_circ_0000478, hsa_circ_0116639, *IRF5* and *MTRNR2L8* might serve as minimally invasive biomarkers of highly active disease.

Keywords: multiple sclerosis; biomarkers; transcriptome; microRNAs; circular RNAs; oligoclonal bands

---

1. Introduction

Multiple sclerosis (MS) is a chronic, inflammatory, neurodegenerative and demyelinating disease of the central nervous system (CNS). It is considered an autoimmune disease, in which peripheral autoreactive lymphocytes enter the CNS and develop an immune response, leading to demyelinating lesions, both in white and grey matter [1]. It is estimated that about 2–3 million people have MS and it typically affects young adults, with an onset between 20 and 40 years of age. Moreover, MS is three times more prevalent in women than men and there is evidence that this ratio has increased in the last 70 years [1], a phenomenon shared with several other autoimmune diseases.

Both the disease course and clinical phenotype of MS are highly variable among patients and also with time in the same individual. For this reason, biomarkers can aid in the diagnosis, the differentiation of MS phenotypes and also in the monitoring of disease progression [2,3].

Disease activity biomarkers can be associated with the different pathophysiological processes of the disease and they could ideally help to distinguish between patients with an aggressive course and those with a more benign form [2]. In this context, the presence restricted to cerebrospinal fluid (CSF) of anti-myelin lipid-specific oligoclonal IgM bands (LS-OCMBs) has been defined as an accurate predictor of an aggressive evolution [4]. However, for this test, cerebrospinal fluid sample is needed, a quite invasive liquid biopsy. Therefore, a great effort has been done towards the discovery of minimally invasive biomarkers such as blood biomarkers [5].

In this context, gene expression profiling studies have been widely used for new biomarker discovery, but also to elucidate the molecular mechanisms underlying the pathogenic processes occurring in the disease [6,7]. In addition to the classical protein-coding transcriptome, non-coding transcriptome has gained great interest in the last decades, and several authors, including our group, have demonstrated that it has a role in MS pathogenesis [8–10]. MicroRNAs are the best studied class of small non-coding RNAs, although others such as small nucleolar RNAs have also been related to MS [11,12]. MiRNAs are single-strand small non-coding RNAs that regulate gene expression at a post-transcriptional level, binding to their target mRNAs, and they participate in almost all known biological processes [13]. More recently, circular RNAs (circRNAs) have emerged as new players in the RNA field, with an important role in the post-transcriptional regulatory mechanisms. They have been found to participate in several processes such as tumor, metabolism and immune-related pathways and consequently, they have also been linked to various diseases such as neurological and autoimmune diseases including a few studies in MS [14–18]. Both miRNA and circRNA have been proposed as promising source of biomarkers in a wide variety of sample types, such as blood, serum, saliva, urine and CSF [19–21].

In light of these evidences, and due to the increasing need for a solid, reproducible and accessible biomarker for MS, we hypothesized that a whole-transcriptome study of peripheral blood mononuclear cells (PBMCs) from patients with LS-OCMBs characterization could reveal new biomarkers that correlate with this stablished CSF marker. Such a biomarker could be used more easily to monitor patients on an ongoing basis, since blood sampling is less invasive, with less adverse effects, than doing a lumbar puncture.

With this in mind, in the present study we analyzed the expression of small non-coding RNA, circRNA and linear RNAs in peripheral blood mononuclear cells (PBMCs), from 89 patients with positive ($n = 42$) and negative ($n = 47$) LS-OCMBs characterization, and found two circular RNAs and two linear RNAs, with differential expression between the two groups, that could serve as future blood biomarkers of highly active disease.

2. Experimental Section

2.1. Patients, Sample Collection and RNA Isolation

MS patients were recruited in the Hospital Ramon y Cajal after giving informed consent. Blood samples were obtained and PBMCs were isolated following a standard Ficol gradient separation protocol and frozen in liquid nitrogen until used. Total RNA was isolated using the miRNeasy mini kit (Qiagen, Hilden, Germany) following the manufacturer's instructions. RNA concentration was measured using the NanoDrop ND-1000 spectrophotometer (ThermoFisher Scientific, Waltham, Massachusetts, MA, USA), and the que quality of the samples included in microarray and RNA-seq experiments was assessed using the Agilent 2100 Bioanalyzer (Agilent Technologies, Santa Clara, CA, USA), obtaining a RNA integrity number higher than 6 in all the samples. CSF was obtained to analyze the status of LS-OCMBs as previously described [4,22].

The main clinical and demographical characteristics of patients are summarized in Table 1. A complete list of samples and the experiment in which each of them was included is available in Table S1. The study was approved by the hospital's ethics committee (MMC-UEM-2018-01, October 2018). The profiling cohort includes only female samples, aiming at reducing the source of variability and considering that MS is three times more prevalent in females than men in this disease [1].

Table 1. Summary of patients' clinical and demographical data.

	Microarrays			**RNAseq**					
	LS-OCMB status	Sex	Age	LS-OCMB status	Sex	Age			
Profiling cohort	P = 5	F = 5 M = 0	35 (23–58)	P = 4	F = 4 M = 0	38 (23–58)			
	N = 6	F = 6 M = 0	34.5 (27–53)	N = 4	F = 4 M = 0	35 (27–44)			
	miRNA validation *			circRNA validation *			linear RNA validation		
	LS-OCMB status	Sex	Age	LS-OCMB status	Sex	Age	LS-OCMB status	Sex	Age
Validation cohort	P = 42	F = 24 M = 18	34 (17–58)	P = 42	F = 24 M = 18	34 (17–58)	P = 30	F = 18 M = 12	33.4 (17–51)
	N = 47	F = 39 M = 8	37 (20–53)	N = 46	F = 38 M = 8	37 (20–53)	N = 30	F = 24 M = 6	36.9 (20–49)

* Including patients in profiling cohort. Age—mean (range). LS-OCMB—lipid-specific oligoclonal IgM bands. P—positive. N—negative. F—females. M—males. There are 7 subjects (1 positive and 6 negative) in validation cohorts for which we do not have age data.

2.2. *Microarray Analysis*

Total RNA (200 ng) was labeled using the FlashTag HSR Biotin labelling kit (Genisphere LLC, Hatfield, Pennsylvania, PA, USA) and hybridized to the GeneChip miRNA 4.0 Array (Affymetrix, Santa Clara, CA, USA), which covers 2578, 2025 and 1996 human mature miRNAs, pre-miRNAs and snoRNAs, respectively. Labeled RNA was hybridized to the array, washed and stained in a GeneChip Fluidics Station 450 and scanned in a GeneChip Scanner 7G (Affymetrix, Santa Clara, CA, USA).

Microarray data analysis was carried out in Transcriptome Analysis Console 4.0 software (Affymetrix, Santa Clara, CA, USA), applying the RMA + DABG algorithm only to human probesets for normalization, detection and summarization purposes. We performed a classical differential expression analysis between patients with positive and negative LS-OCMBs, considering as differentially expressed those probesets showing a p-value lower than 0.01 and an absolute fold-change (FC) value higher or equal to 1.5.

2.3. *RNAseq*

Library preparation and Next Generation Sequencing was performed at CD Genomics (Shirley, New York, NY, USA). The concentration and quality of the RNA samples was again measured using Agilent 2100 Bioanalyzer before library preparation. After normalization, rRNA was depleted from the total RNA sample using the Ribo-Zero rRNA removal kit and followed by purification and fragmentation steps. To construct the sequencing libraries, a strand-specific cDNA synthesis was performed, the 3′ ends were adenylated and adaptors were ligated. The resulting libraries were subjected to a quality control and normalization process. Paired-end sequencing was performed with Illumina HiSeq X Ten PE150 (Illumina, San Diego, CA, USA).

The data presented in this study (raw data of microarray and RNA-seq experiments) are openly available in Gene Expression Omnibus (GEO) under the series reference GSE159036.

2.4. CircRNA Detection and Quantification in RNA-Seq Data

First, quality of the sequencing was checked and, then, reads were mapped to the human genome (hg19, downloaded from UCSC Genome Browser [23]) using STAR version 2.5.4b (https://code.google.com/archive/p/rna-star/) [24] or BWA version 0.7.17-1 (http://maq.sourceforge.net) [25]. Subsequently, circRNA prediction was performed by CIRCexplorer2 version 2.3.3 (https://circexplorer2.readthedocs.io/en/latest/) [26] and CIRI2 version 2.0.5 (https://sourceforge.net/projects/ciri/) [27] adhering to the recommendation by the authors. Moreover, only circRNAs supported by both algorithms were considered as bona fide circRNAs and used in subsequent analyses, a method that has been described in the literature by other authors [28]. CircRNA expression was based on back-spliced junctions-spanning reads according to CIRI2 quantification. After filtering out circRNAs with low expression (sum of reads < 10), differential expression analysis was performed using DESeq2 version 1.28.1 (http://www.bioconductor.org/packages/release/bioc/html/DESeq2.html) [29] package for R (version 3.6.3) (https://www.r-project.org/) in R-studio (Version 1.0.136) (https://rstudio.com/), considering as differentially expressed those circRNA showing a p-value < 0.05 and a fold-change higher than 2. To select a group of candidates for validation purposes, two additional filters were applied: (1) BaseMean value higher than five (BM > 5) and (2) the transcripts having a read count value of zero in any of the samples were removed. Finally, we selected ten candidate circRNAs having the highest absolute fold-change value.

2.5. Linear RNA Detection and Quantification in RNA-Seq Data

After sequencing and quality control, the Kallisto version 0.44.0 (http://pachterlab.github.io/kallisto/) [30] algorithm was used for transcript pseudoalignment, identification and quantification. Differential expression analysis was performed using DESeq2 package. Before running the DESeq2 algorithm, we applied a filter of a minimum number of reads (sum of number of reads higher than or equal to 10) to remove low expression transcripts. For subsequent analysis, due to the large number of transcripts detected and our small sample size, we added a filter to keep only the most robust transcripts regarding their read count. Therefore, we created a detection filter, as follows: (1) Transcripts detected in both groups—transcripts having at least two reads in $\frac{3}{4}$ of samples from each group. (2) Transcripts detected only in one of the groups—transcripts having at least two reads in $\frac{3}{4}$ of samples in the negative group but only in 1 sample from the positive group (detected only in negative group), and transcripts having at least two reads in $\frac{3}{4}$ of positive group but only in 1 from negative group (detected only in positive group). Transcripts selected with this detection filter were considered as consistent linear RNAs. Finally, differentially expressed transcripts were considered those showing a p-value < 0.05 and an absolute fold-change value higher than two. For validation purposes, we selected ten candidate linear RNAs having the highest absolute fold-change value and having an assigned gene name.

All these profiling experiments and data analysis steps, tools and filters are summarized in Figure 1.

2.6. cDNA Synthesis and Quantitative PCR

For the validation of candidate microRNAs, total RNA (10 ng) was reverse transcribed into cDNA using TaqMan™ Advanced miRNA cDNA synthesis kit (Applied Biosystems™, Foster City, CA, USA). To quantify miRNA expression, we used TaqMan Advanced miRNA assays and TaqMan Fast Advanced Master Mix (Applied Biosystems™, Foster City, CA, USA), following the manufacturer's protocol. Assay for hsa-miR-191-5p was used as a reference miRNA for normalization purposes.

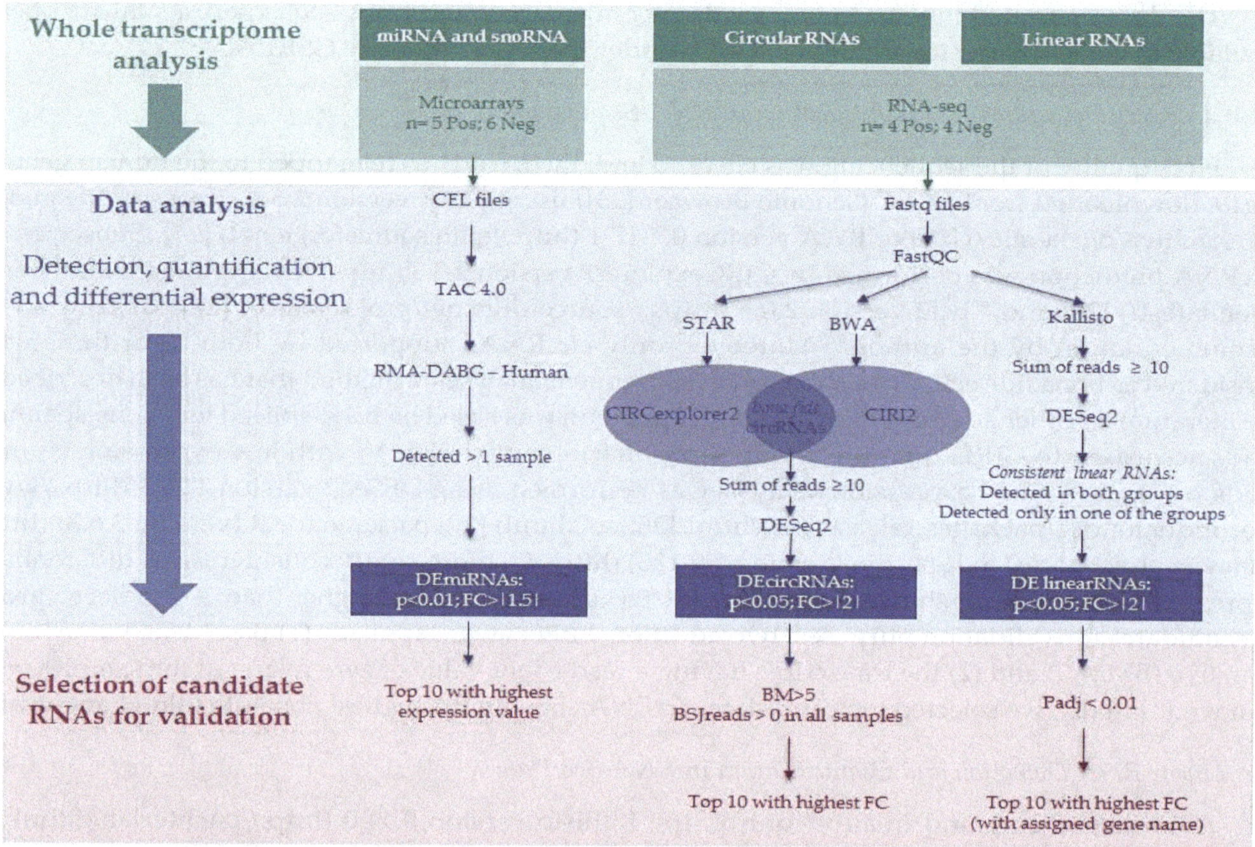

Figure 1. Summary of the study indicating profiling experiments, data analysis tools, filters and candidate selection criteria. Pos—positive. Neg—negative. DE—differentially expressed. FC—fold-change. BM—BaseMean. BSJ—backspliced junction. Padj—adjusted *p*-value. BWA—Burrows-Wheeler Aligner.

For the validation of candidate circRNA, total RNA (500 ng) was reverse transcribed into cDNA with random primers using the High Capacity cDNA Reverse Transcription Kit (Applied Biosystems, Foster City, CA, USA), following the kit protocol. PCR reaction was set up using 10 ng of cDNA as the template and using Power SYBRGreen Master Mix (Applied Biosystems^{TM} Foster City, CA, USA) with the following thermal cycling program: A temperature of 50 °C for 2 min, 95 °C for 10 min, 40 cycles of 95 °C for 15 s and 60 °C for 1 min, followed by a dissociation curve analysis. Divergent primers were used so that the amplicon spans the backspliced junction (BSJ), as described previously [18]. EEF1A1 and B2M were used as the reference genes, using the mean value of both genes for normalization purposes. The presence of a single-peak in the melting curve indicated the specificity of the amplification.

For the validation of candidate linear RNAs, total RNA (500 ng) was reverse transcribed into cDNA with oligo-dT and random primers using the miScript II RT (Qiagen, Hilden, Germany) kit with the HiFlex buffer, as indicated in manufacturer's protocol. PCR reaction was set up using 10 ng of cDNA as template and using miSscript SYBRGreen PCR kit (Qiagen, Hilden, Germany) with the following thermal cycling program: A temperature of 95 °C for 15 min, 40 cycles of 94 °C for 15 s, 55 °C for 30 s and 70 °C for 30 s, followed by a dissociation curve analysis. The amplification of each linear RNA was carried out with QuantiTect primer Assays (Qiagen, Hilden, Germany) (Table S2) and B2M was used as a reference gene for normalization. The presence of a single-peak in the melting curve indicated the specificity of the amplification.

All retrotranscription reactions were run in a Veriti Thermal Cycler (Applied Biosytems, Foster City, CA, USA) and quantitative PCR reactions were performed in a CFX384 Touch Real-Time PCR Detection System (Bio-Rad laboratories, Inc., Hercules, CA, USA).

Prior to run all the validation experiments, a technical validation of the circRNA amplification was carried out. The RT-qPCR amplification products were subsequently purified with the ExoSAP-IT™ PCR Product Cleanup Reagent (Applied Biosystems, Foster City, CA, USA) following the manufacturer's instructions and Sanger sequenced (ABIprism 3130) (Applied Biosystems, Foster City, CA, USA) in order to check for the presence of the BSJ. In addition, the PCR products were also subjected to electrophoresis on agarose gel to confirm the presence of a single amplification product.

The Raw Cq values and melting curves were analyzed in CFX Maestro 1.0 (Bio-Rad laboratories, Inc., Hercules, CA, USA). Expression levels represented as fold-change (FC) were calculated using the 2^DDCq method. Statistical analysis was done by R in RStudio on DCq data. Distribution of data was tested with Shapiro–Wilk test and the difference of the distribution was assessed by Student t-test or non-parametric Wilcoxon Rank sum test. In each circRNA and linear RNA dataset, outlier samples were removed before the statistical analysis, identifying those values using boxplot.stat function in R.

2.7. *Gene Overrepresentation Test*

In order to describe the function of differentially expressed transcripts, the PANTHER overrepresentation test was applied (released 7 November 2019, Panther [31]), based on the Complete Biological Process from Gene Ontology database (released 9 December 2019). As a reference background, we used the list of genes giving rise to detected transcripts defined above. Fisher test was carried out and false discovery rate (FDR) correction was applied to raw *p*-values, taking as a significant threshold FDR values below 0.05.

2.8. *ROC Curve Analysis*

Based on DCq values obtained by RT-qPCR, we performed a receiver operating characteristic curve (ROC curve) analysis in R environment in RStudio. Three different datasets were used: (1) circRNA validation data, (2) linear RNA validation data and (3) samples in both datasets to test different combination of transcripts. This last dataset was smaller given that we needed to include only samples without any missing value (Table S1). The combination of different transcripts was computed with ROC function of "Epi" package.

3. Results

3.1. *microRNA Expression Profile*

Microarray analysis was able to detect 2827 probesets in at least one sample out of the total 6659 human probesets (42.45%) (Figure 2A). Among detected probesets, 33 showed a differential expression between positive and negative patients for LS-OCMBs, and more importantly, the top 10 probesets that show the highest expression are able to group patients according to their LS-OCMBs status (Figure 2B). Among these 10 probesets, we can find five mature miRNA, two pre-miRNA and two small nucleolar RNAs. For validation purposes, we selected the four mature miRNA for which TaqMan Advanced miRNA Assays were available (hsa-miR-6800-5p, hsa-miR-6821-5p, hsa-miR-4485 and hsa-miR-4741). However, RT-qPCR validation results did not confirm the alteration of these four miRNAs (Figure 2C).

3.2. *circRNA Expression Profile*

RNA-seq analysis pipeline of circular transcriptome detected 27,630 bona fide circRNAs and 5431 circRNAs (19.6%) with sum of reads ≥ 10 (Figure 3A). Differential expression analysis revealed that 124 circRNAs are altered ($p < 0.05$; FC > |2|) between the two groups, 72 of them being upregulated, while 52 are downregulated.

We selected ten candidate circRNAs to confirm their differential expression by RT-qPCR in a larger cohort. First, the technical test for primer amplification confirmed a single and specific circRNA amplification for nine out of the 10 circRNA candidates. circMETRNL was the one that did not show a good amplification and a single band in agarose gel, so we discarded it in subsequent validation experiments. Additionally, Sanger sequencing of the PCR product confirmed that the amplicons span the BSJ (Figure S1). As it can be observed in Figure 3C, the lower expression of hsa_circ_0000478 and hsa_circ_0116639 was confirmed by qPCR in PBMCs from patients with positive LS-OCMBs (FC = −1.5 and FC = −1.65, respectively; $p < 0.01$).

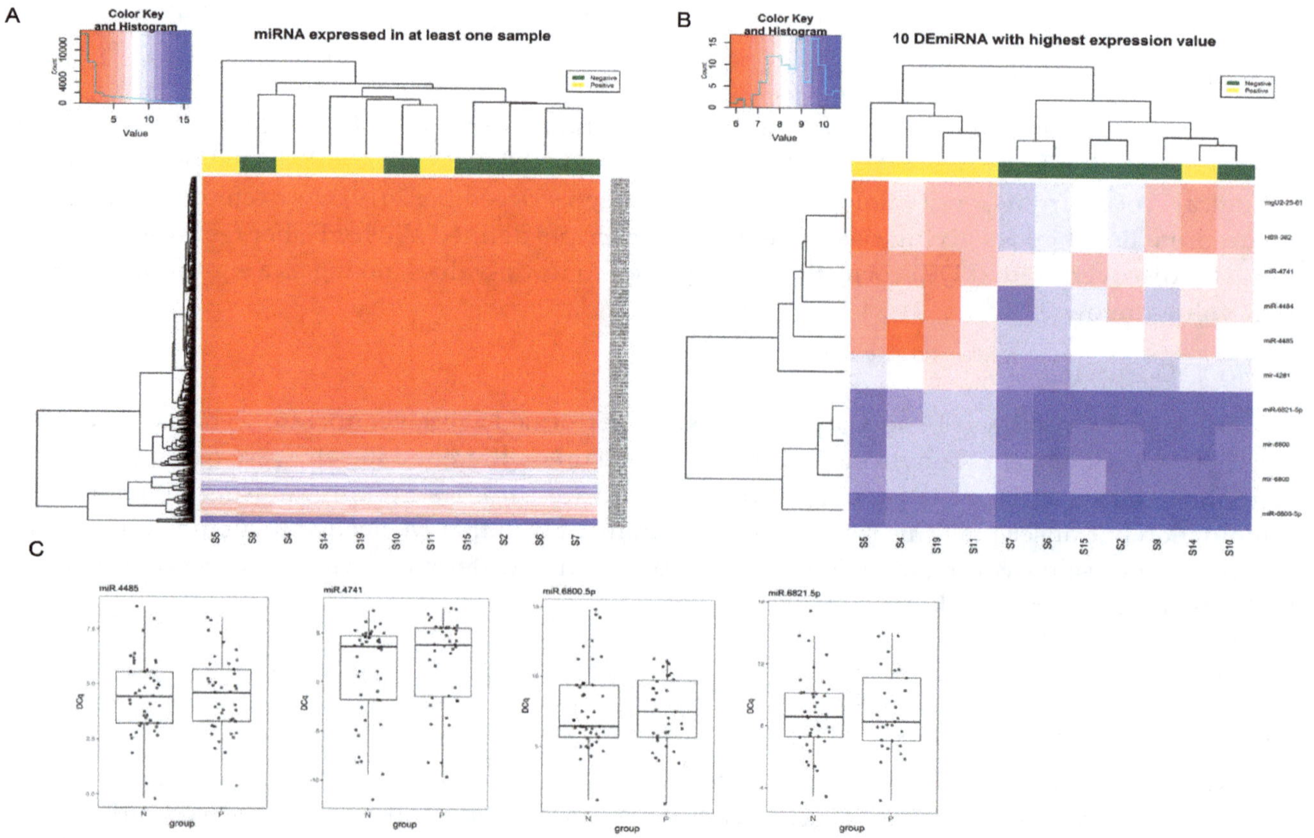

Figure 2. Results of miRNA expression profile by microarrays. (**A**) Heatmap showing the expression (microarray intensity signal) of miRNA that are expressed in at least one sample. (**B**) Heatmap of the expression of the ten DEmiRNAs showing the highest expression. Hierarchical clustering shows that the expression pattern of these ten miRNAs is able to group patients according to their LS-OCMBs status. (**C**) RT-qPCR validation results of selected candidate miRNAs. P—positive LS-OCMB status. N—negative LS-OCMB status. DE—differentially expressed.

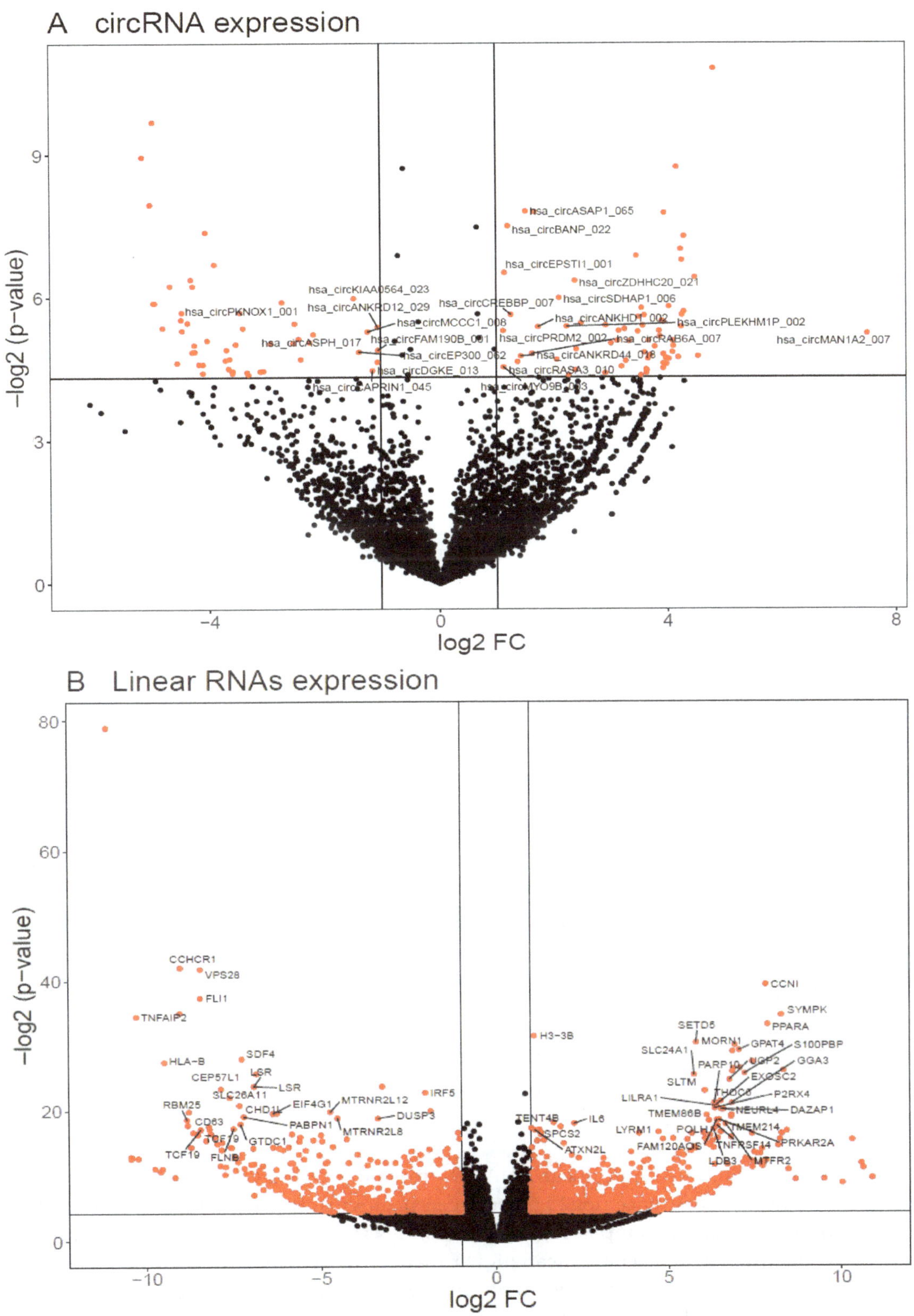

Figure 3. *Cont.*

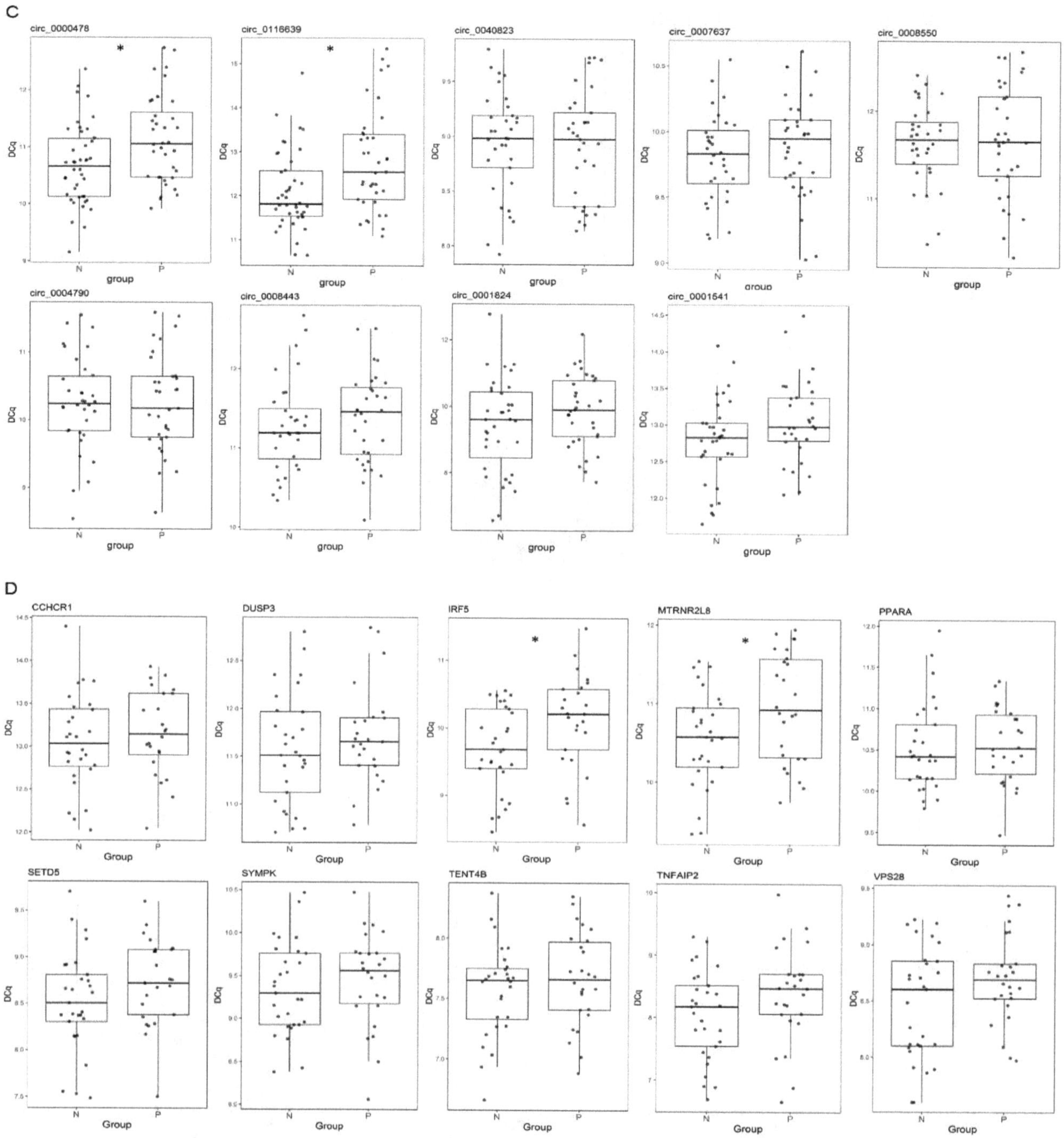

Figure 3. Results of circRNAs and linear RNAs expression profile by RNA-seq. (**A**) Volcano plot showing the expression difference (log2 FC) between positive and negative group of circRNA that show a sum of reads across all samples higher than 10. DEcircRNA are highlighted in red and labels point at those DEcircRNA with a base mean higher than 5. (**B**) Volcano plot showing the expression difference (log2 FC) of linear RNAs between positive and negative groups. Differentially expressed linear RNAs are highlighted in red and labels point at those DE linear RNAs with an adjusted p-value < 0.01. (**C**) RT-qPCR validation results of selected candidate circRNAs. Asterisk indicates a statistically significant difference ($p < 0.01$). circ_0000478 and circ_0116639 validation includes more samples than the rest of the circRNAs because of limitations in sample amount (Table S1). (**D**) RT-qPCR validation results of selected candidate linear RNAs. Asterisk indicates a statistically significant difference ($p < 0.05$). P: positive LS-OCMB status. N: negative LS-OCMB status.

3.3. Linear Transcripts Expression Profile

In the present study, we also analyzed the linear transcriptome by RNA-seq, identifying 115,869 transcripts with ≥10 reads in total. We applied an additional filter using a detection criterion, which permitted to identify 84,863 linear RNAs with a consistent expression pattern, from which 92.8% were detected in both groups. Among them, 2441 transcripts were differentially expressed ($p < 0.05$ and FC >| 2|), from which 1421 were detected in both groups (Figure 3B). The rest of the transcripts are specific to one of the groups, 382 being expressed only in PBMCs from patients with negative LS-OCMBs status while 638 transcripts are only expressed in patients with positive LS-OCMBs.

We selected ten candidate linear RNAs to confirm their differential expression by RT-qPCR in a larger cohort. As it can be observed in Figure 3D, the lower expression of IRF5 and MTRNR2L8 was confirmed in PBMCs from patients with positive LS-OCMBs (FC = −1.33 in both transcripts; $p < 0.05$).

Differentially expressed linear RNAs are enriched in biological processes regarding mainly the immune system. The most significant and enriched terms (FDR < 0.01 and fold-enrichment > 2) are shown in Figure 4. Complement activation, humoral immune response and type I interferon signaling pathway appear among the top enriched terms.

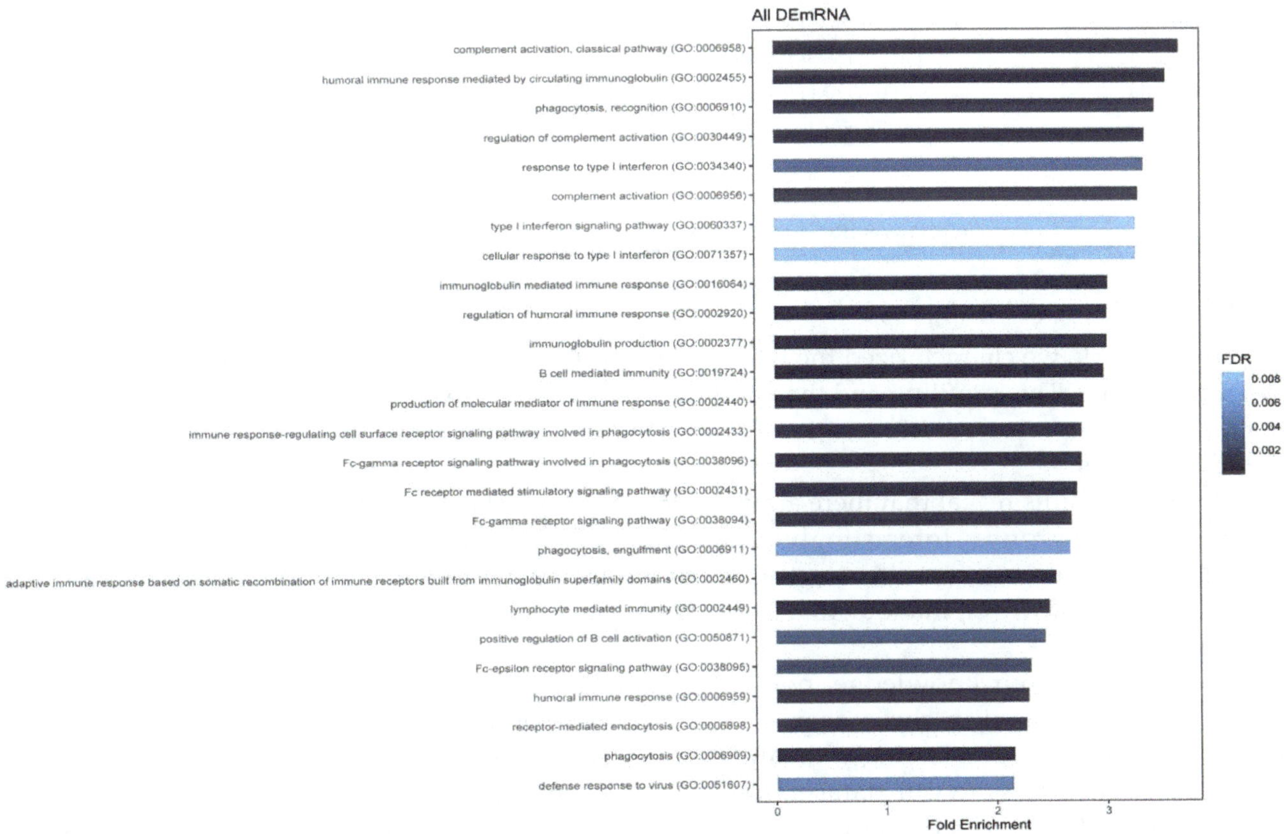

Figure 4. Results from gene overrepresentation test of 2441 DEmRNA. The most significant (fold-enrichment > 2) and enriched (FDR < 0.01) GO biological processes are shown. Bars are colored according to their FDR value. DE—differentially expressed. FDR—false discovery rate.

3.4. Evaluation of circRNA and Linear RNAs as Biomarkers of a Highly Active Disease

In order to assess the potential of the four validated RNAs as blood biomarkers of the LS-OCMB status we performed the ROC curve analysis. As shown in Table 2, different combinations of RNAs were tested to find the best performance in discriminating both groups. We found that different combinations of both circRNAs and linear RNAs improves the performance, reaching AUC values of around 70%.

Table 2. ROC analysis results of the four candidate transcripts and different combinations. ROC—receiver operating characteristic.

Marker/Combination	Transcripts	Sample Size	AUC (%)	CI (%)
circRNA-1	circ_0000478	80 (43 LS-OCMB−; 37 LS-OCMB+)	65.9	53.9–77.9
circRNA-2	circ_0116639		66.4	54.2–78.5
Combi_circ	circ_0000478-circ_0116639		68.9	57.2–80.5
linearRNA-1	IRF5	55 (29 LS-OCMB−; 26 LS-OCMB+)	65.6	50.7–80.6
linearRNA-2	MTRNR2L8		67.0	52.4–81.7
Combi_linear	IRF5-MTRNR2L8		68.6	54.1–83.1
circRNA-1	circ_0000478	51 (26 LS-OCMB−; 25 LS-OCMB+)	65.1	49.8–80.4
circRNA-2	circ_0116639		66.2	50.6–81.7
linearRNA-1	IRF5		67.1	51.8–82.3
linearRNA-2	MTRNR2L8		69.0	54.1–83.9
CombiALL	circ_0000478-circ_0116639-IRF5-MTRNR2L8		69.8	55.3–84.4
combi1	circ_0000478-circ_0116639		66.3	51.1–81.6
combi2	IRF5-MTRNR2L8		70.3	55.6–85.0
combi3	circ_0000478-IRF5		68.3	52.8–83.8
combi4	circ_0000478-MTRNR2L8		68.6	53.7–83.6
combi5	circ_0116639-IRF5		69.8	55.0–84.7
combi6	circ_0116639-MTRNR2L8		67.8	52.8–82.9
combi7	circ_0000478-circ_0116639-IRF5		69.8	55.0–84.6
combi8	circ_0000478-circ_0116639-MTRNR2L8		68.2	53.3–83.0
combi9	circ_0000478-IRF5-MTRNR2L8		68.8	53.7–83.8
combi10	circ_0116639-IRF5-MTRNR2L8		68.8	53.8–83.7

4. Discussion

In this work, we characterized the whole-transcriptome of PBMCs from MS patients with distinct LS-OCMB status. This profiling and the validation experiments revealed that the global transcriptome of PBMCs from patients with positive LS-OCMBs is different from those patients with negative LS-OCMB status.

RNA-seq results reveal that there are 124 circRNAs and 2441 linear RNAs differentially expressed between the two groups. Interestingly, 58% of linear RNAs are detected only in one of the groups, highlighting that there is a specific expression pattern in PBMCs from patients with different LS-OCMB status. It is true; however, that our RNA-seq sample size is limited and these observations should be taken with care.

To the best of our knowledge, none of the circRNAs have been previously related with MS. Circ_0000478 is located in chromosome 13 and its host gene is von Willebrand factor A domain containing 8 (*VWA8*). Interestingly, the linear transcript of this gene is also among the differentially expressed linear RNAs in our dataset, having a fold-change of −3.23 (p = 0.047). This transcript has been recently described and codes a mitochondrial protein with still uncertain function [32]. Regarding circ_0116639, it is located in chromosome 22, overlapping the *EP300* gene. EP300 is a histone acetyltransferase, which is detected in our study but is not differentially expressed. These differences in expression patterns of the circRNA with their host genes reveals that the biogenesis of circRNAs is independently regulated from that of their host genes, as it has been previously described [33].

Of note, interferon regulatory factor 5 (*IRF5*) is one of the confirmed downregulated transcripts, and polymorphisms in this gene has been associated to the risk of developing MS in last genome-wide association analysis, performed by the International Multiple Sclerosis Genetics Consortium, as well as in replication studies in Spanish cohorts [34,35]. Additionally, SNPs in this gene have been related to increased levels of CXCL13 in CSF, a chemokine related to highly active disease [36]. On top of that, it has been shown in animal models that IRF5 is related with the microglial polarization towards a pro-inflammatory state (M1) in response to stroke and in Alzheimer's disease [37,38]. This could suggest microglial implication in a more aggressive disease course, as it has been suggested by other authors in a exome sequencing project [39]. Nonetheless, our findings are made in peripheral PBMCs, so the *IRF5* source might be peripheral monocytes or macrophages. In any case, further research is needed to uncover *IRF5* implication in a highly active MS disease course.

On the other hand, MT-RNR2 like 8 transcript (*MTRNR2L8*), the other validated linear transcript showing lower expression in the LS-OCMB+ group, is coded in chromosome 11, and, interestingly, it spans the location of the miR-4485 stem-loop location, one of the four miRNAs selected for validation in the present study. According to microarray data, miR-4485 is downregulated in LS-OCMB+ groups, as it is *MTRNR2L8*. The fact that *MTRNR2L8* is a host gene for mir-4485 may explain that both transcripts appear downregulated in this group of patients, even if the miRNA could not have been validated. These results point at a possible interaction between these two RNAs that might be related to a more active disease, but further research is needed to confirm this hypothesis. According to UniProt, MTRNR2L8 has a role as a neuroprotective and antiapoptotic factor and it has been found to be increased in a specific area of the brain from patients with major depressive disorder [40]. Although the function of this gene is still unclear, the possible role as a neuroprotective factor is very interesting in the case of MS, since we find this gene downregulated in PBMCs. But again, further studies should be conducted to uncover the possible link between *MTRNR2L8* expression in peripheral blood and disease activity, as well as the mechanisms underlying this relationship.

Gene overrepresentation test shows that biological processes related to complement activation, humoral immune response and type I interferon response are among the most enriched term. Of note, intrathecal synthesis of IgM antibodies has previously been correlated with intrathecal complement activation [41], and its role in demyelination and axonal damage has been clearly demonstrated [42]. Interestingly, different components of the complement system have been related to MS and plasma levels of some of the components have been proposed as MS disease state biomarkers [43]. Of note, these processes are enriched among altered genes in PBMC from patients with a marker of a high activity disease. This analysis may reveal that those patients may have an altered immune response that may explain their higher disease activity, but further and other kind of studies will be needed to explore this hypothesis.

The main aim of this study was to identify in blood a biomarker or a group of them that could differentiate between positive and negative LS-OCMB patients, thus could be used as a more accessible marker of highly active disease. ROC curve analysis revealed that these markers in combination have around 70% of accuracy, which is considered, in general, an acceptable performance [44]. Taking into account that these are measured in blood, they may help in the clinics to perform repeated measurements, while taking serial samples of CSF has serious drawbacks. Efforts are being made to define patients with a highly active disease course, given that their effective therapeutic window might be narrower than a more benign or less active disease form [45]. In line with this, several biomarkers have been proposed to identify individuals with aggressive disease course, such as CSF levels of neurofilament light chain, CXCL13 or CHI3L1 [46–48]. Other authors have also reported differences in non-coding transcriptome between patients with different disease activity. Quintana and colleagues studied the expression in CSF of a panel of miRNAs patients with MS with LS-OCMB characterization and patients with other neurological diseases (ONDs) [49]. They found differences in the expression of miR-30a-5p, miR-150, miR-645 and miR-191 between the OND group and the LS-OCMB+ group, but they could not find any difference between patients with positive and negative LS-OCMBs. Due to differences in the profiling platforms between their study and the present one, we are unable to check the expression of our candidate miRNA in data from Quintana and colleagues. Another study reported that serum levels of miR-24-3p correlate with disease progression index, calculated dividing EDSS value by disease duration, but the status of LS-OCMB is not measured [50]. More recently, the expression in blood of long non-coding RNAs has also been described to show the capacity of discriminating highly active MS patients from others with less active disease course, based on a age-related MS severity score [51].

All these studies highlight the need of biomarkers that are able to identify patients with highly active disease and the effort that the scientific community is doing in this direction. In addition, it is also important to have a consensus on the definition of what is an aggressive disease course, given that each study uses different parameters to measure and classify patients in each of the groups, which makes the comparison between them really challenging [52,53]. An early recognition of a patient in this group could benefit from different therapeutic advice and; therefore, the possibility to improve the long-term outcome of the disease.

Our miRNA profiling study discovered some miRNA differentially expressed between the two groups, although they have not been validated by RT-qPCR experiments. In this regard, other techniques such as droplet digital PCR (ddPCR) may help in reducing variability and discover small differences between groups. Although it has been reported that the sensitivity is not increased with ddPCR in gene expression studies, and that the performance is similar provided that the amount of starting material is enough and there are no contaminants in the reaction [54,55]. Nonetheless, it is a technique that could be considered in future validation projects aiming at definitely discarding or including those miRNAs as biomarkers for a more aggressive MS course.

5. Conclusions

In summary, we have identified two circRNAs and two linear RNAs which are downregulated in patients with positive LS-OCMB status. Our findings are important in the field of biomarkers for multiple sclerosis, given that they could contribute to the identification of patients with highly active disease. Additionally, an important advantage compared to other biomarkers is that they are detected in blood, allowing serial tests to monitor their levels, while this task is not so recommended for lumbar puncture. Future studies in larger cohorts will be needed to confirm their utility, but we consider that they may serve as a first screening tool to decide which patients should go into a lumbar puncture to confirm their LS-OCMB status.

Author Contributions: Conceptualization, D.O. (David Otaegui) and M.M.-C.; methodology, D.O. (David Otaegui), M.M.-C., L.I., T.B., D.O. (Danel Olaverri), and L.M.V.; validation, L.I. and L.S.; formal analysis, L.I., D.O. (Danel Olaverri), T.B., M.M.-C., M.E. and L.C.-F.; investigation, L.I., M.M.-C., M.E., L.C.-F.; resources, A.P., T.C.-T., M.E., L.C.-F., L.M.V. and D.O. (David Otaegui); writing—original draft preparation, L.I., D.O. (David Otaegui) and M.M.-C.; writing—review and editing, D.O. (Danel Olaverri), T.B., Á.P., T.C.-T., L.M.V.; visualization, L.I., D.O. (Danel Olaverri), M.M.-C.; supervision, D.O. (David Otaegui), L.I., M.M.-C. and L.M.V.; project administration, D.O. (David Otaegui) and M.M.-C.; funding acquisition, L.M.V., D.O. (David Otaegui) and M.M.-C. All authors have read and agreed to the published version of the manuscript.

Acknowledgments: Authors want to acknowledge the staff of Genomic Platform at Biodonostia Health Research Institute.

References

1. Filippi, M.; Bar-Or, A.; Piehl, F.; Preziosa, P.; Solari, A.; Vukusic, S.; Rocca, M.A. Multiple sclerosis. *Nat. Rev. Dis. Prim.* **2018**, *4*, 1–27. [CrossRef] [PubMed]
2. Comabella, M.; Montalban, X. Body fluid biomarkers in multiple sclerosis. *Lancet Neurol.* **2014**, *13*, 113–126. [CrossRef]
3. Paul, A.; Comabella, M.; Gandhi, R. Biomarkers in Multiple Sclerosis. *Cold Spring Harb. Perspect. Med.* **2019**, *9*. [CrossRef] [PubMed]
4. Villar, L.M.; Sadaba, M.C.; Roldan, E.; Masjuan, J.; Gonzalez-Porque, P.; Villarrubia, N.; Espino, M.; Garcia-Trujillo, J.A.; Bootello, A.; Alvarez-Cermeno, J.C. Intrathecal synthesis of oligoclonal IgM against myelin lipids predicts an aggressive disease course in MS. *J. Clin. Investig.* **2005**, *115*, 187–194. [CrossRef]
5. Polivka, J.J.P., Jr.; Krakorova, K.; Peterka, M.; Topolcan, O. Current status of biomarker research in neurology. *EPMA J.* **2016**, 1–13. [CrossRef]

6. Kemppinen, A.K.; Kaprio, J.; Palotie, A.; Saarela, J. Systematic review of genome-wide expression studies in multiple sclerosis. *BMJ Open* **2011**, *1*, e000053. [CrossRef]
7. Nickles, D.; Chen, H.P.; Li, M.M.; Khankhanian, P.; Madireddy, L.; Caillier, S.J.; Santaniello, A.; Cree, B.A.; Pelletier, D.; Hauser, S.L.; et al. Blood RNA profiling in a large cohort of multiple sclerosis patients and healthy controls. *Hum. Mol. Genet.* **2013**, *22*, 4194–4205. [CrossRef] [PubMed]
8. Irizar, H.; Muñoz-Culla, M.; Sáenz-Cuesta, M.; Osorio-Querejeta, I.; Sepúlveda, L.; Castillo-Triviño, T.; Prada, A.; Lopez de Munain, A.; Olascoaga, J.; Otaegui, D. Identification of ncRNAs as potential therapeutic targets in multiple sclerosis through differential ncRNA—mRNA network analysis. *BMC Genom.* **2015**, *16*, 250. [CrossRef] [PubMed]
9. Dolati, S.; Marofi, F.; Babaloo, Z.; Aghebati-Maleki, L.; Roshangar, L.; Ahmadi, M.; Rikhtegar, R.; Yousefi, M. Dysregulated Network of miRNAs Involved in the Pathogenesis of Multiple Sclerosis. *Biomed. Pharmacother.* **2018**, *104*, 280–290. [CrossRef]
10. Du, C.; Liu, C.; Kang, J.; Zhao, G.; Ye, Z.; Huang, S.; Li, Z.; Wu, Z.; Pei, G.; Du, C.; et al. MicroRNA miR-326 regulates T H -17 differentiation and is associated with the pathogenesis of multiple sclerosis. *Nat. Immunol.* **2009**, *1259*, 1252–1259. [CrossRef] [PubMed]
11. Muñoz-Culla, M.; Irizar, H.; Sáenz-Cuesta, M.; Castillo-Triviño, T.; Osorio-Querejeta, I.; Sepúlveda, L.; López De Munain, A.; Olascoaga, J.; Otaegui, D. SncRNA (microRNA &snoRNA) opposite expression pattern found in multiple sclerosis relapse and remission is sex dependent. *Sci. Rep.* **2016**, *6*. [CrossRef]
12. De Felice, B.; Mondola, P.; Sasso, A.; Orefice, G.; Bresciamorra, V.; Vacca, G.; Biffali, E.; Borra, M.; Pannone, R. Small non-coding RNA signature in multiple sclerosis patients after treatment with interferon-β. *BMC Med. Genom.* **2014**, *7*, 1–9. [CrossRef] [PubMed]
13. Jonas, S.; Izaurralde, E. Towards a molecular understanding of microRNA-mediated gene silencing. *Nat. Rev. Genet.* **2015**, *16*, 421–433. [CrossRef]
14. Floris, G.; Zhang, L.; Follesa, P.; Sun, T. Regulatory Role of Circular RNAs and Neurological Disorders. *Mol. Neurobiol.* **2017**, *54*, 5156–5165. [CrossRef]
15. Xia, X.; Tang, X.; Wang, S. Roles of CircRNAs in Autoimmune Diseases. *Front. Immunol.* **2019**, *10*, 1–8. [CrossRef] [PubMed]
16. Paraboschi, E.M.; Cardamone, G.; Soldà, G.; Duga, S.; Asselta, R. Interpreting Non-coding Genetic Variation in Multiple Sclerosis Genome-Wide Associated Regions. *Front. Genet.* **2018**, *9*, 1–10. [CrossRef]
17. Cardamone, G.; Paraboschi, E.M.; Rimoldi, V.; Duga, S.; Soldà, G.; Asselta, R. The Characterization of GSDMB Splicing and Backsplicing Profiles Identifies Novel Isoforms and a Circular RNA That Are Dysregulated in Multiple Sclerosis. *Int. J. Mol. Sci.* **2017**, *18*, 576. [CrossRef]
18. Iparraguirre, L.; Muñoz-Culla, M.; Prada-Luengo, I.; Castillo-Triviño, T.; Olascoaga, J.; Otaegui, D. Circular RNA profiling reveals that circular RNAs from ANXA2 can be used as new biomarkers for multiple sclerosis. *Hum. Mol. Genet.* **2017**, *26*. [CrossRef]
19. Kacperska, M.J.; Walenczak, J.; Tomasik, B. Plasmatic microRNA as potential biomarkers of multiple sclerosis: Literature review. *Adv. Clin. Exp. Med.* **2016**, *25*, 775–779. [CrossRef]
20. Stoicea, N.; Du, A.; Lakis, D.C.; Tipton, C.; Arias-Morales, C.E.; Bergese, S.D. The MiRNA Journey from Theory to Practice as a CNS Biomarker. *Front. Genet.* **2016**, *7*, 1–8. [CrossRef]
21. Zhang, Z.; Yang, T.; Xiao, J. Circular RNAs: Promising Biomarkers for Human Diseases. *EBioMedicine* **2018**, *34*, 267–274. [CrossRef] [PubMed]
22. Villar, L.M.; González-Porqué, P.; Masjuán, J.; Álvarez-Cermeño, J.; Bootello, A.; Keir, G. A sensitive and reproducible method for the detection of oligoclonal IgM bands. *J. Immunol. Methods* **2001**, *258*, 151–155. [CrossRef]
23. Kent, W.J.; Sugnet, C.W.; Furey, T.S.; Roskin, K.M.; Pringle, T.H.; Zahler, A.M.; Haussler, A.D. The Human Genome Browser at UCSC. *Genome Res.* **2002**, *12*, 996–1006. [CrossRef] [PubMed]
24. Dobin, A.; Davis, C.A.; Schlesinger, F.; Drenkow, J.; Zaleski, C.; Jha, S.; Batut, P.; Chaisson, M.; Gingeras, T.R. STAR: Ultrafast universal RNA-seq aligner. *Bioinformatics* **2013**, *29*, 15–21. [CrossRef]
25. Li, H.; Durbin, R. Fast and accurate short read alignment with Burrows—Wheeler transform. *Bioinformatics* **2009**, *25*, 1754–1760. [CrossRef]
26. Zhang, X.; Dong, R.; Zhang, Y.; Zhang, J.; Luo, Z.; Zhang, J.; Chen, L.; Yang, L. Diverse alternative back-splicing and alternative splicing landscape of circular RNAs. *Genome Res.* **2016**, *26*, 1277–1287. [CrossRef]

27. Gao, Y.; Zhang, J.; Zhao, F. Circular RNA identification based on multiple seed matching. *Brief. Bioinform.* **2017**, 1–8. [CrossRef]
28. Hansen, T.B. Improved circRNA Identification by Combining Prediction Algorithms. *Front. Cell Dev. Biol.* **2018**, *6*, 1–9. [CrossRef]
29. Love, M.I.; Huber, W.; Anders, S. Moderated estimation of fold change and dispersion for RNA-seq data with DESeq2. *Genome Biol.* **2014**, *15*, 1–21. [CrossRef]
30. Bray, N.L.; Pimentel, H.; Melsted, P.; Pachter, L. Near-optimal probabilistic RNA-seq quantification. *Nat. Biotechnol.* **2016**, *34*, 525–528. [CrossRef]
31. Mi, H.; Thomas, P. PANTHER Pathway: An ontology-based pathway database coupled with data analysis tools. *Nat. Protoc.* **2019**, *14*, 703–721. [CrossRef] [PubMed]
32. Luo, M.; Ma, W.; Sand, Z.; Finlayson, J.; Wang, T.; Diaz, R.; Willis, W.T.; Mandarino, L.J. Von Willebrand factor A domain-containing protein 8 (VWA8) localizes to the matrix side of the inner mitochondrial membrane. *Biochem. Biophys. Res. Commun.* **2020**, *521*, 158–163. [CrossRef]
33. Moldovan, L.I.; Hansen, T.B.; Venø, M.T.; Okholm, T.L.H.; Andersen, T.L.; Hager, H.; Iversen, L.; Kjems, J.; Johansen, C.; Kristensen, L.S. High-throughput RNA sequencing from paired lesional- and non-lesional skin reveals major alterations in the psoriasis circRNAome. *BMC Med. Genom.* **2019**, *12*, 1–17. [CrossRef] [PubMed]
34. International Multiple Sclerosis Genetics Consortium. The Multiple Sclerosis Genomic Map implicates peripheral immune cells and microglia in susceptibility. *Science* **2019**, *365*, 1–10. [CrossRef]
35. Vandenbroeck, K.; Alloza, I.; Swaminathan, B.; Antiguedad, A.; Otaegui, D.; Olascoaga, J.; Barcina, M.G.; de las Heras, V.; Bartolome, M.; Fernandez-Arquero, M.; et al. Validation of IRF5 as multiple sclerosis risk gene: Putative role in interferon beta therapy and human herpes virus-6 infection. *Genes Immun.* **2011**, *12*, 40–45. [CrossRef]
36. Lindén, M.; Khademi, M.; Bomfim, I.L.; Piehl, F.; Jagodic, M.; Kockum, I.; Olsson, T. Multiple sclerosis risk genotypes correlate with an elevated cerebrospinal fluid level of the suggested prognostic marker CXCL13. *Mult. Scler. Jounrla* **2012**, *19*, 863–870. [CrossRef]
37. Al Mamun, A.; Chauhan, A.; Yu, H.; Xu, Y.; Sharmeen, R.; Liu, F. Interferon regulatory factor 4/5 signaling impacts on microglial activation after ischemic stroke in mice. *Eur. J. Neurosci.* **2018**, *47*, 140–149. [CrossRef]
38. Zhu, D.; Yang, N.; Liu, Y.-Y.; Zheng, J.; Ji, C.; Zuo, P.-P. M2 Macrophage Transplantation Ameliorates Cognitive Dysfunction in Amyloid-β-Treated Rats Through Regulation of Microglial Polarization. *J. Alzheimer's Dis.* **2016**, *52*, 483–495. [CrossRef]
39. Gil-Varea, E.; Urcelay, E.; Vilariño-Güell, C.; Costa, C.; Midaglia, L.; Matesanz, F.; Rodríguez-antigüedad, A.; Oksenberg, J.; Espino-paisan, L.; Sadovnick, A.D.; et al. Exome sequencing study in patients with multiple sclerosis reveals variants associated with disease course. *J. Neuroinflamm.* **2018**, *15*, 1–10. [CrossRef]
40. Pantazatos, S.P.; Huang, Y.-Y.; Rosoklija, G.B.; Dwork, A.J.; Arango, V.; Mann, J.J. Whole-transcriptome brain expression and exon-usage profiling in major depression and suicide: Evidence for altered glial, endothelial and ATPase activity. *Mol. Psychiatry* **2017**, *22*, 760–773. [CrossRef]
41. Sellebjerg, F.; Christiansen, M.; Garred, P. MBP, anti-MBP and anti-PLP antibodies, and intrathecal complement activation in multiple sclerosis. *Mult. Scler.* **1998**, *4*, 127–131. [CrossRef] [PubMed]
42. Mead, R.J.; Singhrao, S.K.; Neal, J.W.; Lassmann, H.; Morgan, B.P. The Membrane Attack Complex of Complement Causes Severe Demyelination Associated with Acute Axonal Injury. *J. Immunol.* **2002**, *168*, 458–465. [CrossRef] [PubMed]
43. Ingram, G.; Hakobyan, S.; Hirst, C.L.; Harris, C.L.; Loveless, S.; Mitchell, J.P.; Pickersgill, T.P.; Robertson, N.P.; Morgan, B.P. Systemic complement profiling in multiple sclerosis as a biomarker of disease state. *Mult. Scler. J.* **2012**, *18*, 1401–1411. [CrossRef] [PubMed]
44. Mandrekar, J.N. Receiver Operating Characteristic Curve in Diagnostic Test Assessment. *J. Thorac. Oncol.* **2010**, *5*, 1315–1316. [CrossRef] [PubMed]
45. Iacobaeus, E.; Ryschkewitsch, C.; Gravell, M.; Khademi, M.; Wallstrom, E.; Olsson, T.; Brundin, L.; Major, E. Analysis of cerebrospinal fluid and cerebrospinal fluid cells from patients with multiple sclerosis for detection of JC virus DNA. *Mult. Scler. J.* **2009**, *15*, 28–35. [CrossRef]

46. Håkansson, I.; Tisell, A.; Cassel, P.; Blennow, K.; Zetterberg, H.; Lundberg, P.; Dahle, C.; Vrethem, M.; Ernerudh, J. Neurofilament levels, disease activity and brain volume during follow-up in multiple sclerosis. *J. Neuroinflamm.* **2018**, *15*, 1–10. [CrossRef]
47. Khademi, M.; Kockum, I.; Andersson, M.L.; Iacobaeus, E.; Brundin, L.; Sellebjerg, F.; Hillert, J.; Piehl, F.; Olsson, T. Cerebrospinal fluid CXCL13 in multiple sclerosis: A suggestive prognostic marker for the disease course. *Mult. Scler. J.* **2011**, *17*, 335–343. [CrossRef]
48. Cantó, E.; Tintore, M.; Villar, L.M.; Costa, C.; Nurtdinov, R.; Deisenhammer, F.; Hegen, H.; Khademi, M.; Olsson, T.; Piehl, F.; et al. Chitinase 3-like 1: Prognostic biomarker in clinically isolated syndromes. *Brain* **2015**, *138*, 918–931. [CrossRef]
49. Quintana, E.; Ortega, F.J.; Robles-Cedeño, R.; Villar, M.L.; Buxó, M.; Mercader, J.M.; Alvarez-Cermeño, J.C.; Pueyo, N.; Perkal, H.; Fernández-Real, J.M.; et al. miRNAs in cerebrospinal fluid identify patients with MS and specifically those with lipid-specific oligoclonal IgM bands. *Mult. Scler. J.* **2017**, *23*, 1716–1726. [CrossRef]
50. Vistbakka, J.; Sumelahti, M.; Lehtimäki, T.; Elovaara, I.; Hagman, S. Evaluation of serum miR-191-5p, miR-24-3p, miR-128-3p and miR-376c-3 in multiple sclerosis patients. *Acta Neurol. Scand.* **2018**, 1–7. [CrossRef]
51. Gupta, M.; Martens, K.; Metz, L.M.; Jason, A.P.; Koning, D.; Pfeffer, G. Long noncoding RNAs associated with phenotypic severity in multiple sclerosis. *Mult. Scler. Relat. Disord.* **2019**, *36*, 101407. [CrossRef] [PubMed]
52. Iacobaeus, E.; Arrambide, G.; Amato, M.P.; Derfuss, T.; Vukusic, S.; Hemmer, B.; Tintore, M. Aggressive multiple sclerosis (1): Towards a definition of the phenotype. *Mult. Scler. J.* **2020**, 1031–1044. [CrossRef] [PubMed]
53. Díaz, C.; Zarco, L.A.; Rivera, D.M. Highly active multiple sclerosis: An update. *Mult. Scler. Relat. Disord.* **2019**, *30*, 215–224. [CrossRef]
54. Hindson, C.M.; Chevillet, J.R.; Briggs, H.A.; Gallichotte, E.N.; Ruf, I.K.; Hindson, B.J.; Vessella, R.L.; Tewari, M. Absolute quantification by droplet digital PCR versus analog real-time PCR. *Nat. Methods* **2013**, 1–6. [CrossRef]
55. Taylor, S.C.; Laperriere, G.; Germain, H. Droplet Digital PCR versus qPCR for gene expression analysis with low abundant targets: From variable nonsense to publication quality data. *Sci. Rep.* **2017**, 1–8. [CrossRef] [PubMed]

7

Stem Cell-Based Therapies for Multiple Sclerosis: Current Perspectives

Fernando X. Cuascut * and George J. Hutton *

Baylor College of Medicine, Maxine Mesigner Multiple Sclerosis Center, Houston, TX 77030, USA
* Correspondence: fernando.cuascut@bcm.edu (F.X.C.); ghutton@bcm.edu (G.J.H.);

Abstract: Multiple sclerosis (MS) is an inflammatory and neurodegenerative autoimmune disease of the central nervous system (CNS). Disease-modifying therapies (DMT) targeting inflammation have been shown to reduce disease activity in patients with relapsing–remitting MS (RRMS). The current therapeutic challenge is to find an effective treatment to halt disease progression and reverse established neural damage. Stem cell-based therapies have emerged to address this dilemma. Several types of stem cells have been considered for clinical use, such as autologous hematopoietic (aHSC), mesenchymal (MSC), neuronal (NSC), human embryonic (hESC), and induced pluripotent (iPSC) stem cells. There is convincing evidence that immunoablation followed by hematopoietic therapy (aHSCT) has a high efficacy for suppressing inflammatory MS activity and improving neurological disability in patients with RRMS. In addition, MSC therapy may be a safe and tolerable treatment, but its clinical value is still under evaluation. Various studies have shown early promising results with other cellular therapies for CNS repair and decreasing inflammation. In this review, we discuss the current knowledge and limitations of different stem cell-based therapies for the treatment of patients with MS.

Keywords: multiple sclerosis; stem cells; autologous hematopoietic; mesenchymal; neuronal; induced pluripotent; human embryonic

---

1. Introduction

Multiple sclerosis is an autoimmune condition characterized by demyelination and the loss of CNS neurons. Active inflammation is most evident in early RRMS. A neurodegenerative process may contribute to disability accumulation during later secondary progressive MS (SPMS) [1]. Available disease-modifying therapies (DMT) for MS have been shown to reduce the number and severity of relapses. Despite the broad range of options, there is still a therapeutic challenge in finding an effective treatment to halt disease progression and to reverse established neural injuries [2,3]. A subgroup of MS patients and those with an aggressive subtype may continue to deteriorate despite the use of DMT [4,5].

In the last 20 years, stem cell transplantation has been considered as a potentially effective therapeutic approach for aggressive MS. At least five types of stem cells have been considered as potential therapeutic approaches: autologous hematopoietic (aHSC), mesenchymal (MSC), neuronal (NSC), induced pluripotent (iPSC), and human embryonic (hESC) [6]. Each of these cell-based therapies works through various mechanisms, including replacing the malfunctioning immune system using immunoablation with high-dose immunosuppressive therapy (HDIT), followed by aHSC administration [7]; modifying the immune response and intrinsic repair mechanisms by alteration of cytokines and trophic factors (MSC) [8,9]; replacing damaged or lost neuronal tissue with NSC or iPSC [10,11]; and providing immunosuppressive and neuroprotective mechanisms (hESC) [12].

In this review, we aim to describe the current knowledge and limitations regarding cell-based approaches for treating MS, and discuss the future considerations that are required to optimize the therapeutic parameters regarding treatment efficacy and safety.

2. Immunoablation Followed by Hematopoietic Stem Cell Transplantation

2.1. The Procedure

Immunoablative therapy followed by aHSC therapy (aHSCT) to manage highly active and treatment-refractory MS has been investigated for the last two decades, following reports of the coincidental improvement of autoimmune disease symptoms in patients undergoing transplantation for hematological malignancies [13,14]. The therapeutic effects of immunoablation followed by aHSC transplantation were initially studied in rats with experimental autoimmune encephalomyelitis (EAE)—a rodent model of central nervous system (CNS) inflammation—showing that the procedure can induce remission, prevent relapses, and enhance the recovery of symptoms [15–17]. As discussed below, one rationale behind this method is to eliminate the abnormal immune system cells using HDIT, gradually developing a "new" and more tolerant immune system after aHSC infusion [18,19]. An alternative explanation is that HDIT produces a radical and long-lasting suppression of the inflammatory MS activity [20–22]. The procedure encompasses a series of steps which includes the mobilization, harvesting, ablative conditioning, and transplantation of aHSC [23,24] (Figure 1). First, hematopoietic stem cell (HSC) are mobilized, typically from peripheral blood, by using either granulocyte colony-stimulating factor (G-CSF) or granulocyte-macrophage colony-stimulating factor (GM-CSF), with or without cyclophosphamide (CY). It is preferred to pretreat with CY due to the potential for either a clinical relapse or worsening of pre-existing symptoms with the administration of G-CSF or GM-CSF alone [25]. The HSC are then harvested and cryopreserved until the patient is ready for transplantation. The HSC can be positively selected for $CD34^+$ cells ex vivo, which theoretically reduces the risk of reinfusing potentially autoreactive lymphocytes. However, there is limited evidence indicating any obvious advantage of $CD34^+$ selection, which increases the technical complexity of the transplant procedure [26]. The next step is to eliminate autoreactive cells (ablative conditioning) with HDIT. Different conditioning regimens have been proposed and classified according to the intensity of the ablation. High-intensity regimens typically consist of a high IV dose of busulfan, combined with a high dose of CY, and anti-thymocyte globulin (ATG) for in vivo T cell depletion. Total body irradiation is no longer used due to its severe toxicity [26]. Intermediate-intensity regimens involve a combination of different chemotherapies, which often include BCNU, cytosine arabinoside, etoposide, and melphalan, with or without ATG, referred to as BEAM. Other modified BEAM regimens have also been utilized with similar results [27] (Table 1). The low-intensity regimens, also referred to as nonmyeloablative, use CY and ATG [28].

Currently, there is a debate regarding which conditioning regimen should be used. For instance, high-intensity regimens are associated with more adverse effects and mortality [29–33]. Conversely, low-intensity regimens are associated with reduced toxicity and require less supportive care, but may be associated with the early reappearance of MRI lesion activity post-transplant [34–37]. It is becoming more acceptable to use BEAM or modified BEAM as an intermediate regimen for ablative conditioning [38]. After the conditioning regimen, the cryopreserved cells are thawed and then infused back into the patient. ATG is administered before or after the HSC infusion, to primarily remove any autoreactive T cells that might have escaped prior conditioning procedures. Subsequently, the patient enters an aplastic phase, characterized by an extremely low level of hematopoietic blood cells, requiring prophylactic treatment with antivirals and antibiotics.

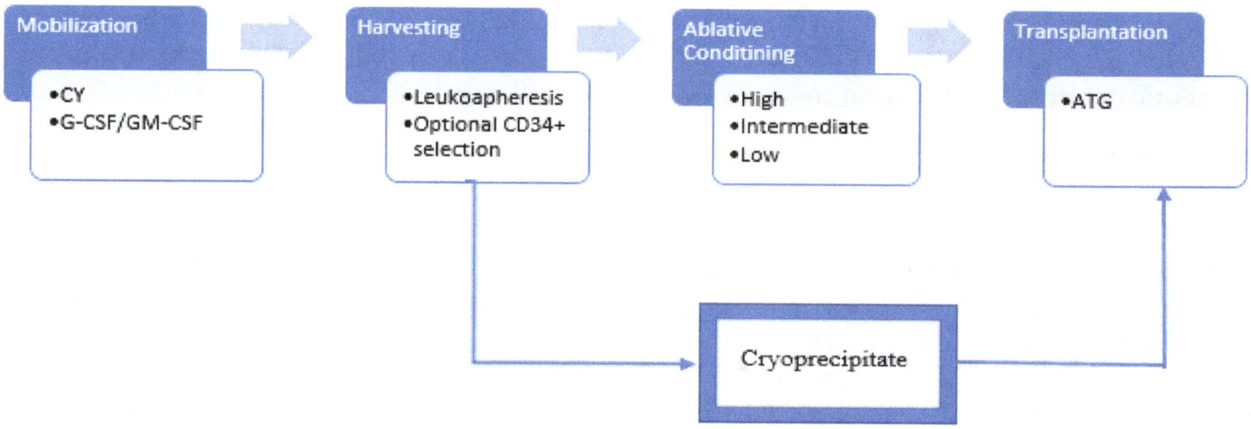

Figure 1. Immunoablation followed by autologous hematopoietic stem cell transplantation. First, HSC are mobilized, typically from peripheral blood, by using granulocyte colony-stimulating factor (G-CSF) or granulocyte-macrophage colony-stimulating factor (GM-CSF), with or without cyclophosphamide (CY). The HSC are then harvested and cryopreserved until the patient is ready for transplantation. The HSC can be positively selected for $CD34^{+}$ cells ex vivo. The next step is to eliminate autoreactive cells (ablative conditioning) using either a high-, intermediate (BEAM), or low-intensity regimen. After the conditioning regimen, the cryopreserved cells are thawed and then infused back into the patient. Anti-thymocyte globulin (ATG) is administered before or after the aHSC infusion to primarily remove any autoreactive T cells that might have escaped prior conditioning procedures. Subsequently, the patient enters an aplastic phase, characterized by an extremely low level of hematopoietic blood cells requiring prophylactic treatment with antivirals and antibiotics.

Table 1. Immunoablation regimens.

Intensity	Regimen
High	High dose of busulfan combined with cyclophosphamide and ATG
Intermediate	BEAM (BCNU, etoposide, cytosine arabinoside, melphalan) +/− ATG
Low (nonmyeloablative)	Cyclophosphamide and ATG

2.2. *Immune Mechanisms*

Although the efficacy of aHSCT in MS is increasingly being validated, the immune mechanisms that account for its therapeutic effects are still unclear. There are at least two basic hypotheses to explain its beneficial effects. First, aHSCT is considered to "reset" the immune system by depleting adaptive immune cells and gradually developing a "new" immune system [7,18,19,39,40]. The naïve T cells reemerge over time and undergo a complex T cell receptor (TCR) rearrangement, leading to an augmentation of the T cell repertoire and clonal diversity [18,19,41]. After immune reconstitution, pathogenic CD4+ Th17 lymphocytes are reduced [42]. On the other hand, T cell clones that recognize and react to myelin basic protein (MBP) are initially depleted by the conditioning regimen but reappear over time, although it has not established whether these cells are pathological [41]. The extent to which aHSCT leads to an immune reconfiguration is not completely clear, and demonstrating how the immune system resets to a pre-pathological state is scientifically challenging. However, the characteristics that the immune system acquires following aHCST certainly suggest that it has become alternatively programmed. Conversely, an alternate explanation of the therapeutic benefits of aHSCT might be that the conditioning regimen severely depletes T cell populations for an extended time, thus inducing a state of long-lasting immunosuppression incapable of mounting an autoimmune response of clinical significance [20–22]. Both of the aforementioned hypotheses may have diverse effects that could be beneficial to MS treatment and, when applied alone, either hypothesis is ineffective or less effective at explaining the benefits of the treatment than when applied in combination. Therefore, the reconciliation of these hypotheses should be achieved in order to obtain optimal therapeutic results [43].

2.3. Current Clinical Knowledge

The initial studies using aHSCT to treat MS were performed over two decades ago [13]. Since then, there has been an increasing number of studies looking into this treatment approach. Typically, the primary endpoint is event-free survival (EFS), which is defined as survival without death, or the patient having no evidence of disease activity (NEDA) (i.e., no disability progression, relapse, and/or new lesions on MRI). Earlier studies were conducted mostly in patients with a high level of disability and progressive disease [13,31,44].

For example, a recent retrospective study evaluated the long-term outcomes of patients with MS treated with aHSCT between January 1995 and December 2006 [45]. In this study, the authors established that most patients had progressive MS (78%), mostly with secondary progressive MS (66%). The median Expanded Disability Status Scale (EDSS) score was 6.5, demonstrating moderately advanced disability, on average. The progression-free survival at 5 years was established for the combined group (46%), RRMS subgroup (73%), and the SPMS subgroup (33%). Also, no statistical difference in the risk of progression between primary progressive MS (PPMS) and SPMS was identified. Furthermore, transplant-related mortality (TRM) occurring in the first 100 days after transplantation was 2.8%. The authors concluded that a younger age, RRMS, and fewer prior disease-modifying treatments were associated with better neurological outcomes.

Recent studies have focused on patients with RRMS with an aggressive disease course, given the evidence that aHSCT is most successful in this population [34,36,46–48]. The HALT-MS study, in which only patients with RRMS were enrolled, demonstrated a 5-year event-free survival of 69.2% [49,50]. Similarly, a phase II multicenter single-arm trial of patients with aggressive MS who underwent aHSCT transplantation reported an event-free survival at 3 years of 69.6% [51]. Both groups also demonstrated an improvement of their EDSS by 0.5 points or more at their latest follow-up. An additional large single-center trial using nonmyeloablative aHSCT in patients with RRMS and SPMS showed a 4-year relapse-free survival of 80% and progression-free survival of 87% [52]. The study also showed improved disability scores 2 years after aHSCT, mainly in those with RRMS and mild to moderate disability. This benefit was not seen in patients with severe disability due to progressive MS. These three major studies concluded that either HDIT or a nonmyeloablative regimen followed by aHSCT was effective in inducing long-term sustained remissions and disability improvement.

The safety of aHSCT has dramatically improved through the years. The European Bone Marrow Transplantation (EBMT) Registry analysis of patients treated from 1995 to 2000 showed a TRM of 7.3%, while the TRM from 2001 to2007 was 1.3%, further decreasing to 0.7% during 2008–2016, and most recently down to 0.2% [24,38,45]. This improvement is likely related to the better selection of patients (younger patients with RRMS and exclusion of older patients with advanced disability), increased experience with aHSCT treatment, and decreased use of high-intensity regimens [31]. For example, high-intensity conditioning regimens were associated with life-threatening infections [32,33]. Furthermore, some clinical trials using nonmyeloablative conditioning report no mortality associated with the procedure [52]. A recent meta-analysis found that TRM was close to zero in studies that included patients who were younger, had RRMS rather than SPMS along with a lower baseline EDSS, and whose procedure was performed in more recent years, although there was no significant association of TRM with regimen intensity [53]. The authors pointed out a few limitations that may contribute to their results. Regardless, growing evidence suggests intense conditioning and/or extensive T cell depletion protocols increase morbidity and mortality rate [24].

3. Mesenchymal Stem Cells

3.1. Preclinical Animal Studies with Mesenchymal Stem Cells

Besides aHSC, the use of MSC has emerged as a potential powerful cellular therapy for inflammatory and neurodegenerative diseases of the CNS, including MS [54,55]. The MSC are multipotent, nonhematopoietic cells that have both immunomodulatory and regenerative properties [56]. Typically, MSC are obtained from the bone marrow, but other tissues have been used, including adipose tissue, umbilical cord blood, and placenta [57,58]. For example, bone marrow MSC (BM-MSC) have been shown to reduce inflammatory responses, stimulate neuronal stem cell differentiation, and promote the regeneration of damaged areas in the CNS [59–63]. These effects are thought to be possible due to peripheral paracrine signals and/or the homing of MSC to injured tissue [64,65].

Studies on EAE have revealed the potential beneficial effects of MSC. EAE mice exhibit multifocal inflammation, variable demyelination, and axonal damage in the CNS via immunization with myelin proteins or immunogenic myelin peptides [65]. The EAE animal model has been helpful in explaining the immunobiological basis of tissue damage in MS and identifying potential therapeutic approaches. When BM-MSC are infused into EAE mice, there is a reduction in the severity of the clinical symptoms and diminished immune cell infiltration, demyelination, and axonal damage [59–63]. These therapeutic effects are seen when MSC are injected intravenously (IV), intraventricular (IVT), and even intraperitoneally (IP) [61,66,67]. However, the optimal route for MSC injection is yet to be determined. Moreover, the therapeutic effects are observed when BM-MSC are injected at disease onset or peak, but are not seen if they are administered during the chronic stage of disease [60].

The exact mechanisms by which BM-MSC mediate their beneficial outcomes are still not completely understood. One potential explanation includes the release of anti-inflammatory and neurotrophic molecules that modulate the immune inflammatory responses targeting the CNS. For instance, EAE mice that received an IVT infusion of exogenous BM-MSC exhibited a significant reduction in disease activity that was associated with the suppression of reactive T cells [67]. In a different study, human BM-MSC infusion in EAE mice was associated with decreased inflammatory myelin-specific Th1 cells and increased anti-inflammatory Th2 cells [59]. These results suggest an immunosuppressive reaction to BM-MSC infusion. Interestingly, IV injection of conditioned media used in MSC (MSC-CM) culture was associated with the symptomatic improvement of EAE mice, suggesting that the beneficial effects were produced by extracellular immunomodulatory molecules secreted by MSC [68].

An additional possibility that may explain the therapeutic effects of MSC is their migration to inflamed tissues. Several studies have tried to describe the ability of MSC to migrate to and repair injured tissue [61,69]. For example, intravenously administered MSC were detected in CNS in proportion to the degree of inflammation [69]. However, the data are limited, and the factors that attract MSC to areas of inflammation have not yet been elucidated.

In addition to their immunomodulatory capabilities, MS might have the potential of influencing neuronal stem cell differentiation and promoting remyelination and axonal survival. For example, MSC promote the differentiation of oligodendrocytes and/or neurons from neuronal stem cells in vitro, in preference to astroglial fate [70]. Similarly, brain dissection and histopathological studies of EAE mice treated with MSC infusion showed an increased number of oligodendrocytes, remyelination of white matter, and improved axonal integrity in injured tissue [59].

By contrast, some studies have reported deteriorative responses and the exacerbation of EAE symptoms with MSC treatment [71]. These findings implicate a different immunobiological mechanism from the previously described possibilities. Moreover, ectopic tissue formation when MS were administered via IVT in an EAE model [72] and malignant transformation are a theoretical concern, although not yet reported in humans [73].

Finally, it is unclear which tissues are the optimal source of MSC. Adipose tissue (AT) has been cited as a superior source because AT-MSC are relatively easier to harvest, have a higher availability, and better expansion capabilities ex vivo than BM-MSC [74]. Further studies are warranted to determine the best source.

3.2. Clinical Trials Using Mesenchymal Stem Cells for the Treatment of Multiple Sclerosis

Based on the results of treating EAE, MSC therapy has advanced to clinical trials. The first publication of a clinical trial using MSC in MS patients was in 2007 by Mohyeddin Bonab and colleagues [75]. Their study assessed the safety and efficacy of autologous BM-MSC transplantation in 10 patients with progressive MS. There were no major adverse events reported with a mean follow-up of 19 months. The preliminary report described varying results of EDSS and MRI progression. The authors pointed out the feasibility of MSC therapy to treat MS patients.

Subsequent studies have investigated the potential of MSC therapy in MS patients. These studies have preliminarily shown beneficial results and the safety of the procedure with no major adverse effects reported [76–78]. However, all studies had an open-label design, and varied in the source dose and administration route.

In 2010, a group of experts formed the International Mesenchymal Stem Cells Transplantation Study Group (IMSCTSG) in order to have a consensus protocol on the use of MSC for the treatment of MS [8]. The protocol established a phase I/II clinical trial to evaluate MS patients treated with autologous MSC who have not responded to at least one year of treatment with conventional immunomodulatory therapy. Patients are randomized to receive either IV infusion of autologous BM-MSC or suspension media. At 6 months, these treatments are switched between the two cohorts. The primary endpoints are to analyze the safety of MSC therapy in MS patients and to measure the reduction in the number and volume of new enhancing lesions over a 6-month period.

The IMSCTSG protocol has been adapted for use in multiple clinical trials with varying results. For example, Llufriu and colleagues completed a randomized placebo-controlled phase II trial with 9 RRMS patients who had failed conventional therapy [79]. At 6 months, patients treated with an IV infusion of BM-MSC had no statistical differences in clinical outcomes, brain MRI findings, and optical coherence tomography (OCT) measures. However, there was a trend towards a lower mean cumulative number of gadolinium-enhancing lesions on MRI. The authors concluded that BM-MSC are safe and may reduce inflammatory MRI parameters.

As mentioned previously, MSC may have a theoretical risk of malignant transformation. Therefore, recent studies have focused on investigating the feasibility of using autologous MSC-derived neuronal progenitors (MSC-NP) in lieu of BM-MSC to reduce pluripotency and to minimize the risk of ectopic differentiation after CNS transplantation [80,81]. A phase I open-label clinical trial showed that autologous IT transplantation of MSC-NP is safe and well tolerated. In addition, the authors reported an improved EDSS median in their cohort of 20 patients with progressive MS after treatment. Lastly, positive trends (e.g., muscle strength, bladder function) were more frequently observed in the subset of SPMS patients when compared to PPMS patients [82]. Other studies have shown similar results in the safety and efficacy of MSC-NP transplantation, demonstrating a potential therapeutic alternative [83]. However, further studies are needed to determine if transplantation of MSC-NP has better outcomes when compared to BM-MSC.

As noted above, MSC-CM has been investigated for its therapeutic potential in preclinical animal models. Recently, Danbour and colleagues assessed the safety and feasibility of IT treatment with BM-MSC followed by MSC-CM in patients with MS [84]. The study was conducted as an open-label prospective phase I/IIa clinical trial. No serious adverse effects were reported after the treatment. However, due to the small number and heterogeneity of enrolled patients, it was not possible to obtain statistically significant differences in the efficacy measurements (e.g., EDSS score, clinical, cognitive, ophthalmological, and radiological).

To date, cell therapy with MSC has been, overall, well tolerated and safe. Still, it is not known whether this treatment is capable of reducing inflammatory MS disease activity or promoting the regeneration of damaged areas in the CNS.

4. Other Stem Cells under Research

4.1. Neuronal Stem Cells (NSC)

In the last decade, there has been particular interest in utilizing NSC as a cellular therapy. Adult NSC are found mostly in two regions of the anterior brain: the subgranular zone (SGZ) within the hippocampal dentate gyrus and the subventricular zone (SVZ) lining the lateral ventricles [85,86]. NSC can give rise to neuronal progenitor cells (NPC) to produce neurons, astrocytes, and oligodendrocytes [87,88]. In EAE, NPC can be activated to migrate to inflammatory demyelinating tissue in the CNS, and differentiate into oligodendrocytes, thus having a potential for therapeutic benefits [10].

One major limitation is the limited number of endogenous NSC available to participate in repair mechanisms [89]. For this reason, therapeutic strategies in animal models are looking into the allogenic infusion of NSC. For example, IVT-transplanted NPC at the peak of EAE migrated exclusively into inflamed white matter and subsequently differentiated into oligodendrocytes; however, their direct implication in myelin repair remains unclear [90]. Additionally, other studies have demonstrated the presence of NPC in some chronically demyelinated lesions [91]. This finding suggests that the absence of NPC in pathological tissue is an unsatisfactory explanation for the clinical symptoms. An alternative proposition to explain this phenomenon is that the prevalent inflammatory setting in EAE produces a non-permissive environment for oligodendrocyte precursor cells (OPC) differentiation and function.

The current clinical trial using NPC comes from MSC-NP, as we previously described.

4.2. Human Embryonic Stem Cells (hESC)

hESC have been considered for cell therapy, owing to their capability to differentiate into all the germ layer derivatives. Specifically, the ability of hESC to differentiate into neural lineage has attracted scientific attention regarding the potential treatment of MS [92]. For example, transplanting hESC-derived neural progenitors into EAE mice led to diminished clinical symptoms. Histological studies revealed the presence of transplanted neural progenitors in mice brains, however, remyelination and the production of mature oligodendrocytes were not observed. The clinical improvement was hypothesized to result from immunosuppressive and neuroprotective mechanisms [12]. Further studies are required to better understand the mechanism of action of hESC in treating CNS demyelinating disease.

There have been a few published case reports using hESC to treat MS with limited data suggesting the safety of the therapy [93]. However, well-designed clinical trials are required to show the long-term efficacy and safety of hESC in the treatment of MS.

4.3. Induced Pluripotent Stem Cells (iPSC)

Lastly, iPSC are pluripotent cells that have been reprogrammed from somatic cells from skin and other tissues. These cells have the potential to become OPC, hence, they may constitute a suitable cellular therapy modality from an autologous source [94]. The therapeutic potential of iPSC is still under research, but some studies suggest that oligodendrocyte precursor-derived iPSC are capable of ameliorating the clinical and pathological features of EAE [95]. However, the therapeutic effect was found to be mostly due to a neuroprotective effect rather than remyelination. Moreover, the efficient differentiation of iPSC toward selected cell phenotypes could represent a great research challenge for directed disease therapy. Finally, recent studies suggest some caution for clinical development due to the potential for malignant transformation and immune rejection [96,97].

5. Conclusions

Immunoablative therapy followed by autologous hematopoietic stem cell transplantation should be considered in aggressive and treatment-refractory MS, since this treatment approach has shown increasing evidence of inducing long-term sustained remission and disability improvement. Further studies are needed to characterize which conditioning regimen should be used. On the other hand, MSC have emerged as a potentially powerful and safe cellular therapy for MS, but the dose, route of administration, and therapeutic effects need further exploration and quantification. Other novel forms of stem cell-based therapies for MS are, at this time, only in the early stages, including those based on hESC, iPSC, and NSC.

References

1. Frischer, J.M.; Steiner, J.P.; Dal-Bianco, A.; Dal-Bianco, A.; Lucchinetti, C.F.; Rauschka, H.; Schmidbauer, M.; Laursen, H.; Sorensen, P.S.; Lassmann, H. The relation between inflammation and neurodegeneration in multiple sclerosis brains. *Brain* **2009**, *132*, 1175–1189. [CrossRef] [PubMed]
2. Reingold, S.C.; Steiner, J.P.; Polman, C.H.; Cohen, J.A.; Freedman, M.S.; Kappos, L.; Thompson, A.J.; Wolinsky, J.S. The challenge of follow-on biologics for treatment of multiple sclerosis. *Neurology* **2009**, *73*, 552–559. [CrossRef] [PubMed]
3. Wingerchuk, D.M.; Carter, J.L. Multiple sclerosis: Current and emerging disease-modifying therapies and treatment strategies. *Mayo Clin. Proc.* **2014**, *89*, 225–240. [CrossRef] [PubMed]
4. Freedman, M.S.; Selchen, D.; Arnold, D.L.; Prat, A.; Banwell, B.; Yeung, M.; Morgenthau, D.; Lapierre, Y. Treatment optimization in MS: Canadian MS Working Group updated recommendations. *Can. J. Neurol. Sci.* **2013**, *40*, 307–323. [CrossRef] [PubMed]
5. Sormani, M.P.; Li, D.K.; Bruzzi, P.; Stubinski, B.; Cornelisse, P.; Rocak, S.; De Stefano, N. Combined MRI lesions and relapses as a surrogate for disability in multiple sclerosis. *Neurology* **2011**, *77*, 1684–1690. [CrossRef] [PubMed]
6. Stem Cells in MS. Available online: https://www.nationalmssociety.org/Research/Research-News-Progress/Stem-Cells-in-MS (accessed on 11 January 2019).
7. Delemarre, E.M.; van den Broek, T.; Mijnheer, G.; Meerding, J.; Wehrens, E.J.; Olek, S.; Boes, M.; van Herwijnen, M.J.; Broere, F.; van Royen, A.; et al. Autologous stem cell transplantation aids autoimmune patients by functional renewal and TCR diversification of regulatory T cells. *Blood* **2016**, *12*, 91–101. [CrossRef] [PubMed]
8. Freedman, M.S.; Bar-Or, A.; Atkins, H.L.; Karussis, D.; Frassoni, F.; Lazarus, H.; Scolding, N.; Slavin, S.; Le Blanc, K.; Uccelli, A.; et al. The therapeutic potential of mesenchymal stem cell transplantation as a treatment for multiple sclerosis: Consensus report of the International MSCT Study Group. *Mult. Scler.* **2010**, *16*, 503–510. [CrossRef] [PubMed]
9. Seo, J.H.; Cho, S.R. Neurorestoration induced by mesenchymal stem cells. *Yonsei Med. J.* **2012**, *53*, 1059–1067. [CrossRef] [PubMed]
10. Picard-Riera, N.; Decker, L.; Delarasse, C.; Goude, K.; Nait-Oumesmar, B.; Liblau, R.; Pham-Dinh, D.; Baron-Van Evercooren, A. Experimental autoimmune encephalomyelitis mobilizes neural progenitors from the subventricular zone to undergo oligodendrogenesis in adult mice. *Proc. Natl. Acad. Sci. USA* **2002**, *99*, 13211–13216. [CrossRef] [PubMed]
11. Thiruvalluvan, A.; Czepiel, M.; Kap, Y.A.; Mantingh-Otter, I.; Vainchtein, I.; Kuipers, J.; Bijlard, M.; Baron, W.; Giepmans, B.; Brück, W.; et al. Survival and functionality of human induced pluripotent stem cell-derived oligodendrocytes in a nonhuman primate model for multiple sclerosis. *Stem Cells Transl. Med.* **2016**, *5*, 1550–1561. [CrossRef] [PubMed]
12. Aharonowiz, M.; Einstein, O.; Fainstein, N.; Lassmann, H.; Reubinoff, B.; Ben-Hur, T. Neuroprotective effect of transplanted human embryonic stem cell-derived neural precursors in an animal model of multiple sclerosis. *PLoS ONE* **2008**, *3*, e3145. [CrossRef] [PubMed]
13. Fassas, A.; Anagnostopoulos, A.; Kazis, A.; Kapinas, K.; Sakellari, I.; Kimiskidis, V.; Tsompanakou, A. Peripheral blood stem cell transplantation in the treatment of progressive multiple sclerosis: First results of a pilot study. *Bone Marrow Transplant.* **1997**, *20*, 631–638. [CrossRef] [PubMed]

14. Snowden, J.A.; Patton, W.N.; O'Donnell, J.L.; Hannah, E.E.; Hart, D.N. Prolonged remission of longstanding systemic lupus erythematous after autologous bone marrow transplant for non-Hodgkin's lymphoma. *Bone Marrow Transplant.* **1997**, *19*, 1247–1250. [CrossRef] [PubMed]
15. Van Gelder, M.; van Bekkum, D.W. Treatment of relapsing experimental autoimmune encephalomyelitis in rats with allogeneic bone marrow transplantation from a resistant strain. *Bone Marrow Transplant.* **1995**, *16*, 343–351. [PubMed]
16. Van Gelder, M.; Kinwel-Bohre, E.P.; van Bekkum, D.W. Treatment of experimental allergic encephalomyelitis in rats with total body irradiation and syngeneic BMT. *Bone Marrow Transplant.* **1993**, *11*, 233–241. [PubMed]
17. Van Gelder, M.; van Bekkum, D.W. Effective treatment of relapsing experimental autoimmune encephalomyelitis with pseudoautologous bone marrow transplantation. *Bone Marrow Transplant.* **1996**, *18*, 1029–1034. [PubMed]
18. Muraro, P.A.; Douek, D.C.; Packer, A.; Chung, K.; Guenaga, F.J.; Cassiani-Ingoni, R.; Campbell, C.; Memon, S.; Nagle, J.W.; Hakim, F.T.; et al. Thymic output generates a new and diverse TCR repertoire after autologous stem cell transplantation in multiple sclerosis patients. *J. Exp. Med.* **2005**, *201*, 805–816. [CrossRef] [PubMed]
19. Muraro, P.A.; Robins, H.; Malhotra, S.; Howell, M.; Phippard, D.; Desmarais, C.; de Paula Alves Sousa, A.; Griffith, L.M.; Lim, N.; Nash, R.A.; et al. T cell repertoire following autologous stem cell transplantation for multiple sclerosis. *J. Clin. Investig.* **2014**, *124*, 1168–1172. [CrossRef] [PubMed]
20. Glastone, D.E.; Peyster, R.; Baron, E.; Friedman-Urevich, S.; Sibony, P.; Melville, P.; Gottesman, M. High-dose cyclophosphamide for moderate to severe refractory multiple sclerosis. *Am. J. Ther.* **2011**, *18*, 23–30. [CrossRef] [PubMed]
21. Krishnan, C.; Kaplin, A.I.; Brodsky, R.A.; Drachman, D.B.; Jones, R.J.; Pham, D.L.; Richert, N.D.; Pardo, C.A.; Yousem, D.M.; Hammond, E.; et al. Reduction of disease activity and disability with high-dose cyclophosphamide in patients with aggressive multiple sclerosis. *Arch. Neurol.* **2008**, *65*, 1044–1051. [CrossRef] [PubMed]
22. Harrinson, D.M.; Gladstone, D.E.; Hammond, E.; Cheng, J.; Jones, R.J.; Brodsky, R.A.; Kerr, D.; McArthur, J.C.; Kaplin, A. Treatment of relapsing-remitting multiple sclerosis with high-dose cyclophosphamide infusion followed by glatimer acetate maintenance. *Mult. Scler. J.* **2012**, *18*, 202–209. [CrossRef] [PubMed]
23. Saccardi, R.; Freedman, M.S.; Sormani, M.P.; Atkins, H.; Farge, D.; Griffith, L.M.; Kraft, G.; Mancardi, G.L.; Nash, R.; Pasquini, M.; et al. A prospective, randomized, controlled trial of autologous haematopoietic stem cell transplantation for aggressive multiple sclerosis: A position paper. *Mult Scler. J.* **2012**, *18*, 825–834. [CrossRef]
24. Mancardi, G.; Saccardi, R. Autologous haematopoietic stem-cell transplantation in multiple sclerosis. *Lancet Neurol.* **2008**, *7*, 626–636. [CrossRef]
25. Openshaw, H.; Stuve, O.; Antel, J.P.; Nash, R.; Lund, B.T.; Weiner, L.P.; Kashyap, A.; McSweeney, P.; Forman, S. Multiple sclerosis flares associated with recombinant granulocyte colony-stimulating factor. *Neurology* **2000**, *54*, 2147–2150. [CrossRef]
26. Snowden, J.A.; Saccardi, R.; Allez, M.; Ardizzone, S.; Arnold, R.; Cervera, R.; Denton, C.; Hawkey, C.; Labopin, M.; Mancardi, G.; et al. Haematopoietic SCT in severe autoimmune diseases: Updated guidelines of the European Group for Blood and Marrow Transplantation. *Bone Marrow Transplant.* **2012**, *47*, 770–790. [CrossRef]
27. Saiz, A.; Blanco, Y.; Berenguer, J.; Gómez-Choco, M.; Carreras, E.; Arbizu, T.; Graus, F. Clinical outcome 6 years after autologous hematopoietic stem cell transplantation in multiple sclerosis. *Neurologia* **2008**, *23*, 405–407. [PubMed]
28. Shevchenko, J.; Kuznestsov, A.N.; Ionova, T.I.; Melnichenko, V.Y.; Fedorenko, D.A.; Kurbatova, K.A.; Gorodokin, G.I.; Novik, A.A. Long-term outcomes of autologous hematopoietic stem cell transplantation with reduced-intensity conditioning in multiple sclerosis: physician's and patient's perspectives. *Ann. Hematol.* **2015**, *94*, 1149–1157. [CrossRef] [PubMed]
29. Bacigalupo, A.; Ballen, K.; Giralt, S.; Lazarus, H.; Ho, V.; Apperley, J.; Slavin, S.; Pasquini, M.; Sandmaier, B.M.; Barrett, J.; et al. Defining the intensity of conditioning regimens: Working definitions. *Biol. Blood Marrow Transplant.* **2009**, *15*, 1628–1633. [CrossRef] [PubMed]

30. Gratwohl, A.; Passweg, J.; Bocelli-Tyndall, C.; Fassas, A.; van Laar, J.M.; Farge, D.; Andolina, M.; Arnold, R.; Carreras, E.; Finke, J.; et al. Autologous hematopoietic stem cell transplantation for autoimmune diseases. *Bone Marrow Transplant.* **2005**, *35*, 869–879. [CrossRef]
31. Saccardi, R.; Kozak, T.; Bocelli-Tyndall, C.; Fassas, A.; Kazis, A.; Havrdova, E.; Carreras, E.; Saiz, A.; Löwenberg, B.; te Boekhorst, P.A.; et al. Autologous stem cell transplantation for progressive multiple sclerosis: Update of the European Group for Blood and Marrow Transplantation autoimmune diseases working party database. *Mult. Scler. J.* **2006**, *12*, 814–823. [CrossRef] [PubMed]
32. Samjin, J.P.; te Boekhorst, P.A.; Mondria, T.; van Doorn, P.A.; Flach, H.Z.; van der Meché, F.G.A.; Cornelissen, J.; Hop, W.C.; Löwenberg, B.; Hintzen, R.Q. Intense T cell depletion followed by autologous bone marrow transplantation for severe multiple sclerosis. *J. Neurol. Neurosurg. Psychiatry* **2006**, *77*, 46–50. [CrossRef] [PubMed]
33. Nash, R.A.; Dansey, R.; Storek, J.; Georges, G.E.; Bowen, J.D.; Holmberg, L.A.; Kraft, G.H.; Mayes, M.D.; McDonagh, K.T.; Chen, C.S.; et al. Epstein-Barr virus-associated posttransplantation lymphoproliferative disorder after high-dose immunosuppressive therapy and autologous CD34-selected hematopoietic stem cell transplantation for severe autoimmune diseases. *Biol. Blood Marrow Transplant.* **2003**, *9*, 583–591. [CrossRef]
34. Mancardi, G.L.; Sormani, M.P.; Di Gioia, M.; Vuolo, L.; Gualandi, F.; Amato, M.P.; Capello, E.; Currò, D.; Uccelli, A.; Bertolotto, A.; et al. Autologous haematopoietic stem cell transplantation with an intermediate intensity conditioning regimen in multiple sclerosis: The Italian multi-centre experience. *Mult. Scler. J.* **2012**, *18*, 835–842. [CrossRef] [PubMed]
35. Curro', D.; Vuolo, L.; Gualandi, F.; Bacigalupo, A.; Roccatagliata, L.; Capello, E.; Uccelli, A.; Saccardi, R.; Mancardi, G. Low intensity lympho-ablative regimen followed by autologous hematopoietic stem cell transplantation in severe forms of multiple sclerosis: A MRI-based clinical study. *Mult. Scler. J.* **2015**, *11*, 1423–1430. [CrossRef] [PubMed]
36. Burt, R.K.; Loh, Y.; Cohen, B.; Stefoski, D.; Balabanov, R.; Katsamakis, G.; Oyama, Y.; Russell, E.J.; Stern, J.; Muraro, P.; et al. Autologous non-myeloablative haemopoeitic stem cell transplantation in relapsing-remitting multiple sclerosis: A phase I/II study. *Lancet Neurol.* **2009**, *201*, 805–816. [CrossRef]
37. Hammerschlak, N.; Rodrigues, M.; Moraes, D.A.; Oliveira, M.C.; Stracieri, A.B.; Pieroni, F.; Barros, G.M.; Madeira, M.I.; Simões, B.P.; Barreira, A.A.; et al. Brazilian experience with two conditioning regimens in patients with multiple sclerosis: BEAM/horse ATG and CY/rabbit ATG. *Bone Marrow Transplant.* **2006**, *45*, 239–248. [CrossRef] [PubMed]
38. Muraro, P.A.; Martin, R.; Mancardi, G.L.; Nicholas, R.; Sormani, M.P.; Saccardi, R. Autologous haematopoietic stem cell transplantation for treatment of multiple sclerosis. *Nat. Rev. Neurol.* **2017**, *13*, 391–405. [CrossRef] [PubMed]
39. Arruda, L.C.; de Azevedo, J.T.; de Oliveira, G.L.V.; Scortegagna, G.T.; Rogrigues, E.S.; Palma, P.V.B.; Brum, D.G.; Guerreiro, C.T.; Marques, V.D.; Barreira, A.A.; et al. Immunological correlates of favorable long-term clinical outcome in multiple sclerosis patients after autologous hematopoietic stem cell transplantation. *Clin. Immunol.* **2016**, *169*, 47–57. [CrossRef] [PubMed]
40. Fassas, A.; Kazis, A. High-dose immunosuppression and autologous hematopoietic stem cell rescue for severe multiple sclerosis. *J. Hematother. Stem Cell Res.* **2003**, *12*, 701–711. [CrossRef]
41. Sun, W.; Uday, P.; Hutton, G.J.; Zang, Y.C.; Krance, R.; Carrum, G.; Land, G.A.; Heslop, H.; Brenner, M.; Zhang, J.Z. Characteristics of T-cell receptor repertoire and myelin-reactive T cells reconstituted from autologous haematopoietic stem-cell grafts in multiple sclerosis. *Brain* **2004**, *127*, 996–1008. [CrossRef] [PubMed]
42. Darlington, P.J.; Touil, T.; Doucet, J.S.; Gaucher, D.; Zeidan, J.; Gauchat, D.; Corsini, R.; Kim, H.J.; Duddy, M.; Jalili, F.; et al. Diminished Th17 (not Th1) responses underlie multiple sclerosis disease abrogation after hematopoietic stem cell transplantation. *Ann. Neurol.* **2013**, *73*, 341–354. [CrossRef]
43. Gosselin, D.; Rivest, S. Immune mechanisms underlying the beneficial effects of autologous hematopoietic stem cell transplantation in multiple sclerosis. *Neurotherapeutics* **2011**, *8*, 643–649. [CrossRef]
44. Bowen, J.D.; Kraft, G.H.; Wundes, A.; Guan, Q.; Maravilla, K.R.; Gooley, T.A.; McSweeney, P.A.; Pavletic, S.Z.; Openshaw, H.; Storb, R.; et al. Autologous hematopoietic cell transplantation following high-dose immunosuppressive therapy for advanced multiple sclerosis: Long-term results. *Bone Marrow Transplant.* **2012**, *47*, 946–951. [CrossRef] [PubMed]

45. Muraro, P.A.; Pasquini, M.; Atkins, H.L.; Bowen, J.D.; Farge, D.; Fassas, D.; Freedman, M.S.; Georges, G.E.; Gualandi, F.; Hamerschlak, N.; et al. Long-term outcomes after autologous hematopoietic stem cell transplantation for multiple sclerosis. *JAMA Neurol.* **2017**, *74*, 459–469. [CrossRef] [PubMed]
46. Krasulová, E.; Trneny, M.; Kozak, T.; Vacková, B.; Pohlreich, D.; Kemlink, D.; Kobylka, P.; Kovárová, I.; Lhtáková, P.; Havrdov, E. High-dose immunoablation with autologous haematopoietic stem cell transplantation in aggressive multiple sclerosis: A single centre 10-year experience. *Mult. Scler. J.* **2010**, *16*, 685–693. [CrossRef]
47. Fassas, A.; Kimiskidis, V.K.; Sakellari, I.; Kapinas, K.; Anagnostopoulos, A.; Tsimourtou, V.; Kazis, A. Long-term results of stem transplantation for MS: A single-center experience. *Neurology* **2011**, *76*, 1066–1070. [CrossRef] [PubMed]
48. Cassanova, B.; Jarque, I.; Gascón, F.; Hernández-Boluda, J.C.; Pérez-Miralles, F.; de la Rubia, J.; Alcalá, C.; Sanz, J.; Mallada, J.; Cervelló, A.; et al. Autologous hematopoietic stem cell transplantation in relapsing-remitting multiple sclerosis: Comparison with secondary progressive multiple sclerosis. *Neurol. Sci.* **2017**, *38*, 1213–1221. [CrossRef] [PubMed]
49. Nash, R.A.; Hutton, G.J.; Racke, M.K.; Popat, U.; Devine, S.M.; Steinmiller, K.C.; Griffith, L.M.; Muraro, P.A.; Openshaw, H.; Sayre, P.H.; et al. High-dose immunosuppressive therapy and autologous HCT for relapsing-remitting MS. *Neurology* **2017**, *88*, 842–852. [CrossRef] [PubMed]
50. Nash, R.A.; Hutton, G.J.; Racke, M.K.; Popat, U.; Devine, S.M.; Griffith, L.M.; Muraro, P.A.; Openshaw, H.; Sayre, P.H.; Stüve, O.; et al. High-dose immunosuppressive therapy and autologous hematopoietic cell transplantation for relapsing-remitting multiple sclerosis (HALT-MS): A 3-year interim report. *JAMA Neurol.* **2015**, *72*, 159–169. [CrossRef] [PubMed]
51. Atkins, H.L.; Bowman, M.; Allan, D.; Anstee, G.; Arnold, D.L.; Bar-Or, A.; Bence-Bruckler, I.; Birch, P.; Bredeson, C.; Chen, J.; et al. Immunoablation and autologous haemopoietic stem-cell transplantation for aggressive multiple sclerosis: A multicentre single-group phase 2 trial. *Lancet* **2016**, *388*, 576–585. [CrossRef]
52. Burt, R.K.; Balabanov, R.; Sharrack, B.; Morgan, A.; Quigley, K.; Yaung, K.; Helenowski, I.B.; Jovanovic, B.; Spahovic, D.; Arnautovic, I.; et al. Association of nonmyeloablative hematopoietic stem cell transplantation with neurological disability in patients with relapsing-remitting multiple sclerosis. *JAMA* **2015**, *313*, 275–284. [CrossRef] [PubMed]
53. Sormani, M.P.; Muraro, P.; Schiavetti, I.; Signori, A.; Laroni, A.; Saccardi, R.; Mancardi, G.L. Autologous hematopoietic stem cell transplantation in multiple sclerosis: A meta-analysis. *Neurology* **2017**, *13*, 391–405. [CrossRef] [PubMed]
54. Uccelli, A.; Laroni, A.; Freedman, M.S. Mesenchymal stem cells for the treatment of multiple sclerosis and other neurological diseases. *Lancet Neurol.* **2011**, *10*, 649–656. [CrossRef]
55. Rice, C.M.; Kemp, K.; Wilkins, A.; Scolding, N.J. Cell therapy for multiple sclerosis: An evolving concept with implications for other neurodegenerative diseases. *Lancet* **2013**, *382*, 1204–1213. [CrossRef]
56. Pittenger, M.F.; Mackay, A.M.; Beck, S.C.; Jaiswal, R.K.; Douglas, R.; Mosca, J.D.; Moorman, M.A.; Simonetti, D.W.; Craig, S.; Marshak, D.R. Multilineage potential of adult human mesenchymal stem cells. *Science* **1999**, *284*, 143–147. [CrossRef] [PubMed]
57. Zhang, X.; Bowles, A.C.; Semon, J.A.; Scruggs, B.A.; Zhang, S.; Strong, A.L.; Gimble, J.M.; Bunnell, B.A. Transplantation of autologous adipose stem cells lacks therapeutic efficacy in the experimental autoimmune encephalomyelitis model. *PLoS ONE* **2014**, *9*, e85007. [CrossRef] [PubMed]
58. Li, D.; Chai, J.; Shen, C.; Han, Y.; Sun, T. Human umbilical cord-derived mesenchymal stem cells differentiate into epidermal-like cells using a novel co-culture technique. *Cytotechnology* **2014**, *66*, 699–708. [CrossRef]
59. Bai, L.; Lennon, D.P.; Maier, K.; Caplan, A.L.; Miller, S.D.; Miller, R.H. Human bone marrow-derived mesenchymal stem cells induce Th2 polarized immune response and promote endogenous repair in animal models of multiple sclerosis. *Glia* **2009**, *57*, 1192–1203. [CrossRef] [PubMed]
60. Zappia, E.; Casazza, S.; Pedemonte, E.; Benvenuto, F.; Bonanni, I.; Gerdoni, E.; Giunti, D.; Ceravolo, A.; Cazzanti, F.; Frassnoni, F.; et al. Mesenchymal stem cells ameliorate experimental autoimmune encephalomyelitis inducing T-cell anergy. *Blood* **2005**, *106*, 1755–1761. [CrossRef] [PubMed]
61. Zhang, J.; Li, Y.; Chen, Y.; Cui, Y.; Lu, M.; Elias, S.B.; Mitchell, J.B.; Hammill, L.; Vanguri, P.; Chopp, M. Human bone marrow stromal cell treatment improves neurological functional recovery in EAE mice. *Exp. Neurol.* **2005**, *195*, 16–26. [CrossRef] [PubMed]

62. Gerdoni, E.; Gallo, B.; Casazza, S.; Musio, S.; Bonanni, I.; Pedemonte, E.; Mantegazza, R.; Frassoni, F.; Mancardi, G.; Pedotti, R.; et al. Mesenchymal stem cells effectively modulate pathogenic immune response in experimental autoimmune encephalomyelitis. *Ann. Neurol.* **2007**, *61*, 219–227. [CrossRef] [PubMed]
63. Kemp, K.; Hares, K.; Mallam, E.; Heesom, K.J.; Scolding, N.; Wilkins, A. Mesenchymal stem cell-secreted superoxide dismutase promotes cerebellar neuronal survival. *J. Neurochem.* **2010**, *114*, 1569–1580. [CrossRef] [PubMed]
64. Wilkins, A.; Kemp, K.; Ginty, M.; Hares, K.; Mallam, E.; Scolding, N. Human bone marrow derived mesenchymal stem cells secrete brain-derived neurotrophic factor which promotes neuronal survival in vitro. *Stem Cell Res.* **2009**, *3*, 63–70. [CrossRef] [PubMed]
65. Krishnamoorthy, G.; Wekerle, H. EAE: An immunologist's magic eye. *Eur. Immunol.* **2009**, *39*, 2031–2035. [CrossRef] [PubMed]
66. Gordon, D.; Pavlovska, G.; Glover, C.P.; Uney, J.B.; Wraith, D.; Scolding, N.J. Human mesenchymal stem cells abrogate experimental allergic encephalomyelitis after intraperitoneal injection, and with sparse CNS infiltration. *Neurosci. Lett.* **2008**, *448*, 71–73. [CrossRef] [PubMed]
67. Kassis, I.; Grigoriadis, N.; Gowda-Kurkalli, B.; Mizrachi-Kol, R.; Ben-Hur, T.; Slavin, S.; Abramsky, O.; Karussis, D. Neuroprotection and immunomodulation with mesenchymal stem cells in chronic experimental autoimmune encephalitis. *Arch. Neurol.* **2008**, *65*, 753–761. [CrossRef] [PubMed]
68. Bai, L.; Lennon, D.P.; Caplan, A.I.; DeChant, A.; Hecker, J.; Kranso, J.; Zaremba, A.; Miller, R.H. Hepatocyte growth factor mediates mesenchymal stem cell-induced recovery in multiple sclerosis models. *Nat. Neurosci.* **2012**, *15*, 862–870. [CrossRef] [PubMed]
69. Karussis, D.; Kassis, I. Use of stem cells for the treatment of multiple sclerosis. *Expert Rev. Neurother.* **2007**, *7*, 1189–1201. [CrossRef] [PubMed]
70. Rivera, F.J.; Couillard-Despres, D.; Pedre, X.; Ploetz, S.; Caioni, M.; Lois, C.; Bogdahn, U.; Aigner, L. Mesenchymal stem cells instruct oligodendrogenic fate decision on adult neural stem cells. *Stem Cells* **2006**, *24*, 2209–2219. [CrossRef] [PubMed]
71. Glenn, J.D.; Smith, M.D.; Calabresi, P.A.; Whartenby, K.A. Mesenchymal stem cells differentially modulate effector CD8+ T cell subsets and exacerbate experimental autoimmune encephalomyelitis. *Stem Cells* **2014**, *32*, 2744–2755. [CrossRef]
72. Grigoriadis, N.; Lourbopoulos, A.; Lagoudaki, R.; Frischer, J.M.; Polyzoidou, E.; Touloumi, O.; Simeonidou, C.; Deretzi, G.; Kountouras, J.; Spandou, E. Variable behavior and complications of autologous bone marrow mesenchymal stem cells transplanted in experimental autoimmune encephalomyelitis. *Exp. Neurol.* **2011**, *230*, 78–89. [CrossRef] [PubMed]
73. von Bahr, L.; Batsis, I.; Moll, G.; Häqq, M.; Szakos, A.; Sunberg, B.; Uzunel, M.; Ringden, O.; Le Blanc, K. Analysis of tissues following mesenchymal stromal cell therapy in humans indicate limited long-term engraftment and no ectopic tissue formation. *Stem Cells* **2012**, *30*, 557–564. [CrossRef] [PubMed]
74. Riordan, N.H.; Ichim, T.E.; Min, W.P.; Wang, H.; Solano, F.; Lara, F.; Alfaro, M.; Rodriguez, J.P.; Harman, R.J.; Patel, A.N.; et al. Non-expanded adipose stromal vascular fraction cell therapy for multiple sclerosis. *J. Transl. Med.* **2009**, *7*, 29. [CrossRef] [PubMed]
75. Mohyeddin Bonab, M.; Yazdanbakhsh, S.; Loftfi, J.; Alimoghaddom, K.; Talebian, F.; Hooshmand, F.; Ghavamzadeh, A.; Nikbin, B. Does mesenchymal stem cell therapy help multiple sclerosis patients? Report of a pilot study. *Iran. J. Immunol.* **2007**, *4*, 50–57.
76. Karussis, D.; Karageorgiou, C.; Vaknin-Dembinsky, A.; Gowda-Kurkalli, B.; Gomori, J.M.; Kassis, I.; Bulte, J.W.; Petrou, P.; Ben-Hur, T.; Abramsky, O.; et al. Safety and immunological effects of mesenchymal stem cell transplantation in patients with multiple sclerosis and amyotrophic lateral sclerosis. *Arch. Neurol.* **2010**, *67*, 1187–1194. [CrossRef] [PubMed]
77. Yamout, B.; Hourani, R.; Salti, H.; Barada, W.; El-Hajj, T.; Al-Kutoubi, A.; Herlopian, A.; Baz, E.K.; Mahfouz, R.; Khalil-Hamdan, R.; et al. Bone marrow mesenchymal stem cell transplantation in patients with multiple sclerosis: A pilot study. *J. Neuroimmunol.* **2010**, *227*, 185–189. [CrossRef] [PubMed]
78. Bonab, M.M.; Sahraian, M.A.; Aghsaie, A.; Karvigh, S.A.; Hosseinian, S.M.; Nikbin, B.; Lotfi, J.; Khorramnia, S.; Motamed, M.R.; Togha, M.; et al. Autologous mesenchymal stem cell therapy in progressive multiple sclerosis: An open label study. *Curr. Stem Cell Res. Ther.* **2012**, *7*, 407–414. [CrossRef] [PubMed]

79. Llufriu, S.; Sepulveda, M.; Blanco, Y.; Marín, P.; Moreno, B.; Berenguer, J.; Gabilondo, I.; Martínez-Heras, E.; Sola-Valls, N.; Arnaiz, J.A.; et al. Randomized placebo-controlled phase II trial of autologous mesenchymal stem cells in multiple sclerosis. *PLoS ONE* **2014**, *9*, e113936. [CrossRef] [PubMed]
80. Harris, V.K.; Yan, Q.J.; Vyshkina, T.; Sahabi, S.; Liu, X.; Sadiq, S.A. Clinical and pathological effects of intrathecal injection of mesenchymal stem cell-derived neural progenitors in an experimental model of multiple sclerosis. *J. Neurol. Sci.* **2012**, *313*, 167–177. [CrossRef]
81. Harris, V.K.; Faroqui, R.; Vyshkina, T.; Sadiq, S.A. Characterization of autologous mesenchymal stem cell-derived neural progenitors as a feasible source of stem cells for central nervous system applications in multiple sclerosis. *Stem Cells Transl. Med.* **2012**, *1*, 536–547. [CrossRef] [PubMed]
82. Harris, V.K.; Stark, J.; Vyshkina, T.; Blackshear, L.; Joo, G.; Stefanova, V.; Sara, G.; Sadiq, S.A. Phase I trial of intrathecal mesenchymal stem cell-derived neural progenitors in progressive multiple sclerosis. *eBioMedicine* **2018**, *29*, 23–30. [CrossRef] [PubMed]
83. Harris, V.K.; Vyshkina, T.; Sadiq, S.A. Clinical safety of intrathecal administration of mesenchymal stromal cell-derived neural progenitors in multiple sclerosis. *Cytotherapy* **2016**, *18*, 1476–1482. [CrossRef] [PubMed]
84. Dahbour, S.; Jamali, F.; Alhattab, D.; Al-Radaideh, A.; Ababneh, O.; Al-Ryalat, N.; Al-Bdour, M.; Hourani, B.; Msallam, M.; Rasheed, M.; et al. Mesenchymal stem cells and conditioned media in the treatment of multiple sclerosis patients: Clinical, ophthalmological and radiological assessments of safety and efficacy. *CNS Neurosci. Ther.* **2017**, *2*, 866–874. [CrossRef] [PubMed]
85. Weiss, S.; Dunne, C.; Hewson, J.; Wohl, C.; Wheatley, M.; Peterson, A.C.; Reynolds, B.A. Multipotent CNS stem cells are present in the adult mammalian spinal cord and ventricular neuroaxis. *J. Neurosci.* **1996**, *16*, 7599–7609. [CrossRef]
86. Morshead, C.M.; Reynolds, B.A.; Craig, C.G.; McBurney, M.W.; Staines, W.A.; Morassutti, D.; Weiss, S.; van der Koou, D. Neural stem cells in the adult mammalian forebrain: A relatively quiescent subpopulation of subependymal cells. *Neuron* **1994**, *13*, 1071–1082. [CrossRef]
87. Ming, G.L.; Song, H. Adult Neurogenesis in the Mammalian Brain: Significant Answers and Significant Questions. *Neuron* **2012**, *70*, 687–702. [CrossRef] [PubMed]
88. Bakemore, W.F.; Hans, S.K. The origin of remyelinating cells in the central nervous system. *J. Neuroimm.* **1999**, *98*, 69–76. [CrossRef]
89. Armstrong, R.C.; Le, Q.T.; Flint, N.C.; Vana, A.C.; Zhou, Y.X. Endogenous cell repair of chronic demyelination. *J. Neuropathol. Exp. Neurol.* **2006**, *65*, 245–256. [CrossRef] [PubMed]
90. Ben-Hur, T.; Einstein, O.; Mizrachi-Kol, R.; Ben-Menachem, O.; Reinhartz, E.; Karussis, D.; Abramsky, O. Transplanted multipotential neural precursor cells migrate into the inflamed white matter in response to experimental autoimmune encephalomyelitis. *Glia* **2003**, *41*, 73–80. [CrossRef] [PubMed]
91. Chang, A.; Tourtellotte, W.W.; Rudick, R.A.; Trapp, B.D. Premyelinating oligodendrocytes in chronic lesions of multiple sclerosis. *N. Engl. J. Med.* **2002**, *346*, 165–173. [CrossRef]
92. Izrael, M.; Zhang, P.; Kaufman, R.; Shinder, V.; Ella, R.; Amit, M.; Itskovitz-Eldor, J.; Chebath, J.; Revel, M. Human oligodendrocytes derived from embryonic stem cells: Effect of noggin on phenotypic differentiation in vitro and on myelination in vivo. *Mol. Cell Neurosci.* **2007**, *34*, 310–323. [CrossRef] [PubMed]
93. Shroff, G. Human embryonic stem cells for the treatment of multiple sclerosis: A case report. *Case Rep. Int.* **2015**, *4*, 38–42. [CrossRef]
94. Czepiel, M.; Balasubramaniyan, V.; Schaafsma, W.; Stancic, M.; Mikkers, H.; Hiusman, C.; Boddeke, E.; Copray, S. Differentiation of induced pluripotent stem cells into functional oligodendrocytes. *Glia* **2011**, *59*, 882–892. [CrossRef] [PubMed]
95. Laterza, C.; Merlini, A.; De Feo, D.; Ruffini, F.; Menon, R.; Onorati, M.; Fredickx, E.; Muzio, L.; Lombardo, A.; Comi, G.; et al. iPSC-derived neural precursors exert a neuroprotective role in immune-mediated demyelination via the secretion of LIF. *Nat. Commun.* **2013**, *4*, 2597. [CrossRef] [PubMed]
96. Zhao, T.; Zhang, Z.N.; Rong, Z.; Xu, Y. Immunogenicity of induced pluripotent stem cells. *Nature* **2011**, *474*, 212–215. [CrossRef] [PubMed]
97. Okano, H.; Nakamura, M.; Yoshida, K.; Okada, Y.; Tsuji, O.; Nori, S.; Ikeda, E.; Yamanaka, S.; Miura, K. Steps toward safe cell therapy using induced pluripotent stem cells. *Circ. Res.* **2013**, *112*, 523–533. [CrossRef] [PubMed]

8

Recent Advances in Antigen-Specific Immunotherapies for the Treatment of Multiple Sclerosis

Olga Kammona [1] and Costas Kiparissides [1,2,*]

1 Chemical Process and Energy Resources Institute, Centre for Research and Technology Hellas, P.O. Box 60361, 57001 Thessaloniki, Greece; kammona@cperi.certh.gr
2 Department of Chemical Engineering, Aristotle University of Thessaloniki, 54124 Thessaloniki, Greece
* Correspondence: costas.lpre@cperi.certh.gr

Abstract: Multiple sclerosis (MS) is an autoimmune disease of the central nervous system and is considered to be the leading non-traumatic cause of neurological disability in young adults. Current treatments for MS comprise long-term immunosuppressant drugs and disease-modifying therapies (DMTs) designed to alter its progress with the enhanced risk of severe side effects. The Holy Grail for the treatment of MS is to specifically suppress the disease while at the same time allow the immune system to be functionally active against infectious diseases and malignancy. This could be achieved via the development of immunotherapies designed to specifically suppress immune responses to self-antigens (e.g., myelin antigens). The present study attempts to highlight the various antigen-specific immunotherapies developed so far for the treatment of multiple sclerosis (e.g., vaccination with myelin-derived peptides/proteins, plasmid DNA encoding myelin epitopes, tolerogenic dendritic cells pulsed with encephalitogenic epitopes of myelin proteins, attenuated autologous T cells specific for myelin antigens, T cell receptor peptides, carriers loaded/conjugated with myelin immunodominant peptides, etc.), focusing on the outcome of their recent preclinical and clinical evaluation, and to shed light on the mechanisms involved in the immunopathogenesis and treatment of multiple sclerosis.

Keywords: multiple sclerosis; autoimmune diseases; antigen-specific immunotherapies; tolerogenic vaccines; tolerance induction; central nervous system; myelin peptides; myelin basic protei; proteolipid protein; myelin oligodendrocyte glycoprotein

---

1. Introduction

Multiple sclerosis (MS) is a chronic inflammatory disease of the central nervous system (CNS) caused by genetically-predisposed hosts by infectious and environmental factors which induce complex autoimmune responses in the CNS resulting in degeneration of the myelin sheath and axonal loss in the brain and spinal cord [1–14] It is the most prominent demyelinating disease leading to progressive clinical disability in MS patients [5,6,15] due to ineffective remyelination [13,15]. More than 2 million people worldwide suffer from MS and it is considered as the leading non-traumatic cause of neurological disability in young adults with a disease onset commonly around 20 and 40 years of age [4,6,15,16]. High prevalence of the disease is reported in North America and Europe [15].

MS exhibits a vastly heterogeneous clinical course [6,17] which varies from a benign disease course that doesn't lead to serious disability, demonstrated by 10–15% of MS patients, to aggressive forms of the disease leading to severe disability and even paralysis. The increased heterogeneity of the disease severity strongly affects the design and duration of therapeutic schemes administered to MS patients [17].

MS features the following stages: a pre-clinical stage, namely, a radiologically-isolated syndrome (RIS), which is then demonstrated as a clinically-isolated syndrome (CIS) [2,3], followed by a relapsing remitting stage (RRMS) which may later advance into secondary progressive disease (SPMS) [2,4,6,16,18]. It should be noted that a minority of MS patients (e.g., 10–15% [3,6,16]) exhibit progressive MS from the disease onset, known as primary progressive MS (PPMS) [2,4,6,18] (Figure 1). The aforementioned classification corresponds to the inflammatory image of MS which can be detected via magnetic resonance imaging (MRI) [2,16].

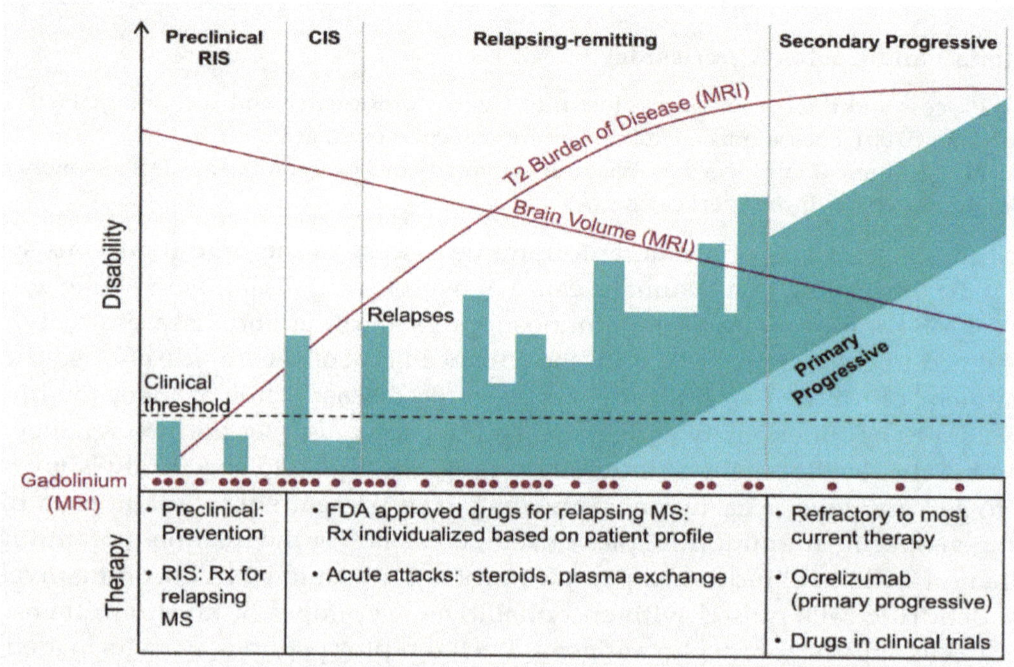

Figure 1. Stages of multiple sclerosis (MS). RIS: radiologically isolated syndrome; CIS: clinically isolated syndrome; FDA: U.S. food and drug administration (with the permission of [2]).

RRMS affects approximately 85% of MS patients [3,6,19] of whom women are twice as many as men [6]. It is characterized by periods of relapses (i.e., episodes of neurologic dysfunction, such as sensory disturbances, optic neuritis, or disturbances of motor/cerebellar function) followed by remission periods (i.e., periods of partial or full clinical recovery) [2,3,6,14,16]. Relapses coincide with CNS inflammation/demyelination visualized by MRI as lesions found mainly in the white matter [3]. In the majority of patients, RRMS advances to SPMS [16] within 10–20 years after diagnosis [3,6].

RRMS involves the movement of immune cells from the peripheral sites to the CNS (mainly in the white matter, even though extensive number of demyelinated plaques can be located in the grey matter [20]) resulting in the formation of localized inflammatory sites. Inflammatory processes in these sites induce killing of oligodendrocytes, myelin damage, and axon injury and loss, resulting in impaired neurological function [20]. On the other hand, the progressive disease implicates the generation of a pathological process within the brain [2]. Thus, the characteristic feature of SPMS is no longer the inflammatory lesions but an atrophic brain attributed to enhanced loss of axons, cortical demyelination, activation of microglia, and inefficient remyelination [2,3]. SPMS patients demonstrate progressive neurological dysfunction resulting in enhanced physical disability (e.g., inability to walk) [2,3].

PPMS is also characterized by gradual neurological decline without relapses [3,6]. In comparison with RRMS, the disease onset for PPMS is usually ten years later and it does not exhibit female predominance [6]. To date, clinical evidence shows significant differences between RRMS and progressive MS [21], reflected by the diverse response to currently existing treatments, but not between SPMS and PPMS. [18].

Currently, there is no cure for MS. Some existing treatments appear to be beneficial for patients with RRMS. However, there is still a lack of effective therapies for the progressive forms of MS [2].

The present paper aims to extensively review the different, recently developed myelin antigen-specific strategies (e.g., myelin peptide based vaccination, vaccination with plasmid DNA encoding myelin epitopes, tolerogenic dendritic cells pulsed with encephalitogenic epitopes of myelin proteins, vaccination with attenuated autologous T cells specific for myelin antigens, T cell receptor vaccination, carrier-aided administration of myelin immunodominant peptides, etc.) for the prevention/treatment of MS, especially with respect to their in vivo and clinical evaluation outcomes and the challenges they face in order to be translated to MS patients. It also seeks to unravel the mechanisms involved in the immunopathogenesis of the relapsing remitting and progressive MS, as well as the mechanisms of action of the developed tolerance-inducing vaccines.

The different antigen-specific immunotherapies are analytically presented in a comparative manner in separate tables providing detailed information about the selected myelin antigen, the vaccination strategy (e.g., prophylactic, preclinical, therapeutic), the administration route (e.g., intravenous, subcutaneous, intraperitoneal, epicutaneous, intradermal, oral, nasal, pulmonary) and the administered dose, the cell type (e.g., tolerogenic dendritic cells, T cells, hematopoietic stem cells, bone marrow cells) and the inductive agent, the carrier type (e.g., polymer particles, soluble antigen arrays, immune polyelectrolyte multilayers, inorganic particles, pMHC-NPs, mannan-conjugated myelin peptides, liposomes, exosomes, antigen-presenting yeast cells), and its characteristics (e.g., size, zeta potential, antigen loading), as well as the vaccination outcome.

The review paper is based on a systematic search of PubMed using the following search terms: multiple sclerosis, antigen-specific immunotherapies, tolerogenic vaccines, nanocarriers, nanomedicine, DNA vaccination, cell-based vaccination, clinical trials. The search covered the time period from 1 January 2000 till today. Publications addressing pre-clinical and clinical evaluation of antigen-specific immunotherapies for multiple sclerosis were selected for inclusion.

2. Immunopathogenesis of MS

Successful preclinical studies and clinical trials for MS which target cells and molecules of the immune system support the idea that the latter has a dominant role in the pathogenesis of MS. These studies have proposed that cells of the adaptive immune system like B cells and various effector T cells, combined with cells of the innate immune system such as natural killer cells and microglia, uniquely contribute to the disease [2]. However, it should be mentioned that while the peripheral adaptive immune system (T lymphocytes) is the primary driver of RRMS, the innate immune system (microglia and astrocytes) together with B lymphocytes is considered to drive progressive MS [2]. The CNS of MS patients has been also found to exhibit infiltration of activated T cells, B cells, plasma cells, dendritic cells (DCs), and macrophages indicating the contribution of both cellular and humoral (i.e., antibody-mediated) immune responses as well as of various immunopathological effector mechanisms to the damage of CNS tissue [22,23].

It has been suggested that two independent types of inflammation, developing in parallel, can occur in multiple sclerosis patients. The first one is related with the focal invasion of T and B cells through BBB leakage, giving rise to classic active demyelinated plaques in the white matter. The second one deals with a slow accumulation of T and B lymphocytes without profound BBB damage in the perivascular Virchow Robin spaces and the meninges, where they form cellular aggregates resembling, in most severe cases, tertiary lymph follicles. The latter can be linked with the development of demyelinated lesions in the cerebral and cerebellar cortex, slow expansion of existing lesions in the white matter, and diffuse neurodegeneration in normal-appearing white and/or grey matter [18]. The presence of the lymphoid follicle-like structures (follicle-like ectopic germinal centers) in the inflamed cerebral meninges of some SPMS patients could indicate that B-cell maturation is sustained locally in the CNS and contributes to the induction of a compartmentalized humoral immune response [2,22].

The role of the various immune cells and the immunopathological effector mechanisms contributing to the development of MS are discussed below.

The ability of the human immune system to respond to an enormous number of encountered antigens comes with the risk that some T cells will be able to recognize self-antigens, such as CNS (e.g., myelin) antigens. Most autoreactive T lymphocytes are usually deleted in the thymus via a process known as negative selection (central tolerance). However, a number of these T cells escape from the thymus to peripheral sites where they are normally kept under control by mechanisms of peripheral tolerance. If these mechanisms fail, due to reduced action of regulatory T cells and/or enhanced resistance of effector T and B lymphocytes to suppression, autoreactive T cells recognizing CNS antigens are activated in the peripheral lymphoid system to become effector cells, via molecular mimicry (i.e., activation by a viral peptide having sufficient sequence similarity [24] or otherwise sharing an immunologic epitope [25] with the CNS antigen), recognition of CNS proteins released in the periphery, presentation of new autoantigens and bystander activation (i.e., T cell receptor (TCR)-independent and cytokine-dependent activation probably due to viral infection [26]). Then the activated T cells (CD8+ T cells, and CD4+ T cells differentiate to T helper 1 (Th1) and Th17 cells) together with B cells and monocytes (cells of the innate immune system) infiltrate the CNS by crossing the blood-brain barrier (BBB) leading to inflammation. There, they are reactivated via encountered resident antigen presenting cells, APCs (e.g., microglial cells) and infiltrating APCs (e.g., dendritic cells, macrophages) presenting CNS autoantigens on the major histocompatibility complex, MHC (also known as human leucocyte antigen, HLA, in humans [11]) molecules. Specifically, CD4+ T cells interact with MHC II expressing cells, like dendritic cells, macrophages and B cells, whereas CD8+ T cells directly interact with MHC I/antigen-expressing cells, like neurons and oligodendrocytes. It should be noted that MHC class II is adequately expressed only on professional APCs, while MHC class I is expressed by all cell types in the CNS inflammatory milieu. Therefore, CD4+ T cells are mainly found in perivascular cuffs, and meninges, whereas CD8+ T cells additionally infiltrate the parenchyma of the irritated lesions. Upon contact with their cognate antigen, CD4+ T cells are thought to secrete cytokines and immune mediators resulting in the attraction of resident immune cells like microglia, macrophages and astrocytes, secretion of proinflammatory cytokines, enhanced APC function, and increased production of reactive oxygen and nitrogen species (ROS/RNS). On the other hand, apart from secreting inflammatory mediators, CD8+ T cells directly attack oligodendrocytes and neurons, thus causing oligodendrocyte death (e.g., via secretion of granzymes and perforin leading to pore formation and stimulation of programmed cell death [2]) and neuronal damage (e.g., release of cytolytic granules leading to axonal dissection [2]) (Figure 2). The above result in inflammation, myelin loss, and axonal injury. This inflammatory cascade leads to the recruitment of monocytes and macrophages into the lesion resulting in the release of more CNS antigens and their presentation to potentially autoreactive T cells. It should be mentioned that epitope spreading could result in a broader autoimmune response involving additional autoantigens [1–3,11,27–33].

CD4+ T cells are considered to have a paramount role in the immunopathogenesis of MS due to the secretion of interferon gamma (IFNγ) and IL-17 [2,20,34]. However, it has been lately revealed that CD8+ T cells are also responsible for the initiation of human MS pathogenesis where, contrary to experimental autoimune encephalomyelitis (EAE), CD8+ T cells are the predominant T lymphocyte infiltrate in acute and chronic MS lesions [1,2]. Compared with CD4+ T cells, CD8+ T cells can be found more frequently in the white matter and in the cortical demyelinating lesions in the grey matter, and their density can be closely correlated with axonal damage [1,3]. Epitope spreading, assisted by cross-presentation of antigens by monocyte-derived DCs, has been found to activate myelin-specific CD8+ T cells also in an EAE model [3]. It has been suggested that CD8+ T cells remain in the CNS (e.g., brain and spinal cord) as tissue-resident cells, and upon re-encounter of their cognate antigen, focally propagate neuroinflammation [18].

Despite the fact that MS is considered a T lymphocyte-mediated disease [35], the important results of anti-CD20 therapy (e.g., rituximab, ocrelizumab) in MS indicate a significant role for B cells in its pathogenesis. B cells can have either a pro- or an anti-inflammatory role, based on their subtype and context. Their pro-inflammatory functions, comprise critical antigen presentation in the context of MHC class II molecules to Th17 and Th1 cells, secretion of pro-inflammatory cytokines (e.g., tumor necrosis factor alpha, TNF-α, interleukin-6 (IL-6) and granulocyte-macrophage colony-stimulating factor, GM-CSF) that promote CNS inflammation and propagate demyelination and neurodegeneration, and production of antibodies [36]. B lymphocytes can traffic out of the CNS to the cervical lymph nodes where they can undergo affinity maturation and then re-enter the CNS and promote further damage [3].

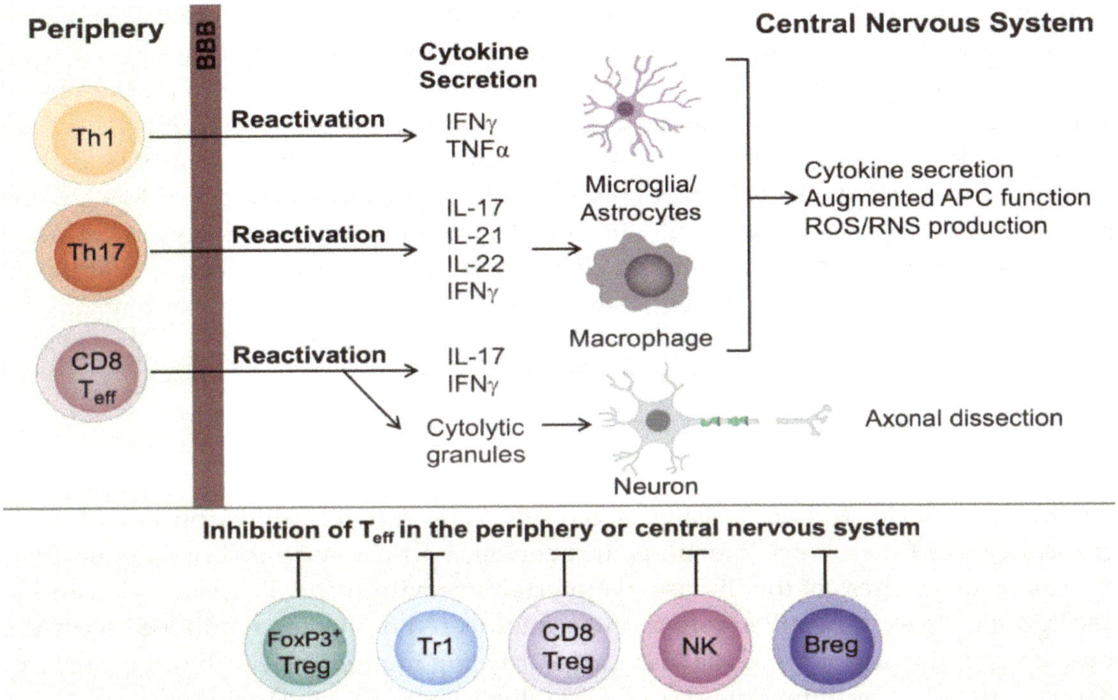

Figure 2. Effector T cells in multiple sclerosis (with the permission of [2]).

B cells are considered a unique population of APCs since, in contrast to other APCs which recognize various exogenous and endogenous antigens, B cells are highly selective (i.e., they specifically recognize only the antigens that are bound to their unique surface B cell receptor). Studies with the EAE model have indicated that some autoantigens, like the highly immunogenic myelin oligodendrocyte glycoprotein (MOG), require their presentation by B cells to activate CD4+ T cells. Accordingly, it can be speculated that the antigen(s) which trigger human MS are likewise B cell dependent [36]. Furthermore, active genes in B cells represent a major component of more than 200 variants known to increase the risk for developing MS. Remarkably, the gene that encodes the MHC class II DR β chain, which is known to be critical for APC function, is considered, genome-wide, the strongest MS predisposition signal. Probably, the net effect of this genetic burden is biased biology of B cells towards a pro-inflammatory phenotype, which promotes the presentation of self-antigens to effector T cells or augments the autoimmune responses through the production of cytokines and other immune mediators [36].

Regulatory T cells (CD4 FoxP3+ Tregs, CD4+ Tr1 regulatory cells, CD8 Tregs), regulatory B cells (Breg) cells and natural killer cells (NK cells) can achieve regulation of effector T cells in the peripheral lymphoid tissue or in the CNS. CD4 FoxP3+ Tregs (<4% of circulating CD4 T cells) express the transcription factor Forkhead box protein 3 (FoxP3) along with numerous inhibitory checkpoint molecules on their surface. They are activated by self-antigens and they suppress the activation of other cell types through a mechanism that requires cell contact [37]. CD4+ Tr1 regulatory cells impede cell proliferation mainly via the secretion of IL-10 [38]. Both Tregs are considered important in MS due to the exhibition of unique characteristics. Subsets of CD8+ Tregs that have been indicated to suppress immune responses and disease progression via distinct mechanisms have been identified by a unique expression of molecules like CD122, CD28, CD102 and HLA-G [2,39,40]. In addition, Th2 cells secreting cytokines like IL-4, IL-5, and IL-13, are considered to be able to downregulate the activity of pro-inflammatory cells [27]. B cells can also regulate various B and T cell mediated effector immune functions via secretion of regulatory cytokines IL-10 and IL-35, transforming growth factor beta (TGF-β), or programmed death-ligand 1 (PD-L1). Specifically, IL-10 secreting B-regs inhibit pro-inflammatory T cell responses, partly mediated via IFNγ and IL17 [2,3,36]. Finally, NK cells are known to suppress immune responses via killing activated, possibly pathogenic, CD4+ T cells.

Immune-modulatory networks are triggered in parallel with the deleterious activity of effector T cells, in order to limit CNS inflammation and initiate tissue repair, resulting in partial remyelination. The modulation of immune activation can be associated with clinical remission. However, it should be mentioned that in the absence of treatment, suppression of autoimmunity cannot be fully achieved. Consequently, additional attacks will normally lead to the progressive form of MS [2]. The action of autoreactive T and B cells in MS could be owed to the defective function of regulatory cells. Disease-associated HLA class II variants might skew the selection in the thymus so that the regulatory T cells which are released into the peripheral sites cannot adequately suppress autoreactive effector T cells [3].

3. MS Therapies

3.1. Disease-Modifying Therapies

Current treatments for MS can be categorized into long-term immunosuppressant drugs, which have significant risks for various infections and cancer, and disease-modifying therapies (DMTs) designed to alter the progress of the disease via interference with B and T cells activity, and reduction of BBB disruption. For example, the more recently engineered monoclonal antibodies (mAbs) act via blocking α4 integrin interactions (e.g., natalizumab) or lysing immune cells exhibiting surface markers like CD20 (ocrelizumab, ofatumumab) [41] or CD52 (alemtuzumab). Due to their different mechanisms of action (Figure 3), DMTs' efficacy and safety profiles [42] vary significantly. Presently, there exist more than 10 FDA (U.S. Food and Drug Administration) approved DMTs for RRMS aiming to reduce relapse level and severity of inflammation in CNS. DMTs can be classified based on the administration route as intravenous, self-injectable and oral formulations (Table 1) [16,23,31,43–49].

Among the FDA-approved DMTs, ocrelizumab, alemtuzumab and natalizumab seem to have the highest anti-inflammatory effect and to efficiently reduce relapses as proven by MRI scans [2,50]. Another approach for the treatment of MS involves the use of low-dose interleukin 2 (IL-2). This treatment is based on the weak in vivo response of effector T cells to low-dose IL-2 compared with Foxp3+ Treg cells which proliferate due to the expression of the high-affinity IL-2 receptor (CD25). This treatment has been shown to be well tolerated but, since non-specific expansion of the Foxp3+ Treg population cannot be excluded, it may effect susceptibility to infections and malignancies in some patients [51]. Interestingly, it has been shown that the more aggressive and less selective targeting of immune cells leads to more effective disease suppression, though at the cost of enhanced risk of side effects like infections and neoplasms due to decreased normal immune surveillance [27].

Despite the noteworthy advancements in the treatment of MS, the observed rates of progressive disability as well as of early mortality are still bothersome. Accordingly, there exists a need for safer, well tolerated and highly efficient treatments. This need is even higher for therapies capable of stopping or slowing the progression, and improving the disability in progressive MS [14,16,52–54]. Till now, only one therapy (ocrelizumab) appeared to be beneficial for the treatment of PPMS [14,16].

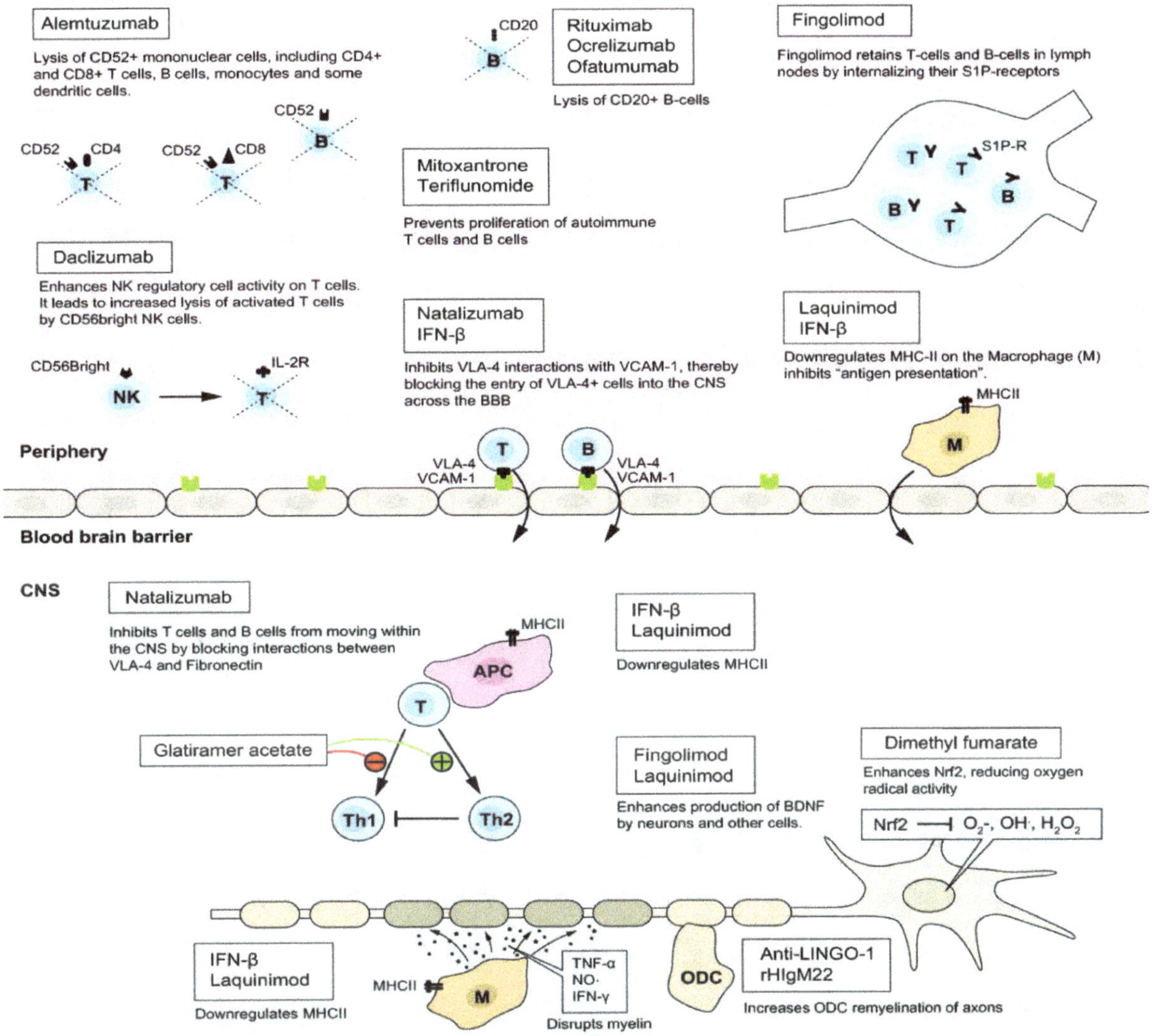

Figure 3. Suggested mechanism of action of several disease-modifying therapies (DMTs) (with the permission of [47]).

Table 1. Disease-modifying-therapies for RRMS (based on [16,23,43,45]).

Therapeutic Molecule	Commercial Name	Year of Approval	Admin. Route	Admin. Frequency	Mode of Action	Side Effects
IFN-β1a	Avonex® Rebif®	1993	i.m. s.c.	Once a week Three times a week	Decrease of proinflammatory and increase of anti-inflammatory cytokines; decreased migration of inflammatory cells across the BBB; decrease of Th17 cells; modulation of T and B cells.	Symptoms similar to those of flu; leukopenia; liver damage.
pegIFN-β1a	Plegridy®		s.c.	Once per two weeks	Decrease of proinflammatory and increase of anti-inflammatory cytokines; decreased migration of inflammatory cells across the BBB; decrease of Th17 cells; modulation of T and B cells	Symptoms similar to those of flu; leukopenia; liver damage.
IFN-β1b	Betaseron® Extavia®	1993	s.c.	Once per two days	Decrease of proinflammatory and increase of anti-inflammatory cytokines; decreased migration of inflammatory cells across the BBB; decrease of Th17 cells; modulation of T and B cells; down regulation of MHC expression on APCs.	Symptoms similar to those of flu; leukopenia; liver damage.
Glatiramer acetate	Copaxone®	1996	s.c.	-	Decrease of proinflammatory and increase of anti-inflammatory cytokines; decrease of Th17 cells; increase of Th2 cells and Tregs; blocking of pMHC.	Erythema; induration; heart palpitations; dyspnea; tightness of chest; flushes/anxiety.
Dimethyl fumarate	Tecfidera®	2013	oral	Twice or three times per day	Anti-inflammatory-Increase of Th2 cells; anti-oxidative stress; neuroprotection through activation of Nrf-2 pathway.	Flushes; vomit; diarrhea; nausea; decrease of WBC.
Teriflunomide	Aubagio®	2012	oral	Once per day	Inhibition of dihydroorotate dehydrogenase; inhibition of T and B cells;	Lymphopenia; nausea; hypertension; fatigue; headache; diarrhea; peripheral neuropathy; acute renal failure; alopecia.
Fingolimod	Glenya®	2010	oral	Once per day	S1P receptor modulator; preventing the circulation of lymphocytes in non-lymphoid tissues including the CNS.	Weakening of heart rate; hypertension; macular edema; increased liver enzymes; decreased lymphocyte levels.
Siponimod [55] Ozanimod [56]	Mayzent® Zeposia®	2019 2020 USA	oral oral		Binding to S1P-1 and S1P-5 S1P receptor agonist	
Laquinimod			Oral		Immunomodulation of T cells, DCs and monocytes; neuroprotection of astrocytes; decrease of proinflammatory and increase of anti-inflammatory cytokines; reduced infiltration of cells into the CNS.	No severe cardiac adverse effects were detected during Phase III clinical trials.
Cladribine [57]	Mavenclad®	2017 EU 2019 USA			Reduction of circulating T and B cells.	Risk of cancer

Table 1. *Cont.*

Therapeutic Molecule	Commercial Name	Year of Approval	Admin. Route	Admin. Frequency	Mode of Action	Side Effects
Mitoxantrone	Novatrone®	2000 USA	i.v.	Once per three months	Cytotoxic for B and T cells; reduction of Th1 cytokines; inhibition of type II topoisomerase.	Cardiotoxicity; leukemia
Methylprednisolone			i.v.	-	Immunosuppression; anti-inflammatory effects.	Risk of infections; retention of sodium; glucose intolerance; mood disturbances.
Dalfampridine	Ampyra®		oral	Twice per day	Blocking of potassium channel; improvement of motor symptoms.	
Natalizumab	Tysabr®	2004	i.v.	Once per 28 days	Targeting α4-integrin	Progressive multifocal leukoencephalopathy.
Ofatumumab	Arzerra®		i.v.	Once per two weeks	Targeting CD20	
Ocrelizumab	Ocrevus®		i.v.	Once per six months	Targeting CD20	
Alemtuzumab	Lemtrada®	2013 EU	i.v.	Once a year	Targeting CD52	High risk of infections Graves' disease
Daclizumab	Zinbryta®		s.c.	Once per month	Targeting CD25	
Rituximab	Rituxan®		i.v.	-	Targeting CD20	Chills; nausea; hypotension
Obinutuzumab	Gazyva®		i.v.	-	Direct cell death	Risk of infections; nausea; thrombocytopenia; neutropenia

IFN: interferon; i.m.: intramuscular; s.c.: subcutaneous; BBB: blood-brain barrier; MHC: major histocompatibility complex; APCs: antigen presenting cells; Nrf-2: nuclear factor erythroid-2; WBC: white blood cell; CNS: central nervous system; i.v.: intravenous.

3.2. Antigen-Specific Immunotherapies

The Holy Grail for the treatment of MS is to specifically suppress the disease while at the same time allow the immune system to be functionally active against infectious diseases and malignancy. This could be achieved via the development of immunotherapies designed to specifically suppress immune responses to self-antigens [43,51,58–60]. Even though the detailed mechanisms of MS induction have not been fully clarified, a dominant hypothesis is that the loss of immune tolerance to myelin proteins like myelin basic protein (MBP), proteolipid protein (PLP) and myelin oligodendrocyte glycoprotein (MOG) leads to the recruitment of myelin-specific CD4+ T cells, resulting in myelin damage [14,61].

Antigen-specific immunotherapies are based on the introduction of self-antigens to APCs in the absence or presence of very low levels of costimulatory molecules (i) acting directly via TCR on effector T cells resulting in immunological anergy and deletion of pathogenic T cell clones (passive tolerance), and (ii) through activation, expansion, and differentiation of antigen-specific regulatory T cells which secrete anti-inflammatory cytokines (active tolerance) [62,63] (Figure 4).

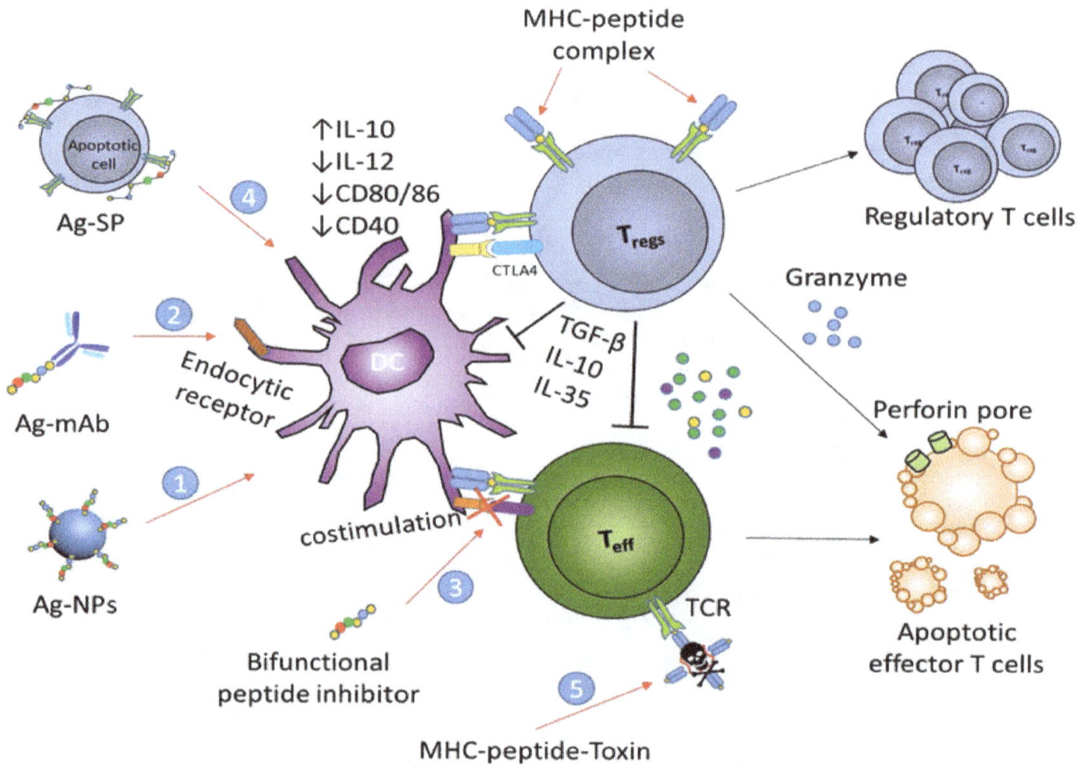

Figure 4. Bioconjugate-based approaches for the induction of Ag-specific tolerance in autoimmune diseases. The engineered bioconjugates target autoantigens and tolerogenic molecules to DCs (1); to facilitate antigen-processing via endocytic receptors (2); to hinder costimulation (3); to link to apoptotic cells for tolerogenic presentation (4); and to deliver toxin to autoantigen-specific T cells (5). These strategic approaches lead to peripheral tolerance as a consequence of anergy and deletion of cognate T cells, and/or induction of Tregs (with permission of [62]).

More specifically, an immunological synapse is established between APCs and T cells that is based on the formation of a trimolecular complex (signal 1) comprising the HLA class II molecule on the APC, the antigen (e.g., immunodominant epitope of a myelin protein) bound to this molecule and the TCR [64,65]. The establishment of the immunological synapse is the most vital process for the activation of effector T cells. In the absence of costimulatory molecules (signal 2), T cells become unresponsive to the antigen stimulation, a state known as anergy [65,66]. The presence of a costimulatory molecule exhibiting inhibitory properties could result to clonal deletion via apoptosis of the T cells. Autoreactivity of T lymphocytes can be also suppressed by the induction of regulatory T cells resulting in stable and long-term immune tolerance [59,65]. In vivo experiments have revealed that antigen-specific regulatory T cells are more effective than polyclonal Tregs regarding the control of organ-specific autoimmune diseases [67]. Finally, immune tolerance can be achieved via cytokine induced immune deviation, i.e., skewing of effector T cell subsets from Th1 and Th17 (proinflammatory phenotype) towards Th2 and Tr1 (anti-inflammatory phenotype) [59,65].

Antigen-specific therapies can be categorized according to the nature of the tolerogen (e.g., peptides derived from MBP, PLP, or MOG, mixtures of myelin derived peptides; altered peptide ligands; plasmids encoding myelin derived peptides, peptides related to TCR regions, attenuated myelin-specific T cells, tolerogenic DCs, antigen-coupled cells), the administration route (e.g., intravenous, subcutaneous, intraperitoneal, mucosal, epicutaneous, infusion of Ag-coupled cells) [14,43,51,59,65] and the antigen dose [68]. Since, antigen-specific therapies are thought to combine maximal efficiency with minimal side effects, they could be considered especially appealing [14]. On the other hand, they need to overcome major challenges in order to be efficiently used for the treatment of MS.

The first challenge is that the target antigens in MS are not known and remain to be identified [14,27,65]. The disease is largely heterogeneous. It involves multiple autoantigens (contrary for example to neuromyelitis optica that involves reactivity to Aquaporin-4, AQP4) that can vary between patients depending on genetic characteristics, age, environmental and/or triggering factors, and duration of the disease [2,27,69,70]. It has been assumed that myelin targets like MBP, PLP and MOG are relevant, but this is mainly based on EAE models and not on MS patients. Furthermore, therapeutic efficiency in EAE cannot always be translated in MS. Accordingly, the interpretation of the above remains a crucial challenge for the translation of antigen-specific therapies from bench to bedside [27].

Furthermore, it should be noted that the clinical/neuropathological features of MS change noticeably with time [5,70]. Thus, not all patients will necessarily have similar responses to myelin antigen-specific immunotherapies [5]. Additionally, in chronic MS, the pattern of recognized autoantigens progressively increases during the course of the disease, due to a spread of the adaptive immunity to related self-antigens, a phenomenon recognized as epitope spreading [69,70]. Epitope spreading has been defined as the broadening of epitope specificity from the initial immunodominant epitope-specific immune response to other subdominant protein epitopes [71]. Epitope spreading can be categorized as "intra-molecular" related to shifting of immune responses between different epitopes of the same protein (e.g., MBP) and "intermolecular" related to the shifting of immune responses between two proteins (e.g., MBP and PLP) [27,72]. The hierarchy of immunodominant and cryptic epitopes is supposed to be dependent on a combination of peptide processing and presentation by various APCs, and also on the availability of epitope-specific T lymphocytes, taking into account the mechanisms of central and peripheral tolerance [71]. Accordingly, identifying the autoantigens that should be included in the therapeutic formulation can be rather challenging. This problem might be partially overcome via tolerance spreading, i.e., a gradual spread of the tolerance to the administered autoantigens also to other self-antigens which are involved in autoimmunity [70]. Elucidation of the cellular and molecular mechanisms involved in epitope spreading in MS is very important in order to design efficient antigen-specific immunotherapies for MS patients [71]. In this respect, therapeutic strategies targeting a broader array of epitopes may need to be pursued. Furthermore, since immune reactivity broadens with disease duration, antigen-specific immunotherapies should ideally be delivered early in the course of the disease when epitope spreading has not yet occurred, according to an optimized dosage and frequency schedule [14,27,65,73]. An alternative approach could be to achieve bystander suppression (i.e., modulation of the responses to one target antigen leads to modulation of the responses to neighboring target antigens). However, limiting evidence exists for such therapies [27].

Finally, another challenge regarding the translation of antigen-specific immunotherapies from bench to bedside is that the administration of tolerogenic vaccines to MS patients with inapparent infections could be immunogenic and worsen the course of the disease due to its presentation in the immune system in a pro-inflammatory environment. This has been the case in clinical trials with APL [74]. Thus, a crucial test for tolerogenic vaccines could be the in vivo assessment of their delivery in a proinflammatory environment, either after EAE onset, or by co-delivery of adjuvants and/or pro-inflammatory stimuli during EAE immunization [63].

Continuing research efforts towards the development of effective and safe antigen-specific therapies for MS gave rise to the epicutaneous administration of antigens (e.g., dermal patch loaded with myelin derived peptides) for the establishment of skin-induced immune tolerance in MS. The ability of skin DCs to induce myelin-specific tolerance has already been demonstrated in both in vivo experiments (Table 2) and early clinical trials [28,58]. Finally, oral tolerance has appeared to be efficient regarding the prevention of EAE, but significantly less efficient concerning the therapy of ongoing EAE and MS [75].

4. In Vivo Assessment of Tolerance-Inducing Vaccination in MS

4.1. Animal Model of MS

The typically used animal model of MS is that of the experimental autoimmune encephalomyelitis (EAE) [3,4,18,76–80]. EAE is an acute or chronic neuro-inflammatory brain and spinal cord disease [18] which can be induced in various animal strains such as mice, rats, guinea pigs, rabbits, and even primates [7], via immunization with spinal cord homogenate or with various myelin proteins (e.g., MBP, PLP, MOG) emulsified in complete Freund's adjuvant (active EAE) [7,78,81]. EAE can be also transferred to naïve mice via adoptive transfer of T cells specific for myelin [8,78]. In EAE, myelin peptides are presented on MHC class II molecules to autoreactive T cells, together with costimulatory molecules (e.g., CD80 and CD86), resulting in activation of the T lymphocytes and, consequently, in an autoimmune attack on the myelin sheath [79]. EAE is principally mediated by myelin specific CD4+ T cells [20,78,82,83]. The clinical course of EAE varies based on the immunized animal species and the encephalitogenic antigen used for the inoculation. Usually the animals experience either an acute monophasic, progressive or not, disease, or a chronic relapsing-remitting disease. Ataxia, weight loss, sagging hind limb and paralysis are among the typical clinical signs of EAE [78]. Interestingly, various effective RRMS therapies (e.g., anti-inflammatory, immunomodulatory therapies) have been developed with the aid of EAE models. However, to date, no EAE model exists, that is capable of reproducing the specific features (e.g., clinical and neuropathological) of progressive MS. Therefore, despite the undeniable value of EAE for basic research concerning the mechanisms of brain inflammation and immune mediated CNS tissue damage, its value as model for MS is limited [18].

4.2. Myelin Peptide-Based Vaccination

4.2.1. Immunodominant Myelin Petides

Myelin is a multilaminar sheath around nerve fibers comprising lipid bilayers and different proteins. The major myelin proteins are MBP and PLP which represent more than 75% of the total myelin protein. Additionally, myelin contains MOG [84] representing ~0.05% of the myelin proteins [7], myelin-associated oligodendrocyte basic protein (MOBP), oligodendrocyte-specific protein (OSP), myelin-associated glycoprotein (MAG), and Nogo-A [85].

While the etiology of MS is not clear yet, a favored hypothesis supported by experimental evidence indicates that the cross-reactive immune response between myelin derived epitopic peptides and viral or bacterial components can be considered as an important factor that contributes to the development of autoimmune T cells which initiate a demyelinating inflammatory response. Thus, the determination of the main epitopes of the encephalitogenic myelin and/or neuronal proteins that are implicated in MS is considered of major significance both for the development of antigen-specific therapies for MS and the elucidation of MS pathophysiology and etiology [85].

In recent decades, extensive studies have been performed aiming to identify the immunodominant epitopes recognized by T lymphocytes in MS. These studies have revealed that only the myelin proteins MBP, PLP, MOG, MOBP, and OSP can induce clinical EAE in laboratory animals and that autoimmune T cells against these proteins can be detected in MS patients. Other myelin proteins, like MAG and Nogo-A have been also identified as encephalitogenic proteins. Finally, some neuronal components (e.g., β-Synuclein, Neurofilament) have been found to exhibit encephalitogenic potential [85]. Antigen recognition takes place in the setting of a trimolecular complex formed by HLA, myelin peptide and TCR [64,86,87]. The immunodominant PLP epitopes which can be processed by human APCs lie within the PLP regions 30–60 and 180–230. Similarly, the PLP epitopes that activate T lymphocytes in EAE are within the 40–70, 90–120 and 180–230 regions of the protein [5]. Immunodominant epitopes of MOG that are recognized by encephalitogenic T cells in MS as foreign antigens are MOG_{1-22}, MOG_{35-55} and MOG_{92-106} with the 35–55 epitope being the major immunodominant region of MOG [86]. Analysis of T-cell responses to MOBP in SJL/J mice indicated $MOBP_{15-36}$ as the main encephalitogenic epitope of MOBP [85].

A cyclic analogue of MBP_{87-99} has been designed by Matsoukas and coworkers taking into consideration HLA (His^{88}, Phe^{90}, Ile^{93}) and T-cell (Phe^{89}, Lys^{91}, Pro^{96}) contact side-chain information. cyclo(87-99)MBP_{87-99} was shown to induce EAE, bind HLA-DR4, and enhance CD4+ T-cell proliferation, similarly to the linear MBP_{87-99} peptide [83]. Additionally, peptide analogues derived from the encephalitogenic peptide MBP_{82-98}, the altered peptide ligand MBP_{82-98} (Ala^{91}) and their cyclic analogues were synthesized by Deraos and coworkers and assessed regarding their binding to HLA-DR2 and HLA-DR4 alleles involved in the presentation of myelin epitopes to T cells. The cyclic MBP_{82-98} was shown to bind strongly to HLA-DR2 and to have a lower affinity to the HLA-DR4 allele. Both the cyclic and APL analogues of MBP_{82-98} were found to be promising and were selected to be further evaluated regarding their ability to modulate the responses of autoreactive T cells in MS [88]. In addition to the abovementioned studies, Tapeinou and coworkers developed a peptide compound comprising the MBP_{85-99} immunodominant epitope coupled to an anthraquinone derivative (AQ) via a disulfide (S-S) and six amino hexanoic acid (Ahx) residues. AQ-S-S-(Ahx)6MBP_{85-99} was found to bind reasonably to HLA II DRB1*-1501 antigen indicating the possibility of eliminating encephalitogenic T lymphocytes through generation of a toxic, thiol-containing moiety (AQ-SH) [89].

Yannakakis and coworkers used molecular dynamic simulations to study the interactions of the MOG epitope MOG_{35-55} with the HLA and TCR receptors during the formation of the trimolecular complex TCR-hMOG_{35-55}-HLA DR2 [64]. They also used robust computational methods (e.g., molecular dynamics, pharmacophore modeling, molecular docking) to rationally design non-peptide mimetic molecules capable of binding with enhanced affinity to the T-cell receptor and not to the MHC-peptide complex, thus impeding the formation of the trimolecular complex [90].

To date various studies have assessed different myelin epitopes, as single peptides or mixtures of them, regarding their ability to induce antigen-specific tolerance in EAE animal models (Table 2).

4.2.2. Altered Peptide Ligands (APLs)

Altered peptide analogues (APLs) of the immunodominant myelin protein epitopes have been successfully synthesized and applied in antigen-specific immunotherapies in vivo (Table 2). They are molecules where one or more amino acids in the sequence of the native immunodominant peptides, crucial for the interaction with the TCR, have been substituted. Depending on the substitutions, APLs can induce protective or therapeutic immune responses against EAE [91]. APLs can change agonist peptides into antagonist ones. Antagonistic peptides participating in the trimolecular complex MHC-peptide-TCR and causing suppression of EAE exhibit loss of their side chain interactions with the complementarity determining region 3 (CDR3) loop of the TCR. Substitution of large side chains interacting with the TCR with small side chain amino acids (e.g., Ala) causes antagonism and, therefore, inhibition of EAE symptoms. Moreover, APLs can switch Th1 cell response towards Th2 thus leading to disease suppression. Finally, APLs might activate regulatory T cells capable of antagonizing the deleterious actions of encephalitogenic cells in the CNS [83,87]. Accordingly, mutant cyclic peptides of MBP87-99 (e.g., cyclo(91-99)[Ala96]MBP87-99 and cyclo(87-99)[Arg91Ala96]MBP87-99) were shown to suppress the proliferation of a CD4 T-cell line from a MS patient, bind to HLA-DR4 and exhibit an increased Th2/Th1 cytokine ratio in peripheral BMCs derived from MS patients [83].

Molecular dynamics were applied by Mantzourani and coworkers to study the interactions of the MBP_{87-99} epitope and its antagonistic APLs (e.g., [Arg^{91}, Ala^{96}] MBP_{87-99} and [$Ala^{91,96}$] MBP_{87-99}) with the receptor HLA-DR2b [92].

4.2.3. Y-MSPc

Kaushansky and coworkers [93,94] pursued a "multi-epitope-targeting" approach aiming to simultaneously neutralize T lymphocytes reactive against various major encephalitogenic epitopes. In this respect, they designed a recombinant synthetic protein comprising multiple epitopes of the human myelin protein (Y-MSPc). Y-MSPc was shown to efficiently inhibit the development of EAE induced in mice by a single epitope of myelin protein (classical EAE) or by a cocktail of five different encephalitogenic peptides (complex EAE) and suppress its progression, outperforming the single disease-specific epitope and the.mixture of peptides (Table 2).

4.2.4. Cytokine-Neuroantigen (NAg) Fusion Proteins

Fusion proteins consisting of a cytokine (N-terminal domain) fused with or without an appropriate linker to a neuroantigen (C-terminal domain) represent an emerging platform for antigen-specific vaccination [95,96]. Regarding their mechanism of action, the cytokine domain of the vaccine exhibits high affinity binding to specific surface cytokine receptors on certain subsets of APCs. This results in highly efficient uptake of the neuroantigen domain by these APCs, and its processing and presentation on MHC class II molecules to NAg-specific T lymphocytes. NAg tolerogenic presentation is assumed to induce regulatory responses and results in the establishment of antigen-specific immunological tolerance (Figure 5) [96,97].

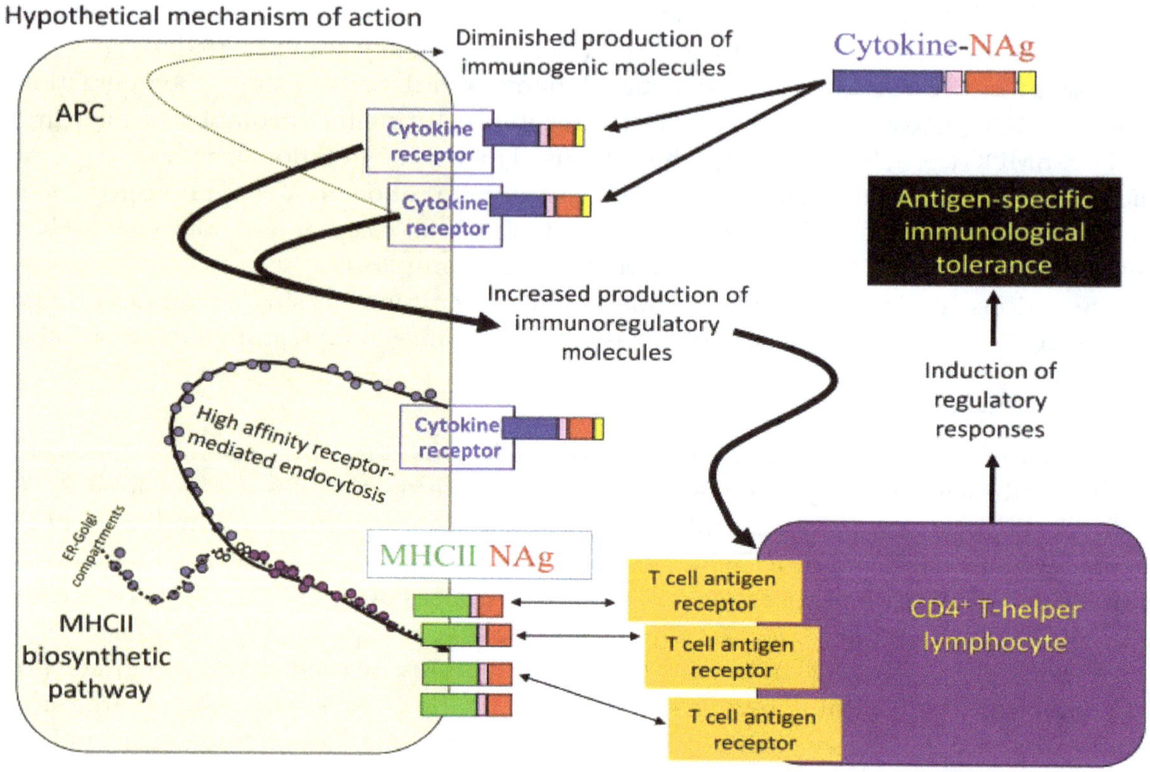

Figure 5. Mechanism of action of cytokine-NAg fusion proteins [96].

Various single-chain cytokine-neuroantigen (NAg) fusion proteins (e.g., granulocyte-macrophage colony-stimulating factor (GMCSF)-NAg, IFNβ-NAg, IL16-NAg, IL2-NAg), where NAg comprises self-myelin epitopes, have been examined as potential tolerogenic and/or therapeutic antigen-specific vaccines in EAE mouse models (Table 2). The developed fusion proteins have been found to target APCs and to effectively prevent the induction of EAE when administered prophylactically as well as to suppress pre-developed EAE. Due to their combined preventive and therapeutic activities, the cytokine-NAg vaccines were characterized as both tolerogenic and therapeutic.The ranking order with respect to their inhibitory activity was the following: GMCSF-NAg, IFNβ -NAg > NAgIL16 > IL2-NAg > MCSF-NAg, IL4-NAg, IL-13-NAg, IL1RA-NAg. [96].

Apart from the aforementioned cytokine-NAg fusion proteins, the macrophage colony stimulating factor (MCSF)-NAg fusion protein was used in order to increase the presentation of NAg by macrophages. However, it was found to be less tolerogenic than GMCSF-Nag, thus indicating the latter fusion protein as the most suitable for antigen-specific vaccination [95,98]. Additionally, it was revealed that GMCSF-MOG does not require a non-inflammatory quiescent environment to effectively prevent the development of EAE which contradicts the previous knowledge regarding tolerogenic vaccines [95,98].

4.2.5. Antibodies Coupled with Myelin Peptides

The dendritic and epithelial cell receptor with molecular weight equal to 205 kDa (DEC205) is expressed by DCs and enables antigen presentation. Injection of antigens (Ags) coupled to antibodies (Abs) specific for DEC205 into mice, at a low dose (e.g., ≤ 0.1 μg of fusion mAb [99]) leads to Ag presentation by nonactivated DCs, resulting in induction of regulatory T lymphocytes. In this respect, fusion of αDEC-205 Abs with MOG_{35-55} [100] and $PLP_{139-151}$ [101] ameliorated EAE in mice. Similarly, Ring and coworkers synthesized single chain fragment variables (scFv) specific for DEC205. scFvs were subsequently fused with MOG (scFvDEC:MOG) and administered to mice both before and after induction of EAE. Significant prevention of EAE was observed by vaccination with scFv DEC:MOG before immunization. In addition, administration of scFv DEC:MOG post immunization led to substantial alleviation of the clinical symptoms of the disease [102]. On the other hand, Tabansky and coworkers targeted the dendritic cell inhibitory receptor 2 (DCIR2) receptor with αDCIR2 Abs fused to $PLP_{139-151}$ and observed significant alleviation of EAE clinical symptoms [79]. In another approach, Kasagy and co-workers demonstrated that administration of anti-CD4 and anti-CD8 Abs followed by injection of $PLP_{139-151}$ resulted in substantially lower EAE scores and reduced rate of relapses in chronic disease in mice [103] (Table 2).

4.2.6. Recombinant T-cell Receptor Ligands (RTLs)

Antigen-specific immunosuppression can be induced via the utilization of MHC-peptide complexes as specific TCR ligands interacting with autoimmune T cells in the absence of co-stimulatory molecules. A recombinant TCR ligand (RTL) typically comprises a single polypeptide chain encoding the β1 and α1 domains of MHC class II molecules linked to a self-antigen [104] and represents the minimal interactive surface with antigen-specific TCR. RTLs fold in a similar manner to native four-domain MHC/peptide complexes but they deliver qualitatively different, suboptimal signals which cause a "cytokine change" to anti-inflammatory factors in targeted autoreactive T cells. Treatment with RTLs could reverse the clinical/histological signs of EAE in different experimental cases (e.g., MBP-induced monophasic disease, MOG peptide-induced chronic EAE, PLP-induced relapsing remitting EAE) and even promote recovery of myelin and axons in mice with chronic disease [105–107] (Table 2).

Alternatively, RTLs could involve natural or recombinant $\alpha_1\alpha_2$ and $\beta_1\beta_2$ MHC class II domains covalently or noncovalently linked with encephalitogenic or other pathogenic peptides. These specific RTLs could bind both to the TCR and the CD4 molecule on the T cells surface via the β_2 MHC domain and were shown to hinder the activation of T cell and thus prevent EAE in rodents [108].

Table 2. Myelin protein/peptide-based vaccination.

Vaccine	Antigen	Targeting Ligand/Drug	Vaccination Type	Admin. Route	Admin. Dose	Animal Model	Vaccination Outcome
Myelin Proteins/Peptides							
MBP [112]	Guinea pig MBP	-	Prophylactic: seven days b.i.	e.c.		SJLxB10.PL female mice (6–8 weeks old) with EAE induced with MBP	Protection from RR form of EAE Reduction of disease incidence to 58%
MBP [113]	Guinea pig MBP	-	Prophylactic: seven and three days b.i. Therapeutic: at initial signs of EAE and after four days	e.c.		B10.PL female mice (6–8 weeks old) with EAE induced with MBP	Prophylactic vaccine: protection from EAE Therapeutic vaccine: suppression of EAE
MBP [114]	Guinea pig MBP	-	Prophylactic: seven and three days b.i.	e.c.		B10.PL and SJLxB10.PL female mice (6–8 weeks old) with acute or RR EAE respectively, induced with MBP Knock out mice: TCRδ-/-, CD1d-/- and β_2m-/- on H-2^u background.	Vaccination with MBP prior to EAE induction prevented the development of the disease (incidence reduction by 50%) and reduced the severity of the clinical symptoms in the mice that developed EAE. Experiments with knock out mice showed that the disease could not be completely suppressed only in β_2m-/- mice.
$MOG_{35–55}$ [115]	$MOG_{35–55}$	-	Preclinical/Therapeutic: 3, 5, and 7 days p.i.	i.v.		C57BL/6 female mice (8–10 weeks old) with EAE induced with $MOG_{35–55}$	Dramatic suppression of EAE development
c-$MOG_{35–55}$ [116]	$MOG_{35–55}$ and cyclic-$MOG_{35–55}$	-	Preclinical/Therapeutic on the same day with immunization and seven days p.i.	s.c.		C57BL/6 female mice (6–10 weeks old) with EAE induced with $MOG_{35–55}$	Amelioration of EAE clinical course and pathology. Reduction of clinical severity of acute phase of EAE and reduction of overall EAE burden.
ATX-MS-1467 [117]	Mixture of $MBP_{30–44}$, MBP $_{131–145}$, $MBP_{140–154}$, $MBP_{83–99}$	-	Prophylactic Preclinical/Therapeutic	s.c.	100 μL of ATX-MS-1467 twice a week	(ObxDR2)F1 mice with EAE induced with spinal cord homogenate	ATX-MS-1467 was shown to effectively prevent and treat EAE. The inhibition of the disease was found to be dose-dependent.
Pool of MBP peptides [118]	$MBP_{68–86}$ and $MBP_{87–99}$		Therapeutic: secen and 11 days p.i.	i.n.	500 μg of each MBP peptide /rat	Lewis female rats (9 weeks old) with EAE induced with $MBP_{68–86}$	Tolerization to a pool of MBP peptides was found to result in amelioration of clinical symptoms of EAE.
$MOG_{35–55}$ [119]	$MOG_{35–55}$	-	Prophylactic: every other day, for 10 days b.i.	oral	200 μg of $MOG_{35–55}$	C57BL/6 male mice (6–8 weeks old) with EAE induced with $MOG_{35–55}$.	Oral vaccination with $MOG_{35–55}$ was found capable of efficiently suppressing pathogenic cells.
MBP [120]	MBP	-	Prophylactic: one day b.i.	oral	100 mg of MBP	Euthymic and adult thymectomized Tg mice with EAE induced with MBP.	Euthymic Tg mice were shown to be protected from EAE after oral administration of MBP contrary to thymectomized mice, thus indicating the key role of thymus in oral tolerance induction.

Table 2. *Cont.*

Vaccine	Antigen	Targeting Ligand/Drug	Vaccination Type	Admin. Route	Admin. Dose	Animal Model	Vaccination Outcome
Altered peptide ligands (APLs)							
APL [121]	P1: $MBP_{87–99}$, P2: $(Ala^{91},Ala^{96})MBP_{87–99}$ P3: cyclo(87–99) $(Ala^{91},Ala^{96})MBP_{87–99}$	-	Prophylactic: on the day of immunization	s.c.		Female Lewis rats (6–8 weeks old) with EAE induced with $MBP_{74–85}$	Suppression of EAE was detected 8 days post P2 and P3 administration. P1 was not found to suppress EAE. P2 was shown to suppress EAE between 8–16 days whereas P3 suppressed EAE until the end of the experiment (e.g., day 18 or 20).
APL [87]	$[Ala^{41}]MOG_{35–55}$, $[Ala^{41,46}]MOG_{35–55}$ and $[TyrOMe^{40}]MOG_{35–55}$ cyclo(46–55)$MOG_{35–55}$ and cyclo(41–55)$MOG_{35–55}$	-	Prophylactic: on the day of immunization.	s.c.		C57BL/6 female mice (12–18 weeks old) with EAE induced with rat $MOG_{35–55}$	Significant reduction of EAE incidence and symptons with the administration of $[Ala^{41,46}]MOG_{35–55}$ or $[Ala^{41}]MOG_{35–55}$ as compared with the delivery of $[TyrOMe^{40}]MOG_{35–55}$, cyclo(46–55)$MOG_{35–55}$ and cyclo(41–55)$MOG_{35–55}$
Y-MSPc							
Y-MSPc [94]	$MOG_{34–56}$ $MBP_{89–104}$ $OSP_{55–80}$ $OSP_{179–201}$ $MOBP_{15–36}$ $PLP_{139–151}$ $PLP_{178–191}$	-	Preclinical/Therapeutic: 3, 5, 7, and 21 days p.i.	i.v.	75 µg of Y-MSPc/mouse	SJL/J female mice (2–3 months old) with EAE induced with $PLP_{139–151}$	Y-MSPc was revealed to be more efficient in inhibiting the development of the disease and suppressing its progression in comparison with a single encephalitogenic peptide or a cocktail of peptides.
Y-MSPc [93]	$OSP_{55–74}$ $MOBP_{55–77}$ $MOBP_{15–36}$ $MOG_{34–56}$ $PLP_{175–194}$ $PLP_{139–151}$ $MBP_{89–104}$		Preclinical/Therapeutic: administration post immunization	i.v.	75 µg of Y-MSPc/mouse	(C57Bl/6J6SJL/J)F1 mice with EAE induced with $PLP_{139–151}$ or rhMOG (active classical EAE), or a mixture of $hMOG_{34–56}$, $hPLP_{139–151}$, $hMOBP_{15–36}$, $hMBP_{89–104}$, $hOSP_{55–80}$ (active complex EAE), or via transfer of line T cells specific for $phMOG_{34–56}$ or $phPLP_{139–151}$ (passive EAE)	Y-MSPc was shown to be more efficient in inhibiting the development of classical or complex EAE, suppressing the disease course and reversing the chronic disease, compared with a single encephalitogenic peptide or a cocktail of peptides. Additionally, Y-MSPc appeared to be more effective in suppressing passive EAE.

Table 2. *Cont.*

Vaccine	Antigen	Targeting Ligand/Drug	Vaccination Type	Admin. Route	Admin. Dose	Animal Model	Vaccination Outcome
Cytokine-neuroantigen (NAg) fusion proteins							
GMCSF-NAg and MCSF-NAg [60]	Guinea pig $MBP_{69–87}$	GM-CSF M-CSF cytokines	Therapeutic: Exp.1: 9, 10, 12, and 14 days p.i.; exp. 2: 10, 11, and 13 days p.i.; exp. 3: eight and 11 days p.i.	s.c.	1 nmol of fusion protein(s) per injection (exp. 1 and 2), 4 nmol on day 8 and 1 nmol on day 11 (exp. 3)	Lewis rats with EAE induced with DHFR-NAg fusion protein	GMCSF-NAg was found to potently target $MBP_{69–87}$ to subsets of myeloid APCs and to successfully induce antigen-specific tolerance.
GMCSF-NAg MCSF-NAg [98]	$MBP_{69–87}$	GMC-SF MCSF	Prophylactic: 21, 1,4 and 7 days b.i. Therapeutic: 9, 10, 12 and 14 days p.i. (exp. 1), or 10, 11, and 13 days p.i. (exp. 2), or eight and 11 days p.i. (exp. 3)	s.c.	Prophylactic: 4 nmol of fusion protein(s) per injection Therapeutic: 1 nmol (exp. 1 & 2), 4 nmol on day 8 and 1 nmol on day 11 (exp. 3)	Lewis rats with EAE induced with DHFR-NAg fusion protein	Prophylactic vaccination with GMCSF-NAg resulted in attenuation of EAE severity. Furthermore, treatment with GMCSF-NAg successfully inhibited EAE progression to more severe stages.
GMCSF-NAg [122]	$MOG_{35–55}$	GM-CSF	Preclinical/Therapeutic: p.i.	s.c.	2 or 1 nmol of GMCSF-NAg	C57BL/6 mice with EAE induced with MOG $_{35–55}$ (active EAE) or with activated MOG-specific Th1 T cells (passive EAE). SJL mice with EAE induced with $PLP_{139–151}$. B cell deficient, CD4-deficient, IFN-γR1-deficient, and 2D2	GMCSF-NAg was shown to suppress the established disease especially in passive EAE models. It also proved to be an efficient therapy for *Cd4*−defficient mice and to exhibit tolerogenic activity in B cell deficient mice.
Cytokine-NAg [97]	$MOG_{35–55}$ $PLP_{139–151}$	GM-CSF	Prophylactic: 21, 14 and 7 days b.i. Therapeutic: 13, 15, 17, and 20 days p.i.	s.c.	Prophylactic: 2 nmol of cytokine-NAg Therapeutic: 4 nmol on days 9 and 11, and 2 nmol on day 14 p.i.	C57BL/6 with EAE induced with $MOG_{35–55}$ (active EAE) or with transfer of activated $MOG_{35–55}$-specific T lymphocytes. In order to provoke another bout of EAE on day 42, mice were challenged with $MOG_{35–55}$. SJL mice with EAE induced with $PLP_{139–151}$.	Fusion of GM-CSF with myelin protein epitopes was found to lead to efficient antigen uptake by myeloid APCs resulting in blocking of the development and progression of EAE.
Cytokine-NAg [96]	$MBP_{69–87}$ $MBP_{73–87}$ $PLP_{139–151}$ $MOG_{35–55}$	GMCSF IFN-β IL16 IL2	Prophylactic: 21, 14, and 7 days b.i. Therapeutic: 13, 15, 17, and 20 days p.i. or alternatively after the onset of paralysis	s.c.		C57BL/6 mice with EAE induced with $MOG_{35–55}$. SJL mice with RR EAE induced with $PLP_{139–151}$. Lewis rats with EAE (acute monophasic form) induced with $MBP_{73–87}$	The developed cytokine-NAg fusion proteins were shown to target APCs and to successfully prevent the induction of EAE when administered prophylactically as well as to suppress on-going EAE.
Cytokine-NAg [123]	Guinea pig MBP	rat IL-2 or IL-4	Prophylactic: 21, 14 and 7 days b.i. Preclinical/Therapeutic: five days p.i. and on every other day through days 9, 11, or 13 p.i.	s.c.	Prophylactic: 0.5-1 nmol per injection	Lewis rats with EAE induced with guinea pig MBP fusion protein	Prophylactic or therapeutic vaccination with IL-2/NAg resulted in attenuation of EAE course, whereas administration of IL4-NAg indicated lack of tolerogenic activity.

Table 2. *Cont.*

Vaccine	Antigen	Targeting Ligand/Drug	Vaccination Type	Admin. Route	Admin. Dose	Animal Model	Vaccination Outcome
GMCSF-NAg [95]	MOG_{35-55}	GM-CSF	C57BL/6 mice: Prophylactic 21, 14, and 7 days b.i. 2D2-FIG mice: Preclinical/Therapeutic: 0, 7, and 14 days, or 7 and 14 days, or 14 days p.i.	C57BL/6 mice: s.c. 2D2-FIG mice: i.v.	C57BL/6 mice: 2 nmol GMCSF-MOG_{35-55} per injection 2D2-FIG mice: 4 nmol per injection	C57BL/6 mice with EAE induced with MOG $_{35-55}$ 2D2-FIG mice with a transgenic MOG-specific repertoire of T cells and a GFP reporter of FOXP3 expression	The pretreatment with the GMCSF-MOG fusion protein elicited CD25+ Tregs which were required for the induction of tolerance. Vaccination of 2D2-FIG with GMCSF-MOG elicited circulating FOXP3+ Tregs the number of which was maintained with multiple boosters.
MOG_{35-55}/I-A^b dimer [107]	MOG_{35-55}	I-A^b dimer	Therapeutic: nine days p.i. (treatment duration: four days).	i.p.	12 nM MOG_{35-55}/I-A^b dimer (1 μg/mouse/day)	C57BL/6 female mice (6–8 weeks old) with EAE induced with MOG_{35-55}	The administration of MOG_{35-55}/I-A^b dimer resulted in the reduction of antigen-specific T cells and amelioration of EAE symptoms.
Antibodies coupled with myelin peptides							
α-receptor–MOGp mAbs [100]	DNA for MOG_{29-59} (MOGp)	α-DEC mAbs α-Langerin mAb	Prophylactic: transfer of MOG-specific CD4+ T cells 15 days b.i. and admin. of α-receptor–MOGp mAbs 14 days b.i.	s.c.	3 μg of α-receptor mAbs	C57BL/6 (B6) mice with EAE induced with MOG_{35-55}	Prophylactic vaccination with α-DEC- and a-Langerin–MOGp mAbs led to reduction of disease incidence, onset delay and amelioration of clinical scores.
αDEC205-$PLP_{139-151}$ mAb [Stern et al., 2010]	$PLP_{139-151}$	anti-DEC205	Prophylactic: 10 or 15 days b.i.	i.p.	1 μg of fusion mAb	SJL/J female mice (6–10 weeks old) with EAE induced with PLP $_{139-151}$	Administration of αDEC205-$PLP_{139-151}$ mAb was found to alleviate the disease symptoms.
scFv DEC:MOG [102]	MOG	scFv specific for DEC205	Prophylactic: seven and three days b.i. Therapeutic: oje and four days after disease onset, signified by a clinical score equal to 1	i.v.	10 μg of scFvDEC:MOG	C57/Bl6 mice with EAE induced with WSCH	Almost complete prevention of EAE (90% of mice) was observed by administration of scFv DEC:MOG b.i. Moreover, vaccination with scFv DEC:MOG p.i. resulted in significant alleviation of the clinical symptoms in 90% of the mice.
αDCIR2-$PLP_{139-151}$ fusion mAb [79]	$PLP_{139-151}$	αDCIR2	Prophylactic: 10 days b.i.	i.p.	1 μg of fusion mAbs	SJL/J female mice (6–10 weeks old) with EAE induced with $PLP_{139-151}$ (active EAE) or via adoptive transfer of splenocytes from αDCIR2-$PLP_{139-151}$-treated mice (passive EAE)	Vaccination with αDCIR2+-$PLP_{139-151}$ fusion mAb was shown to decrease the severity of the disease and to delay its onset. Mice receiving splenocytes from αDCIR2-$PLP_{139-151}$-treated mice exhibited substantially lower clinical scores in comparison to those receiving cells from αDCIR2 mAb-treated mice.

Table 2. *Cont.*

Vaccine	Antigen	Targeting Ligand/Drug	Vaccination Type	Admin. Route	Admin. Dose	Animal Model	Vaccination Outcome
αCD4/CD8+$PLP_{139–151}$ [123]	$PLP_{139–151}$	Anti-CD4, anti-CD8a Ab	Prophylactic: admin. of mAb 21 days b.i. followed by $PLP_{139–151}$ delivery every other day for 16 days. Therapeutic: Mice treated with αCD4/CD8 Abs on day 11 p.i. were injected with αCD4/CD8+$PLP_{139–151}$ every other day from day 12–26.	i.p.	100 µg of CD4-/mouse) 100 µg of CD8a-/mouse 25 µg $PLP_{139–151}$ per injection	SJL female mice (seven weeks old) with EAE induced with $PLP_{139–151}$	αCD4/CD8+$PLP_{139–151}$-treated mice exhibited substantially lower EAE scores and reduced rate of relapses in chronic disease
Recombinant T-cell receptor ligands (RTLs)							
RTL342M [124]	$MOG_{35–55}$	HLA-DR2 peptide-binding domains	Therapeutic (s.c. or i.v.): admin. on the day that the clinical score for each mouse was ≥ 2. Daily admin. for mice receiving multiple doses. Prophylactic (s.c.): admin. of 4, 9, or 14 doses within 15 days. EAE was induced 2 days after the admin. of the final dose.	i.v. s.c.	50 µg of RTL342M	HLA-DR2 positive male/female mice (8–12 weeks old) with EAE induced with $MOG_{35–55}$	RTL treatment was revealed to be more efficient in reducing paralysis when administered in the form of multiple doses instead of a single dose, independently of the administration mode. Furthermore, the treatment with RTL342M could treat or prevent relapses. Pretreatment with RTL342M was shown to prevent the disease.
RTL401 [125]	$PLP_{139–151}$	$\alpha 1$ and $\beta 1$ domains of the I-A^s class II molecule	Upon EAE onset, daily i) i.v. admin. for 3–4 days and ii) s.c. admin. for 8 days.	i.v. s.c.	100 µg of RTL401	SJL mice (6–7 weeks of age) with EAE induced with $PLP_{139–151}$ or $PLP_{178–191}$ or $MBP_{84–104}$. C57BL/6 X SJL) F1 mice (6–7 weeks of age) with EAE induced with $MOG_{35–55}$ or $PLP_{139–151}$.	i.v. or s.c. vaccination with RTL401 resulted in prevention of relapses and long-term reduction of clinical severity only in SJL mice and C57BL/6 X SJL) F1 mice with EAE induced with $PLP_{139–151}$.
RTL401 [126]	$PLP_{139–151}$	$\alpha 1$ and $\beta 1$ domains of the I-A^s class II molecule	Upon EAE onset, daily (i) i.v. admin. for five days and (ii) s.c. for eight days.	i.v. s.c.	100 µL of 1 mg/mL RTL401	SJL female mice (7–8 weeks old) with EAE induced with $PLP_{139–151}$ (active EAE) or via transfer of activated $PLP_{139–150}$-specific T cells (passice EAE)	i.v. or s.c. vaccination with RTL401 was shown to effectively discontinue passive EAE progression, reverse its clinical severity and reduce the infiltration of cells into the CNS, as in the treatment of active EAE. Injury to axons was also prevented.
RTL551 [127]	$MOG_{35–55}$	$\alpha 1$ and $\beta 1$ domains of the I-A^b class II molecule	Upon EAE onset (days 12–14 for active EAE and days 7–12 for passive EAE), daily i.v. admin. for five days.	i.v.	100 µL of 1 mg/mL RTL551	C57BL/6 male mice (6–7 weeks of age) with EAE induced with $MOG_{35–55}$ (active EAE) or via transfer of activated cells (passive EAE).	RTL551 treatment of actively or passively induced EAE resulted in significant reduction of clinical symptoms and spinal cord lesions.

Table 2. *Cont.*

Vaccine	Antigen	Targeting Ligand/Drug	Vaccination Type	Admin. Route	Admin. Dose	Animal Model	Vaccination Outcome
RTL401, RTL402, RTL403 [128]	$PLP_{139–151}$ $PLP_{178–191}$ $MBP_{84–104}$	$\alpha1$ and $\beta1$ domains of the I-A^s class II molecule	At EAE onset (days 10-11), when the clinical score was ≥2, daily s.c. admin. for 8 days.	s.c.	100 µL of 1 mg/mL RTL	SJL/J female mice (7–8 weeks old) with EAE induced with WSCH or with a mixture of $PLP_{139–151}$ and $PLP_{178–191}$.	A single RTL was found capable of successfully treating ongoing disease induced with a mixture of encephalitogenic epitopes as long as the cognate T cell specificity was present.
RTL551 [106]	rhMOG, $hMOG_{35–55}$, $mMOG_{35–55}$	$\alpha1$ and $\beta1$ domains of the I-A^b class II molecule	At EAE onset (days 10–13), when the clinical score was ≥2, daily i.v. admin. for eight days.	i.v.	100 µL of 1 mg/mL RTL551	C57BL/6 male mice (7–8 weeks old) with EAE induced with rhMOG or $mMOG_{35–55}$.	Vaccination with RTL551 could reverse the progression of EAE, reduce demyelination and damage of axons without however induce suppression of anti-MOG Ab response.
RTL401 [129]	$PLP_{139–151}$	$\alpha1$ and $\beta1$ domains of the I-A^s class II molecule	Upon EAE onset (days 10–11), daily admin. for 1, 2, or 5 days.	s.c.	100 µL of 1 mg/mL RTL401	SJL/J female mice (7–8 weeks old) with EAE induced with $PLP_{139–151}$ (active EAE) or via transfer of activated cells (passive EAE). TCR Tg 5B6 mice with EAE induced with $PLP_{139–151}$ B cell deficient (µMT knock-out, KO) mice on C57BL/6 background (7–8 weeks old) with EAE induced with $MOG_{35–55}$.	A new interaction between cells was revealed via which the RTL-equipped myeloid APCs reverse EAE progression by transferring tolerogenic signals to cognate T lymphocytes. It was also found that splenocytes incubated with RTL401 exhibited reduced ability to passively transfer EAE. Finally, it was shown that EAE can be treated by RTL551 in the absence of B cells.
VG312, VG303, VG311 [108]	$MOG_{35–55}$, $MBP_{85–99}$, CABL	$\alpha1$ and $\beta1$ domains of DR2	Therapeutic: i.v. administration for eight consecutive days, 2–4 days after the disease onset.	i.v.	100 µL of VG312, VG303, VG311	Tg HLA-DR2 male and female mice (8–12 weeks old) with EAE induced with $MOG_{35–55}$	Vaccination with VG312 led to peptide- and dose-dependent induction of long-term tolerance to the encephalitogenic epitope $MOG_{35–55}$ and reversal of the clinical/histological symptoms of EAE
RTL401 [130]	$PLP_{139–151}$	$\alpha1$ and $\beta1$ domains of the I-A^s class II molecule	Therapeutic: (i) i.v. admin. for five consecutive days (days 20–24) and (ii) s.c. admin. for 3 days (days 32–34).	i.v. s.c.	100 µg of RTL401	SJL/J female mice (7–8 weeks old) with EAE induced with $PLP_{139–151}$.	Administration of RTL401 post the relapsing EAE peak resulted in prevention of disease relapses, reduction of demyelination and axonal damage.

Table 2. *Cont.*

Vaccine	Antigen	Targeting Ligand/Drug	Vaccination Type	Admin. Route	Admin. Dose	Animal Model	Vaccination Outcome
Bifunctional peptide inhibitor (BPI)							
PLP-B7AP [131]	$PLP_{139–151}$	B7 antisense peptide (AP) derived from CD28 receptor	Prophylactic 11, 8, and 5 days b.i. Preclinical/Therapeutic: 4, 7, and 10 days p.i.	s.c.	Prophylactic: 50 or 100 nmol PLP-B7AP/injection Therapeutic: 100 nmol PBI/injection	SJL/J female mice (5–7 weeks old) with EAE induced with $PLP_{139–151}$	Both prophylactic and therapeutic vaccination with PLP-B7AP resulted in efficient suppression of EAE. Mice treated with PLP-B7AP exhibited significantly low demyelination.
PLP-LABL [132]	$PLP_{139–151}$	LABL	Prophylactic: 11, 8, and 5 days b.i.	s.c.	100 nmol/injection/day	SJL/J female mice (5–7 weeks old) with EAE induced with PLP	The vaccination with PLP-LABL inhibited the inflammatory response resulting in prevention of BBB disruption and thus inhibition of EAE onset and progression.
PLP-LABL derivatives [110]	$PLP_{139–151}$	LABL	Therapeutic: admin. on disease onset, signified by a clinical score ≥1, and for three consecutive days until the score was <1)	i.v.	100 nmol/mouse	SJL/J (H-2S) female mice (5–7 weeks old)	Vaccination with the synthesized BPI derivatives was shown to efficiently inhibit EAE severity, and incidence.
PLP-LABL [133]	$PLP_{139–151}$	LABL	Preclinical/Therapeutic: 4, 7, 10, and 14 days p.i.	i.v.	100 mol/mouse	SJL/J female mice (5–7 weeks old) with EAE induced with $PLP_{139–151}$	Low disease scores and incidence could be observed in mice vaccinated with PLP-LABL.
PLP-LABL derivatives [134]	$PLP_{139–151}$	LABL	Therapeutic: admin. on disease onset, signified by a clinical score ≥1, and for three consecutive days until the score was <1)	i.v.	100 nmol/mouse	SJL/J female mice (5–7 weeks old) with EAE induced with $PLP_{139–151}$	The synthesized BPI derivatives were revealed to suppress EAE progression after intravenous administration more efficiently in comparison with unmodified BPI.
BPI-Fc fusion peptides LABL-Fc-ST-PLP and LABL-Fc-ST-MOG [109]	$PLP_{139–151}$ $MOG_{38–50}$	LABL-Fc-ST	Preclinical/Therapeutic: four and seven days p.i.	i.v.	25 nmol per dose	SJL/J mice (5–7 weeks old) with EAE induced with $PLP_{139–151}$	BPI-Fc fusion peptides were revealed to be highly efficient in suppressing EAE. The vaccinated mice were not found to exhibit weight loss, and featured benign clinical symptoms and reduced demyelination.
PLP–cIBR Derivatives [135]	$PLP_{139–151}$	cIBR7 peptide	Studies I and II: 4, 7, and 10 days p.i. Study III: admin. on disease onset, signified by a clin. score ≥1, and for 3 consecutive days until the score was <1	i.v.	Study I: 100 nmol/injection/day Study II and III: 50 nmol/injection/day	SJL/J (H-2S) female mice (5–7 weeks old) with EAE induced with $PLP_{139–151}$	Vaccination with PLP–cIBR, even at low dose or less frequent i.v. injections, resulted in significant amelioration of EAE and protected CNS against demyelination.

Table 2. *Cont.*

Vaccine	Antigen	Targeting Ligand/Drug	Vaccination Type	Admin. Route	Admin. Dose	Animal Model	Vaccination Outcome
Multivalent BPI ($MVB_{MOG/PLP}$) [111]	MOG_{38-50} $PLP_{139-151}$	LABL	Preclinical/Therapeutic 4, 7, and 10 days p.i.	s.c.	100 nmol/mouse	SJL/J female mice (5–7 weeks old) with EAE induced with $PLP_{139-151}$ C57BL/6 mice (4–6 weeks old) with EAE induced with MOG_{38-50}	$MVB_{MOG/PLP}$ was found to significantly suppress EAE in both animal models despite the evidence of epitope spreading in the C57BL/6 mice.
Antigen-drug conjugates							
$PLP_{139-151}$-DEX [61]	$PLP_{139-151}$	DEX	Preclinical/Therapeutic: 4, 7, and 10 days p.i.	s.c.		SJL/J female mice (4–6 weeks old) with EAE induced with $PLP_{139-151}$	Vaccination with $PLP_{139-151}$-DEX efficiently protected the SJL/J mice from the onset of clinical symptoms compared with DEX treatment.

MBP: myelin basic protein; b.i.: before immunization; EAE: experimental autoimmune encephalomyelitis; e.c.: epicutaneous; RR: relapsing-remitting; MOG: myelin oligodendrocyte glycoprotein; p.i.: post immunization; i.n.: intranasal; APL: altered peptide ligand; Y-MSPc: recombinant synthetic protein comprising multiple epitopes of the human myelin protein; OSP: oligodendrocyte-specific protein; MOBP: myelin associated oligodendrocyte basic protein; PLP: proteolipid protein; GMCSF: Granulocyte-macrophage colony-stimulating factor; MCSF: macrophage colony stimulating factor; DHFR: dihydrofolate reductase; i.p.: intraperitoneal; IFN: interferon; IL: interleukin; mAbs: monoclonal antibodies; scFv: single chain fragment variables; WSCH: whole spinal cord homogenate; RTL: recombinant T-cell receptor ligand; HLA: human leucocyte antigen; rhMOG: recombinant human MOG; mMOG: murine MOG; BPI: bifunctional peptide inhibitor; LABL: ICAm-I binding peptide; DEX: dexamethasone.

4.2.7. Bifunctional Peptide Inhibitors (BPIs)

Bifunctional peptide inhibitors (BPIs) are a promising novel class of peptide conjugates which are designed to selectively impede the maturation of myelin specific T cells. They comprise an immunodominant myelin protein epitope tethered to a signal-2-blocking peptide derived from lymphocyte function-associated antigen-1, LFA-1 (i.e., a T cell protein binding to intercellular adhesion molecule-1, ICAM-1) [109] (Figure 6). It is hypothesized that they bind at the same time to MHC-II and ICAM-1 on APCs thus inhibiting the immunological synapse formation during APC and T cell interactions [110]. The development of molecules that could target more than one epitope is crucial for the application of BPI technology in MS [111]. The performance of BPIs with respect to the induction antigen-specific immune tolerance has been studied in EAE animal models (Table 2).

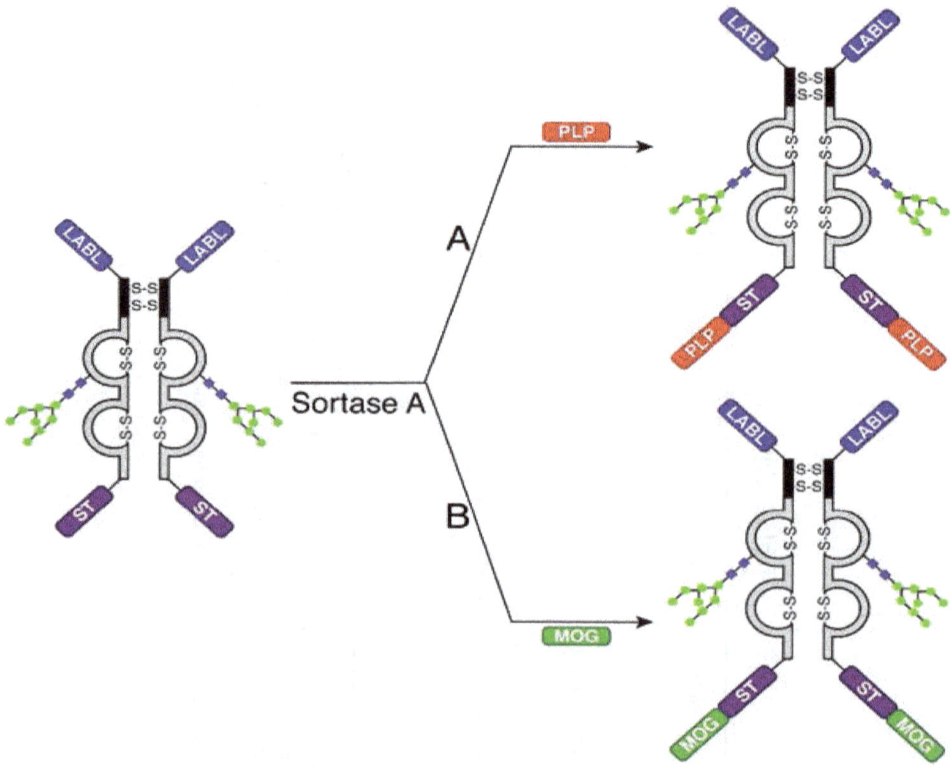

Figure 6. Sortase-mediated addition of two different antigens (A) PLP and (B) MOG to the C-terminus of LABL-Fc-ST (with permission of [109]).

4.2.8. Antigen-Drug Conjugates

Antigen drug conjugates (AgDCs) combine two therapeutic approaches (e.g., antigen-specific immunotherapies and immunomodulatory agents) to treat autoimmune diseases. Via chemical conjugation, the Ag could target the immunomodulatory agent to diseased cells thus minimizing side effects. AgDCs are assumed to exhibit increased affinity specificity through targeting cognate B cell receptors or endogenous autoantibodies. AgDCs formation entails the selection of an appropriate pair of antigen and immune modulator, and a linking scheme. An AgDC combing $PLP_{139-151}$ and dexamethasone ($PLP_{139-151}$-DEX) was administered to mice induced with EAE. It was shown that the AgDC protected the mice from developing clinical symptoms during the 25-day study [61] (Table 2).

4.3. DNA Vaccination

Deoxyribonucleic acid (DNA) vaccination is considered a promising antigen-specific approach for the treatment of MS [91,136–138]. DNA plasmid vaccines for tolerance induction in MS comprise a bacterial plasmid encoding myelin antigen(s). Expression is controlled by a mammalian promoter and a transcription terminator. They are administered either as naked DNA or with the aid of carriers (e.g., cationic lipids, cationic liposomes, polymeric particles), via the intramuscular or intradermal (e.g., "gene gun" delivering gold particles coated with pDNA vaccines) administration routes. Vaccination leads to DNA uptake and gene expression by the cells at the injection site [139,140]. Induction of immune tolerance is achieved via the following potential mechanisms (Figure 7). After intramuscular injection, myocytes are the main transfected cells, as well as few APCs. Antigens are then presented by the following mechanisms: i) myocytes process and present the antigen to T cells leading to T cell anergy ii) myocytes produce and secrete antigen that is taken up by APCs, which subsequently activate T cells. This results in loss of T cell co-stimulation through CD28, downregulation of IL-2, production of IFN-γ and reduced T cell proliferation. Intramuscular injection can also induce IFN-β via TLR9 activation due to the presence of CpG in the plasmid backbone [140], leading to downregulation of IL-12, IFN-γ, and Th17 cell responses. Following intradermal administration, DNA is delivered directly into the resident APCs (e.g., Langerhans and dermal cells). Intradermal vaccination leads to the secretion of regulatory cytokines (e.g., IL-4, IL-10, and TGF-β) thus resulting in the induction of anti-inflammatory Th2 immune responses [139,141]. Balance between tolerance induction and inflammatory immune response can be controlled by the administration route, antigen dose, and modification of the DNA-encoded antigen [141]. Numerous data from in vivo studies with the EAE animal model (Table 3), have demonstrated the efficiency of DNA plasmid vaccines at inhibiting MS via inducing T regulatory cells or anergy, clonal deletion, and immune deviation [139].

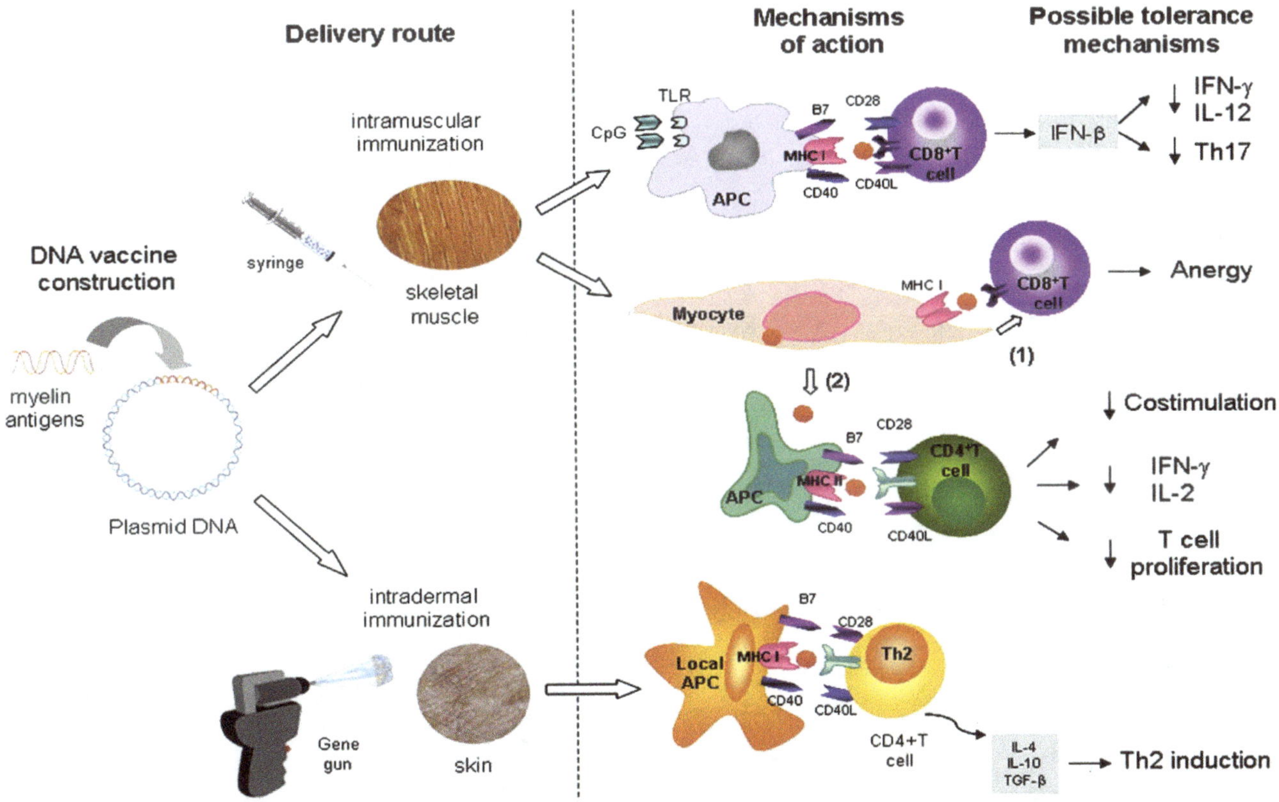

Figure 7. Mechanisms of immune tolerance induction by DNA plasmid vaccines (with permission of [139]).

Table 3. DNA vaccination.

Vaccine	Antigen/Immunosuppr.	Vaccination Type	Admin. Route	Admin. Dose	Animal Model	Vaccination Outcome
pDNA encoding IL-4 pDNA encoding $PLP_{139–151}$ pDNA encoding *MOG* [142]	$PLP_{139–151}$	Prophylactic: 17 and 10 days b.i. Therapeutic: 14 and 21 days p.i Co-vaccination with IL-4 plasmid and MOG plasmid on days 18 and 27 p.i.	i.m	100 µg of plasmid per injection	SJL/J mice with EAE induced with $PLP_{139–151}$ C57BL/6 mice with EAE induced with $MOG_{35–55}$	Co-vaccination with IL-4 and $PLP_{139–151}$ plasmids significantly protected against induction of EAE. Co-vaccination with IL-4 plasmid and MOG plasmid reversed ongoing EAE.
pMOG $_{91–108}$ pK0-$MOG_{91–108}$ (lacking CpG motifs) [143]	$MOG_{91–108}$	Prophylactic: three weeks b.i.	i.m.	200 µg DNA/injection	LEW.1AV1 (RT1av1) female rats (4–5 weeks old) with EAE induced with $MOG_{91–108}$	Vaccinated rats were protected against EAE.
pDNA encoding IL-10 pDNA encoding $MBP_{68–86}$ [144]	$MBP_{68–86}$	Admin. at the disease onset			Female Lewis rats (~6 weeks old) with EAE induced with $MBP_{68–86}$ or $MBP_{87–99}$, or with EAN induced with $P2_{57–81}$	Rats co-vaccinated with IL-10 and $MBP_{68–86}$ plasmids went into rapid remission. Co-administration of pDNA encoding IL-10 and pDNA encoding $MBP_{68–86}$ were shown to suppress EAE in rats induced either with $MBP_{68–86}$ or $MBP_{87–99}$ but not EAN.
pZZ/$MOG_{91–108}$ p$MOG_{91–108}$ pK0-$MOG_{91–108}$ pK3-$MOG_{91–108}$ [145]	$MOG_{91–108}$	Prophylactic: 3–4 weeks b.i.	i.m.	200 µg DNA/injection 100 µg of CpG DNA were added to p$MOG_{91–108}$ before the injection	Female LEW.1AV1 (RT1av1) rats (4–5 weeks old) and female DA rats with EAE induced with $MOG_{91–108}$	Vaccination with pDNA encoding $MOG_{91–108}$ (lacking the ZZ gene) reduced clinical symptoms of EAE and mortality in rats with different genetic background sharing the same MHC.
DNA encoding MBP, PLP, MOG, MAG and IL-4- [10]	MBP, PLP, MOG, MAG/GpG ODN	Therapeutic: admin. at the peak of acute EAE, when mice exhibited paralysis	i.m. i.p.	0.025 mg of each myelin peptide plasmid, 0.05 mg of IL-4 plasmid and 0.05 mg of GpG ODN	Female SJL/J and C57BL/6 (B6) mice (8–12 weeks old) with EAE induced with $PLP_{139–151}$ or $MOG_{35–55}$	Administration of myelin cocktail/IL-4 plasmids and the immunosuppressant GpG ODN resulted in dramatic improvement of the disease in mice having either chronic relapsing or chronic progressive EAE.
pMOG $_{91–108}$ pMOG-IFN-β pMOG-scr [146]	$MOG_{91–108}$	Prophylactic: three weeks b.i.	i.m.	200 µg DNA/injection	Female LEW.1AV1 (RT1av1) rats (4–5 weeks old) and female DA rats with EAE induced with $MOG_{91–108}$	The suppressive ability of DNA vaccination was found to be abrogated via silencing IFN-β.
p2MOG35 [147]	$MOG_{35–55}$/Tacrolimus (FK506)	Preclinical/Therapeutic: three and 17 days p.i.	i.m.	100 µg of p2MOG35/mouse 10 µg of FK506/mouse	Female C57BL/6 mice (6–8 weeks old) with EAE induced with $MOG_{35–55}$	Co-administration of p2MOG35 with FK506 was shown to effectively meliorate EAE in mice.

Table 3. *Cont.*

Vaccine	Antigen/Immunosuppr.	Vaccination Type	Admin. Route	Admin. Dose	Animal Model	Vaccination Outcome
pVAX-PLP, pVAX-MOG [148]	PLP, MOG	Prophylactic: four or 12 weeks b.i.	i.m.	20µg pVAX-PLP, pVAX-MOG	Female SJL/J (9H-2) mice (6 weeks old) with EAE induced with $PLP_{139–151}$ C57/B6 mice with EAE induced with $MOG_{35–55}$	EAE was found to be exacerbated in mice vaccinated with pVAX-PLP 4 weeks prior to immunization whereas both clinical and pathological symptoms were suppressed in mice vaccinated 12 weeks prior to EAE induction. In mice vaccinated with pVAX-MOG, either four or 12 weeks prior to immunization, EAE was shown to be significantly suppressed.

pDNA: plasmid DNA; IL: interleukin; MOG: myelin oligodendrocyte glycoprotein; b.i.: before immunization; p.i.: post immunization; PLP: proteolipid protein; i.m.: intramuscular; EAE: experimental autoimmune encephalomyelitis; MBP: myelin basic protein; EAN: experimental autoimmune neuritis; i.p.: intraperitoneal; GpG: GpG oligonucleotide; DA rats: dark agouti rats; IFN: interferon; pVAX: expressing vector.

4.4. *Cell-Based Vaccination*

4.4.1. Antigen-Specific Tolerogenic Dendritic Cells (tolDCs)

Dendritic cells (DCs) have a critical role in initiating adaptive immune responses in order to eliminate invading pathogens as well as in inducing tolerance towards innocuous components so as to maintain immune homeostasis [149]. Tolerogenic dendritic cells (TolDCs) are considered an attractive therapeutic approach for the induction of antigen-specific tolerance in autoimmune diseases [150,151]. To date various protocols have been developed for the in vitro generation of clinical-grade tolerogenic DCs ([35,152] (Figure 8) [153]) for antigen-specific immunotherapies. Autologous peripheral blood mononuclear cells (PBMCs) or bone marrow derived cells (BMDCs) are differentiated into tolDCs by numerous pharmacologic agents (e.g., immunosuppressive drugs such as rapamycin, cytotoxic T-lymphocyte-associated protein 4 (CTLA-4) Ig, corticosteroids; cyclic AMP inducers such as prostaglandin E2 and histamine; chemicals like vitamin D3, aspirin, etc.; proteins and neuropeptides like HLA-G, vasoactive intestinal peptide, etc.) and immunomodulatory cytokines (e.g., IL-10, TGF and low doses of GM-CSF) [150,153] and are further pulsed in vitro with autoantigens, encephalitogenic peptides, apoptotic cells, etc. [153]. tolDCs can display an immature or a semi-mature phenotype which is characterized by altered cytokine production and low expression of MHC and co-stimulatory molecules [150].

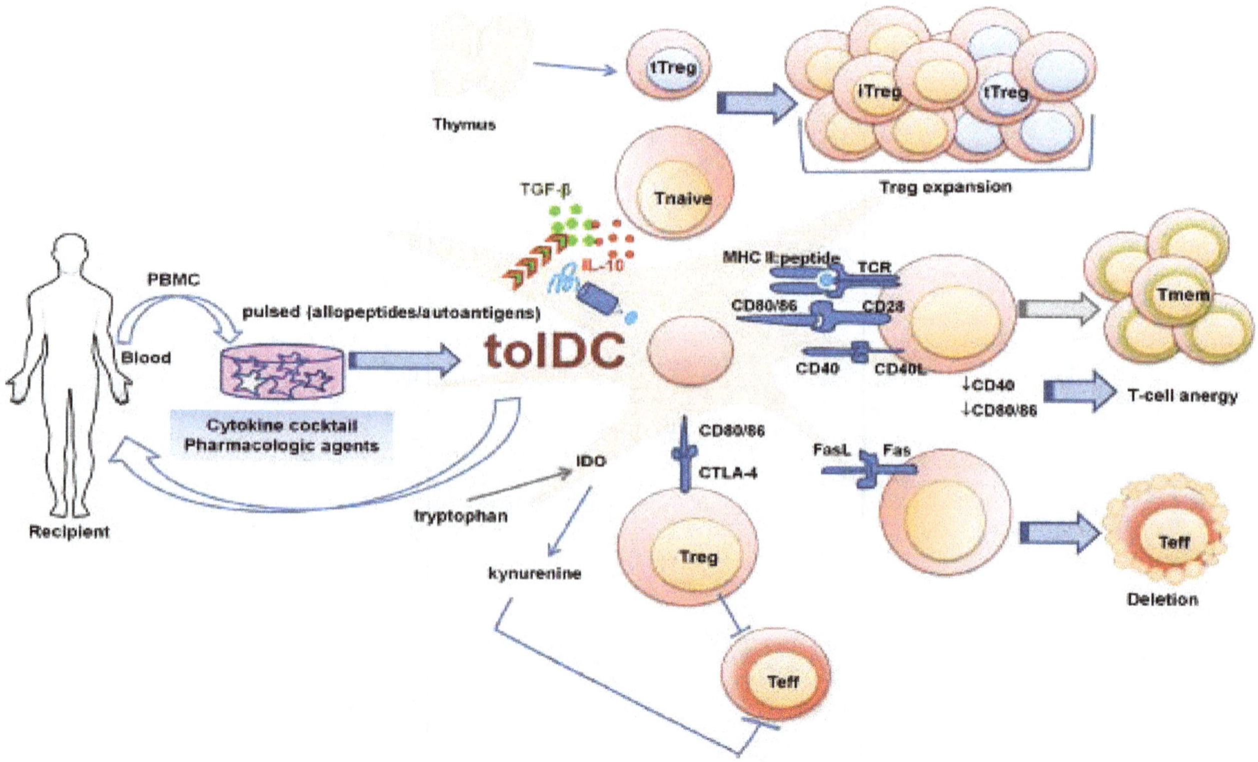

Figure 8. Strategies to generate tolDCs for clinical therapeutics [153].

Depending on the experimental protocol, the molecules used to induce tolerogenic properties, and the targeted cell population, tolDCs use different mechanisms of regulation to induce tolerance (Figure 8), including conversion to a regulatory T cell phenotype, induction of anergy, and antigen-specific deletion of T cell clones [19,35,150,152–154]. Lately, their ability to induce regulatory B cells secreting IL-10 has been also demonstrated [152]. TolDCs can be categorized into induced tolDCs (itDCs) (i.e., those acquiring their tolerogenic features in vitro or in vivo as described above and contribute to the maintenance of tolerance even under proinflammatory conditions) and natural tolDCs (ntDCs) (i.e.,

DCs present in the spleen and other lymphoid sites which inherently aid to establish tolerance in the absence of danger signals) [155].

The therapeutic potential of tolDCs has been demonstrated in the EAE model of MS (Table 4) (Figure 9). A key challenge is the translation of the in vivo results to humans. In this respect, it will be critical to correlate clinical efficiency with variation of immunological parameters and, accordingly, to define the best administration route and the effective dose of cells for this route [152]. Progress in the scientific areas of recombinant protein expression, genome editing and nanotechnology-based drug delivery systems, combined with improved immunization protocols, could further improve the promising tolDC vaccination in the furure [150].

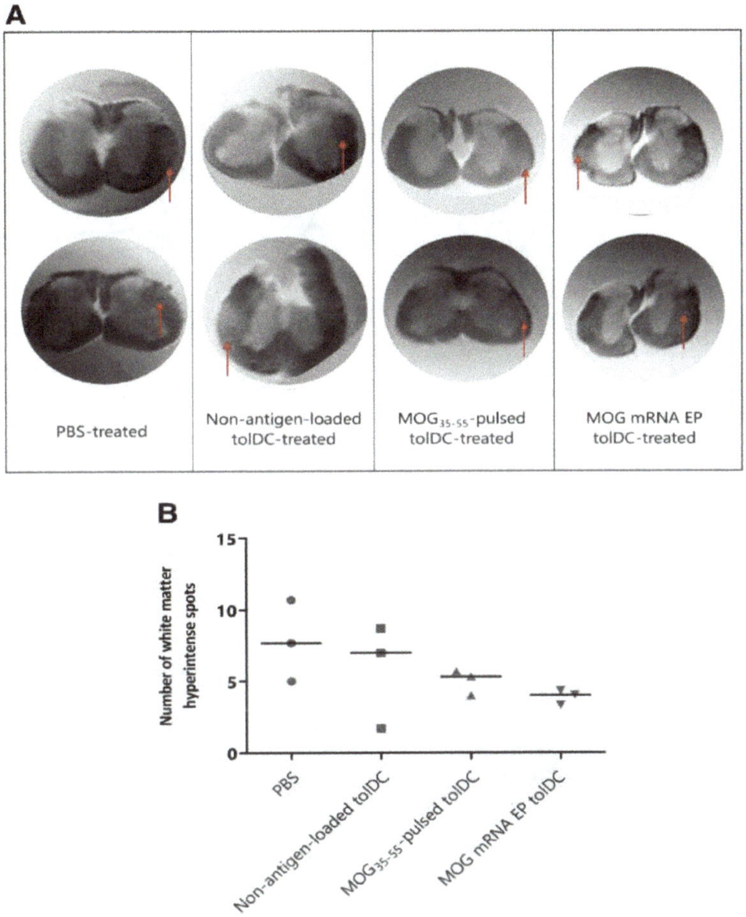

Figure 9. Evaluation of inflammatory lesion load within the spinal cord of tolDC-treated and PBS-treated mice using ex vivo MRI imaging. (**A**) Representative MRI of spinal cord with hyperintense white matter spots marked with a red arrow. Two representative axial slices are shown per treatment group. (**B**) The total number of hyperintense white matter spots along the entire spinal cord was quantified as a measure of lesion load in three mice per treatment group. Results are presented as individual scores for hyperintense spots with median [154].

4.4.2. T Cell Vaccination (TCV)

T cell vaccination involves the extraction of myelin reactive T cells from MS patients and their re-injection after irradiation in order to induce protective immunity [12,80,141,156]. To prepare T-cell vaccines, CSF mononuclear cells or blood PBMC's are stimulated with myelin antigen, and are then expanded specifically for the selected myelin peptide till an adequate population of cloned T cells is available. The latter are activated with antigen, and attenuated via exposure to radiation (6–12,000 Rads) to avoid proliferation after injection [156,157]. In clinic, the TCV protocol also involves multi-epitope TCR peptides [80]. TCV has been found to specifically suppress autoreactive T cells in MS via induction of a complicated anti-ergotypic and anti-idiotypic regulatory network or T cell deletion [80,91,156]. Various typical cytokines and lymphocyte phenotype transfer have been shown to participate in the depletion of the autoreactive T cells and the reversion of abnormal autoimmune responses [80] (Figure 10).

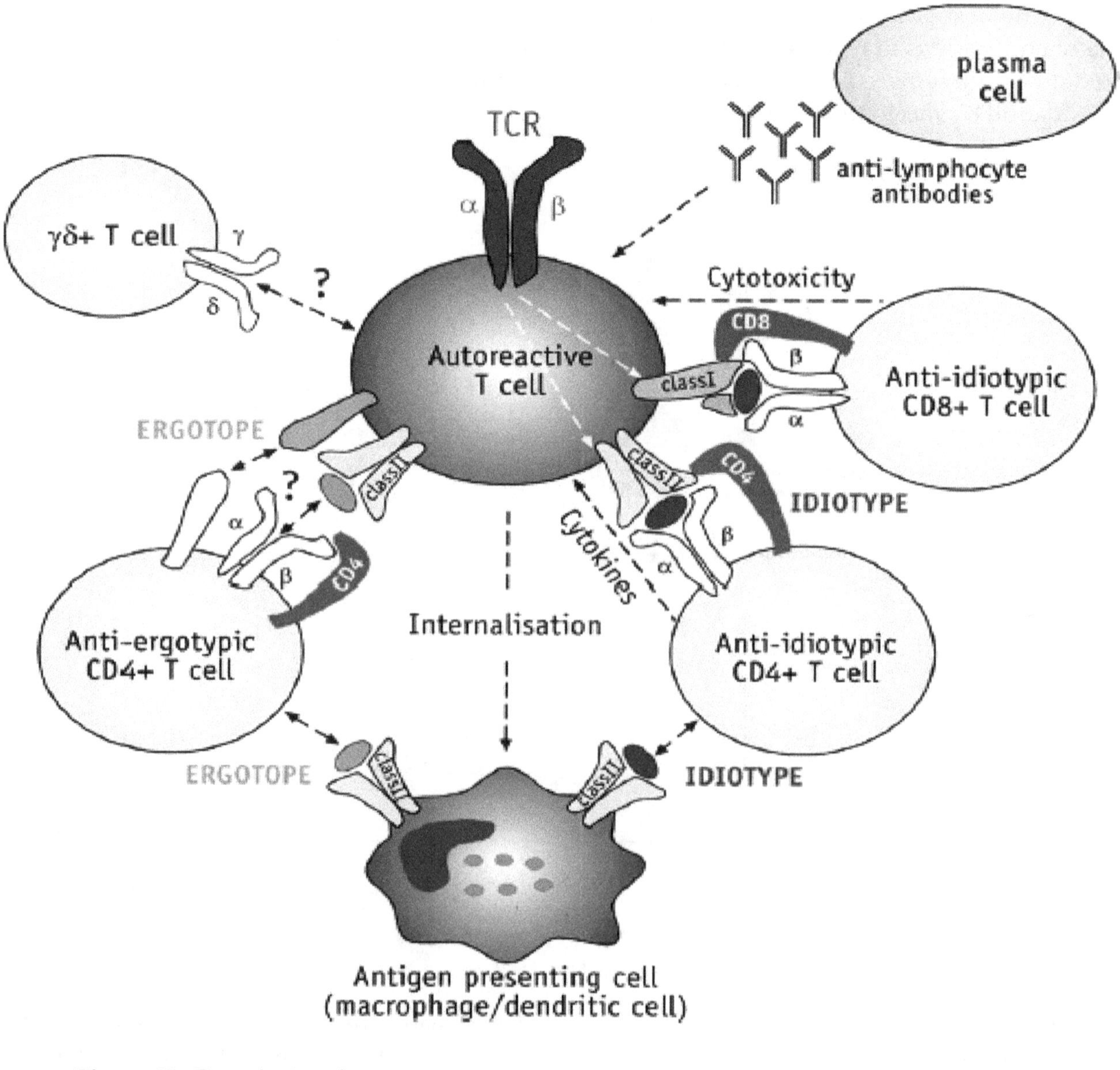

Figure 10. Complexity of anti-vaccine responses induced by TCV (with permission of [29]).

4.4.3. Antigen-Coupled Cells

Intact proteins (e.g., myelin proteins) as well as multiple peptides (e.g., MBP, PLP, and MOG derived peptides) can be coupled to a single cell (e.g., splenocyte [158,159], erythrocyte [67,160]) [86] (Table 4), thus permitting concurrent targeting of various T-cell specificities. This could be critical for antigen-specific immunotherapy in MS, where immune tolerance to multiple T-cell epitopes is considered necessary for the disease treatment due to epitope spreading. Contrary to protein/peptide-induced tolerance, vaccination with protein/peptide-coupled cells lowers the risk of anaphylaxis, since the antigen is chemically crosslinked to the cell surface. Vaccination with antigen-coupled cells has been found to prevent the active- and passive-transfer. Finally, tolerance induction with Ag-coupled cells can help define immunodominant myelin antigens, since the disease progression can be impeded by cells coupled with the spread epitope [75].

Table 4. Cell-based vaccination.

Cells	Inductive Agent/Peptide	Vaccination Type	Admin. Route	Admin. Dose	Animal Model	Vaccination Outcome
Tolerogenic Dendritic cells (tolDCs)						
BMDCs from C57BL/6 mice [161]	Atorvastatin/$MOG_{35–55}$	Preclinical/Therapeutic: days five and 13 p.i.	i.p.	1×10^6 cells per injection	Female C57BL/6 mice (8–10 weeks old) with EAE induced with $MOG_{35–55}$	$MOG_{35–55}$—specific tolDCs successfully ameliorated clinical Symptoms in mice with EAE.
BMDCs [162]	mytomycin C/$MOG_{196–204}$	Admin. of MOG196-pulsed Kb−/−Db−/− DCs to C57BL/6 (B6) mice one week b.i. and one p.i. Admin. of MOG196-pulsed B6 DCs to C57BL/6 mice three days b.i. and two and seven days p.i.	s.c.	1×10^6 cells per injection	Female C57BL/6 (B6) (8–10 weeks old) with EAE induced with $MOG_{35–55}$	Administration of MOG196-pulsed Kb−/−Db−/− DCs or MOG196-pulsed DCs ameliorated EAE in mice.
Murine BMDCs [154]	1α, 25-dihydroxy-vitamin D3/MOG-encoding mRNA or $MOG_{35–55}$	Therapeutic: 13, 17, and 21 days p.i.	i.v.	1×10^6 cells per injection	Female C57BL/6JOlaHsd mice (8–10 weeks old) with EAE induced with $MOG_{35–55}$	Vaccination with tolDCs electroporated with MOG-encoding mRNA or $MOG_{35–55}$ stabilized the clinical signs of the disease already from the first injection. MRI examination of hyperintense spots present along the spinal cord of mice was found to be in line with the clinical score (Figure 9).
BMDCs [163]	CD40-specific and p19-specific shRNA encoding lentiviral vectors/pyromycin/$MOG_{35–55}$	Preclinical/Thereapeutic: 3, 5, and 7 days p.i.	i.v.	2×10^6 cells per injection	C57BL/6 mice with EAE induced with $MOG_{35–55}$	Administration of MOG35–55-pulsed and lentiviral transduced BMDCs led to significant decrease in the clinical symptoms of EAE in mice. The highest decrease in the clinical scores was observed with the administration of co-transduced BMDCs (BoLV-DCs).
BMDCs [164]	Vitamin D3/$MOG_{40–55}$	Preclinical/Therapeutic: two and five days p.i., or five and nine days p.i. or 15, 19, 23, and 33 days p.i.	i.v.	2 or 4×10^6 cells	Female C57BL/6J mice (8–10 weeks old) with EAE induced with $MOG_{40–55}$	$MOG_{40–55}$—specific TolDCs were found to succeed in reducing EAE incidence and ameliorating its clinical signs.
BMDCs [165]	Vitamin D3/$MOG_{40–55}$/cryopreserved		i.v.	2 or 4×10^6 cells	Female C57BL/6J mice (8–10 weeks old) with EAE induced with $MOG_{40–55}$	It was shown that $MOG_{40–55}$—specific TolDCs maintain their tolerogenic properties and can efficiently ameliorate the clinical symptoms of EAE.
Murine BMDCs [166]	Tofacitinib/$MOG_{35–55}$	Therapeutic: 7, 11, and 15 days p.i.	i.v.		Twelve-week Female C57BL/6 mice (12 weeks old) with EAE induced with $MOG_{35–55}$	$MOG_{35–55}$—specific TolDCs efficiently dampened EAE severity and progression.

Table 4. *Cont.*

Cells	Inductive Agent/Peptide	Vaccination Type	Admin. Route	Admin. Dose	Animal Model	Vaccination Outcome
BMDCs [167]	1,25-dihydroxyvitamin $D_3/MOG_{35–55}$	Therapeutic: 10, 13, and 16 days p.i.	i.v.		Female C57BL/6 mice (6–8 weeks old) with EAE induced with $MOG_{35–55}$	Vitamin D3 treated $MOG_{35–55}$—specific. TolDCs succeeded in postponing the disease onset and reducing its clinical scores.
DCs [168]	Estriol (E3)/$MOG_{35–55}$	Prophylactic: one day b.i.	i.v.	$8–10 \times 10^6$ cells per mouse	Female C57BL/6 (H-2b) mice (4–6 weeks old) with EAE induced with $MOG_{35–55}$	Mice vaccinated with E3 $MOG_{35–55}$—specific TolDCs exhibited a reduced cumulative clinical score and EAE severity. They also avoided relapses and development of chronic disease.
BMDCs matured with TNF-α [169]	/$MOG_{35–55}$	Prophylactic: 7, 5, 3, and 1 days b.i. Preclinical: one day p.i.	i.v.	$2–2.5 \times 10^6$ cells per injection Rat anti–mouse IL-10R mAb: 0.5 mg equivalents per mouse	C57Bl/6 mice with EAE induced with $MOG_{35–55}$	Vaccination with $MOG_{35–55}$—specific TNF/DCs improved the clinical disease score. Pulsing of TNF-α/DCs with an unrelated peptide did not succeed in preventing the disease.
DCs [170]	/in vivo pulsing in Lewis rats with EAE induced with $MBP_{68–86}$	Prophylactic: four weeks b.i.	s.c.	1×10^6 cells per rat	Male Lewis rats with EAE induced with $MBP_{68–86}$	Injection of EAE DCs to rats resulted in induction of immune tolerance against the disease as demonstrated by delayed onset and marked decrease of the mean clinical score.
T cell-based vaccination						
Ob2F3 Tregs [171]	Retrovirally transduced pre-stimulated naïve CD4+ Tcells from peripheral blood mononuclear cells (PBMCs) of healthy donors using Ob2F3.	Preclinical/Therapeutic: seven days p.i.	i.v.	2×10^6 cells	Male and female HLA-DR15 transgenic mice (4.5–7.5 months old) with EAE induced with $MOG_{35–55}$	Ob2F3 Tregs were shown to significantly ameliorate $MOG_{35–55}$ induced EAE via bystander suppression.
MBP-specific T-cell lines (e.g., B12 and B12-GFP) [157]		Prophylactic: admin. three times at weekly intervals, with the last injection 10 or seven days b.i.	s.c.	1×10^7 activated and irradiated T cells	Female Lewis rats (6–8 weeks old) with EAE induced via i.v. injection of antigen stimulated T cells.	Vaccination with MBP-specific T cell lines inhibited the development of EAE clinical symptoms.

Table 4. *Cont.*

Cells	Inductive Agent/Peptide	Vaccination Type	Admin. Route	Admin. Dose	Animal Model	Vaccination Outcome
Hematopoietic stem cells (HSCs)						
DC-MOG vector-transduced BM-HSC [172]	Ex vivo modification of HSCs with SIN lentivirus vectors which transcriptionally target the expression of myelin peptides to DCs.	Prophylactic: Lethally Irradiated (10.5 Gy) mice were transplanted with DC-MOG transduced BM-HSCs eight weeks b.i. BM chimeras received neomycin treatment for three weeks post transplantation.	i.v.	1–3 × 10^6 cells per mouse	C57BL/6 mice with EAE induced with MOG peptide.	The transplantation of DC-MOG vector-transduced BM-HSC was found to completely protect mice from developing EAE even in cases of transplantation 6 months b.i. In agreement with the clinical observations, no histological signs of the disease such as demyelination, damage of axons, etc. could be detected in the tolerized mice.
Bone marrow cells (BMC)						
BMCs expressing $MOG_{40–55}$ [173]	liMOG	Prophylactic: mice were transplanted with BMCs transduced with liMOG 21 days b.i. Therapeutic: mice were transplanted with transduced BMCs 15–17 days p.i.	i.v.	0.7–1.6 × 10^6 cells per mouse	Female C57BL/6J mice (5–10 weeks old) with EAE induced with $MOG_{40–55}$	Transplantation of BMCs expressing $MOG_{40–55}$ was shown to protect mice from developing EAE and reduce the disease severity in mice with established EAE.
Myeloid-derived suppressor cells (MDSCs)						
MDSCs isolated via positive selection from BMCs expressing $MOG_{40–55}$ [174]	liMOG	Prophylactic: mice were transplanted with MDSCs transduced with liMOG seven days b.i. Therapeutic: mice were transplanted with transduced MDSCs 13–14 days p.i.	i.v.	0.5–1 × 10^6 cells per mouse	Female C57BL6/J mice (6–8 weeks old) with EAE induced with $MOG_{40–55}$	$MOG_{40–55}$ -expressing MDSCs were found to exhibit both preventive and therapeutic effects in EAE induced with $MOG_{40–55}$

Table 4. *Cont.*

Cells	Inductive Agent/Peptide	Vaccination Type	Admin. Route	Admin. Dose	Animal Model	Vaccination Outcome
Antigen-cell conjugates						
Ag-SP [158]	Chemically treated Ag-coupled SPs	Administration on day −7 b.i. or at peak of disease in actively induced EAE, or two days p.i.	i.v.	50×10^6 Ag-SPs per mouse	Wild-type C57BL/6 (I-Ab), B10.S (I-As), and BALB/c (I-Ad) female mice (5–6 weeks old) with EAE induced with myelin peptide or via adoptive transfer.	It was revealed that syngeneic or allogeneic Ag-SPs can effectively protect mice against ongoing clinical EAE.
Ag-SP [159]	Chemically treated Ag-coupled SPs	Prophylactic: at indicated time points b.i.	i.v.	50×10^6 Ag-SPs or 15–20 μg Ag per mouse	SJL and C57BL/6 mice with EAE induced with myelin peptide or via adoptive transfer.	i.v. infusion of peptide antigens coupled to syngeneic splenic leukocytes (Ag-SP) was found to efficiently induce antigen-specific T cell tolerance.
Ag-RBC [160]	Genetically engineerd Kell-LPETGG RBCs, coupled with MOG $_{35-55}$ through enzymatic surface modification with sortase transpeptidase.	Prophylactic: transfusion seven days b.i. Preclinical: transfusion five days p.i. Therapeutic: Transfusion on the day of EAE onset	i.v.	200 μL RBC-MOG$_{35-55}$	C57BL/6J (CD45.2+), B6.SJL-Ptprc (CD45.1+), BALB/c Female C57BL/6 mice (10–12 weeks old) with EAE induced with MOG$_{35-55}$	The transfusion of RBC-MOG$_{35-55}$ was shown to significantly improve the clinical signs of EAE in mice.

BMDCs: Bone marrow-derived dendritic cells; p.i.: post immunization; i.p.: intraperitoneal; EAE: experimental allergicencephalomyelitis; tolDCs: tolerogenic dendritic cells; s.c.: subcutaneous; b.i.: before immunization; i.v.: intravenous; MBP: myelin basic protein; Tregs: regulatory T cells; Ob2F3: recombinant T-cell receptor (TCR) isolated from a MBP specific Tcell clone of a multiple sclerosis patient; HSCs: hematopoietic stem cells; SIN: selfinactivating; SP: splenocytes; RBCs: red blood cells; liMOG: vector encoding the murine invariant chain (Ii) containing MOG$_{40-55}$ and enhanced green fluorescent protein (EGFP).

4.5. *Carrier-Aided Vaccination*

In recent decades, different strategies have been pursued for the development of carriers [175–179] loaded/conjugated with myelin antigens or combinations of myelin peptides and immunomodulating agents. The developed carriers have been designed to target TCR signaling pathways, as well as cytokines and co-signaling molecules, aiming to enhance TCR-mediated tolerance [30,62,177]. Various biomaterials (e.g., polymers, lipids) have been formulated into micro- or nanoparticles, self-assembled into different structures, or formed molecular conjugates with self-antigens (e.g., conjugation of self-antigens with polymers, antibodies, small molecules). Both nanoparticles (NPs) and microparticles (MPs) can be uptaken by APCs thus enhancing the intracellular delivery of myelin antigens and imunnomodulators [180,181].

4.5.1. Polymer Particles

Polymer micro- and nanoparticles loaded with self-antigens and/or immunomodulatory molecules have recently emerged as ideal carriers for tolerogenic vaccines since their properties (e.g., particle size, composition, antigen/immunomodulator loading) can be fine-tuned to induce peripheral tolerance. Furthermore, NPs can be employed as platforms to regulate the doses and delivery times not only of the self-antigens but also of the tolerogenic adjuvants that are required to promote tolerance [70].

Poly(lactic-co-glycolic acid) (PLGA) NPs are non-toxic, biodegradable/biocompatible and have the advantage of being FDA approved for various clinical uses including drug delivery, diagnostics, etc. Additionally, surface functionalization strategies may improve their interaction with cells, thus optimizing cell targeting and vaccine performance. PLGA NPs are the most extensively assessed nanocarriers in pre-clinical models of autoimmune diseases and their effectiveness regarding antigen-specific immunotherapies (Table 5) represents a proof-of-concept of the feasibility of nanoparticle-aided tolerogenic vaccination. Furthermore, their successful application in animal models appears encouraging concerning potential translation to humans [70].

4.5.2. Soluble Antigen Arrays

Soluble antigen arrays (SAgAs) are synthesized by co-grafting the immunodominant epitope $PLP_{139-151}$ and LABL peptide (i.e., ligand of the intercellular adhesion molecule 1, ICAM-1) to hyaluronic acid (HA) via a hydrolysable oxime bond [182,183]. Their size can be fine-tuned to allow them to drain to the lymph nodes [183]. Another key factor affecting their drainage is the injection site and the molecular weight of HA. For example, following s.c. injection, HA can drain to the lymphatics and its retention time can be affected by its molecular weight [183].

The efficiency of the hydrolysable $SAgA_{PLP-LABL}$ to suppress disease in mice with EAE has been reported in various studies (Table 5) and has been attributed to the simultaneous delivery of the myelin derived antigen and the cell adhesion signal [182]. Furthermore, earlier in vitro studies indicated that SAgAs demonstrate Ag-specific binding with B lymphocytes, target the B cell receptor (BCR) and reduce BCR-mediated signaling [184]. Based on the abovementioned experimental results indicating BCR engagement as the mechanism of action of $SAgA_{PLP-LABL}$ Hartwell and coworkers developed a novel version of $SAgA_{PLP-LABL}$, the cSAgAPLP:LABL (click SAgA), employing non-hydrolysable conjugation chemistry (e.g., copper-catalyzed azide-alkyne aycloaddition) [184,185]. cSAgAPLP:LABL was found to significantly reduce or inhibit BCR-mediated signaling and to exhibit enhanced in vivo efficiency in comparison with the hydrolytically unstable $SAgA_{PLP-LABL}$ [184,185] (Figure 11).

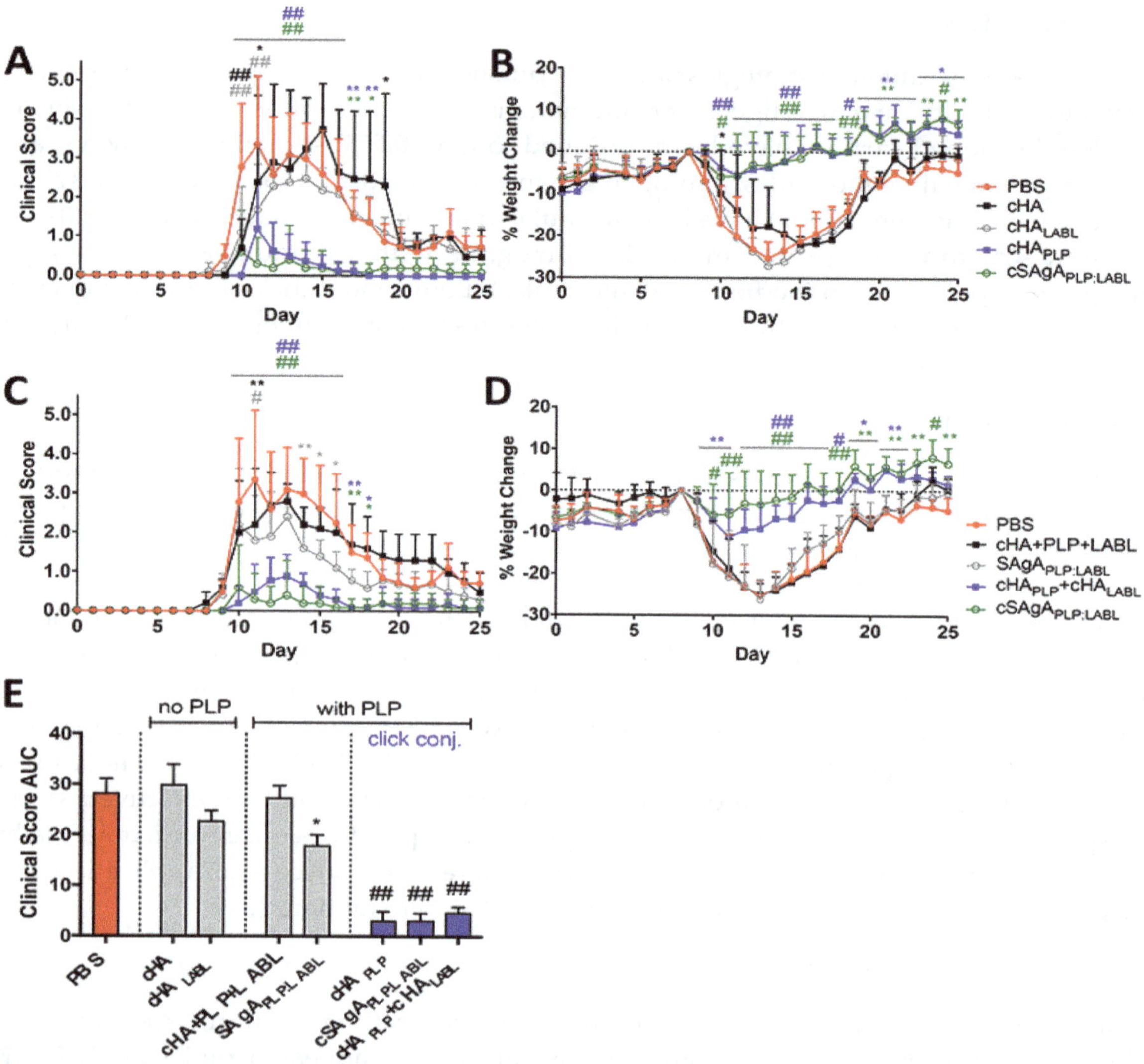

Figure 11. EAE in vivo response to click conjugates (cHA, cHALabl, cHAPLP, and cSAgAPLP:LABL) as measured by (**A**) clinical disease score and (**B**) percent weight loss. EAE in vivo response to groups containing both PLP and LABL (cHA+PLP+LABL, SAgAPLP:LABL, cHAPLP+cHALABL, and cSAgAPLP:LABL) as measured by (**C**) clinical disease score and (**D**) percent weight loss. Data represent mean ± SD ($n = 5$); statistical significance compared to PBS negative control was determined by two-way ANOVA. (**E**) Cumulative EAE in vivo response as measured by clinical disease score area under the curve (AUC) derived from subfigures A and C. Data represent mean ± SEM ($n = 5$); statistical significance compared to PBS negative control was determined by ordinary one-way ANOVA followed by Dunnett's post hoc test. (* $p < 0.05$, ** $p < 0.01$, # $p < 0.001$, ## $p < 0.0001$, color coded according to group) (with permission of [185]).

4.5.3. Immune Polyelectrolyte Multilayers (iPEMs)

It has been recently shown that excess signaling via inflammatory pathways such as toll-like receptors (TLRs) is involved in the pathogenesis of autoimmune diseases. Accordingly, the co-delivery of immunodominant myelin peptides with GpG oligonucleotide, a regulatory ligand of TLR9, could potentially limit TLR signaling during the differentiation of myelin-specific T lymphocytes, thus redirecting their differentiation towards a tolerogenic phenotype like the regulatory T cells. In this respect, immune polyelectrolyte multilayers (iPEMs) were formed using a layer-by-layer approach to co-assemble modified myelin peptides with GpG oligonucleotide. These nanostructures have key characteristics of biomaterial-based nanocarriers, such as tunable physicochemical properties and loading capacity, ability to deliver various active ingredients, etc., lacking, however, synthetic components that could exhibit inflammatory properties.

In in vitro studies, iPEMs have been shown to limit TLR9 signaling, decrease activation of DCs, and polarize myelin-specific T lymphocytes towards a tolerogenic phenotype. Additionally, they have been found to reduce inflammation and induce tolerance in mice with EAE [186,187] (Table 5).

4.5.4. pMHC-Nanoparticles (pMHC-NPs)

The "two signal theory" states that two different signals are required for the activation of naive T cells: (i) engagement of the TCR with its cognate pMHC target, and (ii) a co-stimulatory signal from molecules selectively expressed on professional APCs' surface. It is well known that engagement of the TCR on the surface of a naive T cell without co-stimulation results in the induction of apoptosis or anergy.

The development of pMHC-nanoparticles (pMHC-NPs) for the treatment of autoimmune diseases was based on the hypothesis that pMHC-coated NPs would diminish the responses of autoreactive T cells more efficiently compared with soluble pMHC complexes. This could be due to (i) their multimeric valency, (ii) their potentially superior TCR cross-linking properties compared with "artificial APCs", and (iii) the protection of the NP-bound pMHC molecules from degradation [104]. The ability of pMHC-NPs to stop the progression of EAE was assessed with in vivo experiments in mice (Table 5).

4.5.5. Mannan-Peptide Conjugates

Based on previous studies with the yeast polysaccharide, mannan, Tseveleki and coworkers, examined mannan conjugation with immunodominant myelin epitopes as an approach to divert the differentiation of myelin-specific T lymphocytes towards a regulatory phenotype, thus decreasing the mice susceptibility to EAE. It was shown that the administration of the synthesized conjugates to mice in both prophylactic and therapeutic vaccination protocols resulted in the induction of antigen-specific T cell tolerance and significant amelioration of EAE clinical and histopathological symptoms. [188] (Figure 12) (Table 5). According to these results, it was speculated that conjugation of MOG epitopes to mannan may modulate the autoimmune response in humans, thus potentially reducing the symptoms of MS [188].

4.5.6. Liposomes

Liposomes are tiny vesicles featuring an aqueous core surrounded by a lipid bilayer. They can encapsulate both hydrophilic and hydrophobic drugs and target them to specific cell surfaces via appropriate functionalization. Various types of liposomes have been already approved for clinical use (e.g., delivery of therapeutics, vaccination) and can be designed to induce or tolerate immune responses [189]. Pujol-Autonell and coworkers reported the beneficial effect of MOG peptide loaded liposomes in treating mice with EAE. Liposomes successfully delayed the onset, suppressed the severity and decreased the incidence of the disease [190]. Similarly, Belogurov and co-workers demonstrated that mannosylated liposomes containing MBP_{46-62} could significantly reduce EAE clinical signs in Dark Agouti (DA) rats [189]. Interestingly liposomes loaded with MBP_{46-62}, $MBP_{124-139}$, and $MBP_{147-170}$ and targeting CD206 were proven to be safe and well-tolerated and to normalize cytokine levels in RRMS and SPMS patients [191,192].

4.5.7. Microneedle Patches

Pires and coworkers proposed the use of minimally invasive microneedle patches for the delivery of myelin peptides, as an alternative therapeutic strategy for skin mediated antigen-specific immune tolerance in MS [178].

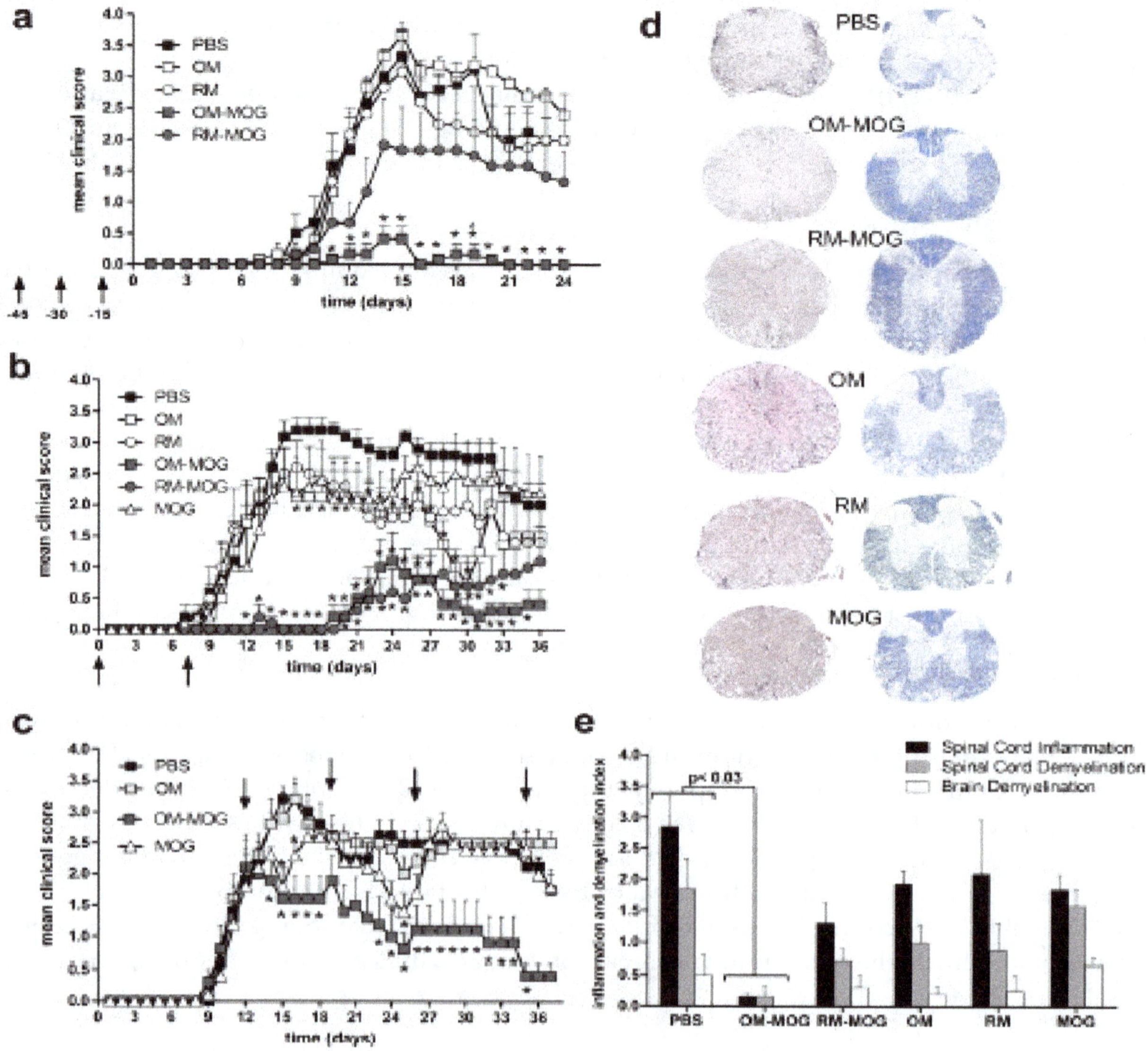

Figure 12. (**a**) Mean clinical scores of MOG-EAE in groups of mice vaccinated i.d. with OM-MOG, RM-MOG, OM, RM, or PBS at indicated time points (arrows) before immunization for EAE induction. (**b**) Mean clinical scores of MOG-EAE in groups of mice vaccinated i.d. at indicated time points (arrows) relative to immunization. (**c**) Mean clinical scores of MOG-EAE in groups of mice injected i.d. at indicated time points (arrows) after immunization. The results shown are from one representative of two (**b**,**c**) or three (**a**) independent experiments. (**d**,**e**) Vaccination with OM-MOG protects C57BL/6 mice from spinal cord inflammation and demyelination during MOG-EAE. (**d**) Inflammatory cell infiltration (left column) and demyelination (right column) were visualized on day 24 following immunization. (**e**) Quantification of spinal cord inflammation (black bars) and demyelination (grey bars) as well as brain demyelination (white bars) in all experimental groups. Representative data from five animals per group are shown. Statistical significance after comparisons between groups of mice (using the Kruskal-Wallis test) or histopathology indices (using Student's t test) is shown (*, $p < 0.05$). Triangles (**a**) indicate time points where pair-wise comparison between OM-MOG and RM-MOG groups also show significant differences (with permission of [188]).

Table 5. Carrier-aided vaccination.

Carrier	Particle Size (nm)	Zeta Potential (mV)	Antigen	Ag Loading (wt%)/Enc. Eff. (%)	Immunomodul. Agent	Vaccination Type	Admin. Route	Dose	Animal Model	Vaccination Outcome
Polymer particles										
PLGA NPs [193]	-	-	$MOG_{35–55}$	-	(r) IL-10	Prophylactic: 31 and 15 days b.i. Therapeutic: eight and 22 days p.i.	s.c.		Female C57BL/6 mice with EAE induced with $MOG_{35–55}$	Vaccination with mixed PLGA-$MOG_{35–55}$ and PLGA-IL10 both in a prophylactic and therapeutic setting resulted in significant protection, decrease of EAE severity and reduction of histopathological lesions in spinal cord.
PLGA NPs [194]	-	-	$PLP_{139–151}$	8μg/mg NP	TGF-β (166ng/mg NP)	Prophylactic: seven days b.i. Therapeutic: 13 days p.i.	i.v. s.c.	2.5, 1.25, 0.0625 mg NPs	Female SJL/J mice (6–8 weeks old) with EAE induced with $PLP_{139–151}$	i.v. vaccination with PLGA-$PLP_{139–151}$-TGF-β demonstrated improved efficiency at lower doses. s.c. delivery of TGF-β-coupled to PLGA- $PLP_{139–151}$ NPs reduced the severity of relapses in EAE.
PLGA MPs [195]	800, 55,000		$MOG_{35–55}$	-/48.6	Vitamin D3 TGF-β1 Recombinant mouse GM-CSF	Preclinical/Therapeutic: 4, 7, and 10, days p.i.	s.c.		Female C57BL/6 mice (10–11 weeks old) with EAE induced with $MOG_{35–55}$	Delivery of various immunomodulators combined with $MOG_{35–55}$ via a dual size MP platform resulted in the induction of enhanced antigen-specific autoimmune protection.
PLGA NPs [196]	151.2, 521.7	−14.1, −5.65	$MOG_{35–55}$	2.58, 0.96 /25.85, 9.65	-	Prophylactic: seven days b.i.	i.v. s.c.	2 mg NPs containing 20 μg $MOG_{35–55}$	Female C57BL/6 mice (6–8 weeks old) with EAE induced with $MOG_{35–55}$	The intravenous injection of PLGA-$MOG_{35–55}$ was shown to delay EAE incidence and enhance antigen-specific immune tolerance.

Table 5. *Cont.*

Carrier	Particle Size (nm)	Zeta Potential (mV)	Antigen	Ag Loading (wt%)/Enc. Eff. (%)	Immunomodul. Agent	Vaccination Type	Admin. Route	Dose	Animal Model	Vaccination Outcome
PLGA-PEMA NPs [197]	429.9	−67.4	$PLP_{139–151}$ $PLP_{178–191}$	0.85/10.61	-	Prophylactic: 7, 25, and 50 days b.i. Preclinical/Therapeutic: 4, 14, and 18 days p.i.	i.v. i.p. s.c. oral	0.0625 0.125 0.625 1.25	Female SJL/J mice (6-8 weeks old) with EAE induced with $PLP_{178–191}$	Vaccination with PLP epitope-coupled PLGA-PEMA NPs was shown to both prevent and treat relapsing-remitting EAE. Tolerance induction was antigen-specific. The i.v. administration route was the most effective.
PLGA/PLA-PEG NPs [198]	-	-	$PLP_{139–151}$		rapamycin	Prophylactic: 14 and 21 days b.i. Therapeutic: 13 days p.i.	s.c. i.v.		SJL mice with EAE induced with $PLP_{139–151}$	s.c. vaccination with the tolerogenic NPs inhibited paralysis. Therapeutic s.c. treatment completely inhibited EAE relapses. A single therapeutic dose of tolerogenic NP sadministered i.v. near the peak of EAE resulted in complete prevention of relapses.
PLGA-PEMA NPs [199]	377.9, 621.5–834.8	−72.8, −50 to −43.7	$PLP_{139–151}$ $PLP_{178–191}$	0.58, 0.24–0.83/7.2, 4.4–16.5	-	Prophylactic: seven days b.i. Therapeutic: 18 days p.i.	i.v.		SJL/J mice with EAE induced with $PLP_{139–151}$ or $PLP_{178–191}$	Antigen-specific immune tolerance was successfully induced by PLP encephalitogenic epitopes, encapsulated in or conjugated with PLGA-PEMA NPs.
PLGA NPs [181]	217	-	MOG40–54/H-2Db-Ig dimer, MOG35–55/I-Ab multimer	-	anti-Fas, PD-L1-Fc TGF-β1CD47-Fc	Therapeutic: 8, 18, 28, and 38 days p.i.	i.v.	1 mg NPs/ mouse/ injection	Female C57BL/6J mice (8–10 weeks old) with EAE induced with MOG35–55	Four i.v. injections of the developed NPs resulted in long-lasting amelioration of the disease by markedly reducing neuroinflammation, clinical EAE score and demyelination

Table 5. *Cont.*

Carrier	Particle Size (nm)	Zeta Potential (mV)	Antigen	Ag Loading (wt%)/Enc. Eff. (%)	Immunomodul. Agent	Vaccination Type	Admin. Route	Dose	Animal Model	Vaccination Outcome
PLGA NPs PLA NPs [200]	PLGA: 351.3–436.2 PLA: 443.2	PLGA: −40.6 to −39.8 PLA: −40.2	$PLP_{139-151}$	PLGA: 0.25–0.28 PLA: 0.25	-	Preclinical/Therapeutic: seven days p.i.	i.v.	2.5, 2.0, 1.5 or 1.0 mg NPs/mouse	Female SJL/J mice (8–10 weeks old) with EAE induced with $PLP_{139-151}$	Low dose vaccination with PLA NPs resulted in long-lasting (>200 days post immunization) significant reduction of the clinical score at the chronic stage of EAE contrary to vaccination with PLGA NPs.
PLGA MPs PEI-coated PLGA-MPs [201]	PLGA: 5080	PLGA: 45.3	MOG_{35-55} MOG_{40-54} MOG_{40-54}/H-2Db-Ig dimer, MOG35–55/I-Ab multimer		anti-Fas, PD-L1-Fc TGF-β1 CD47-Fc	Therapeutic: 8, 18, 28, and 38 days p.i.	i.v. i.p. s.c.		Female C57BL/6J mice with EAE induced with MOG_{35-55}	Four injections of the multipotent particles resulted in long-lasting suppression of EAE and reduction of neuroinflammation in an antigen-specific manner.
PLGA MPs [202]	8000		Ac-PLP-BPI-NH2-2	24/8.2		Preclinical/Therapeutic: 4, 7, 10, and 14 days p.i.	s.c.		Female SJL/J mice (5–7 weeks old) with EAE induced with PLP139–151	Administration of PLGA MPs resulted in slightly less efficient reduction of EAE symptoms compared with the administration of the peptide solution, but without toxicity.
PLGA [203]	400–656	−51.3 to −38.0	PLP $_{139-151}$ PLP $_{178-191}$	0.26–0.8		Prophylactic: seven and one days b.i.	i.v.		Female SJL/J mice (6–8 weeks old) with EAE induced with $PLP_{139-151}$ or both $PLP_{139-151}$ and $PLP_{178-191}$	PLGA NPs coupled with a PLP encephalitogenic epitope were shown to efficiently induce antigen-specific tolerance in a mouse model of relapsing-remitting EAE induced either by $PLP_{139-151}$ or by both $PLP_{139-151}$ and $PLP_{178-191}$

Table 5. *Cont.*

Carrier	Particle Size (nm)	Zeta Potential (mV)	Antigen	Ag Loading (wt%)/Enc. Eff. (%)	Immunomodul. Agent	Vaccination Type	Admin. Route	Dose	Animal Model	Vaccination Outcome
PLGA NPs [204]	363–420	-	$PLP_{139–151}$		LABL	Preclinical/Therapeutic: 4, 7, and 10 days p.i.	s.c.	100 nmol PLP per injection	SJL/J female mice (5–7 weeks old) with EAE induced with $PLP_{139–151}$	It was shown that efficient suppression of EAE required the co-administration of PLP peptide and LABL.
PLGA [205]	538	−43	$PLP_{139–151}$	0.41–0.98	-	Preclinical/Therapeutic: seven days p.i.	i.v.	1 to 100 µg/mL NPs per injection	SJL/J mice with EAE induced with $PLP_{139–151}$	Antigen-specific, dose-dependent tolerance was successfully induced in an EAE model via the administration of PLGA NPs couple with a PLP peptide.
PLGA [206]	500	-	$PLP_{139–151}$	-	IL2	Prophylactic: secen days b.i. Therapeutic: 11 days p.i.	i.v.		SJL/J mice with EAE induced with $PLP_{139–151}$	Vaccination with PLGA NPs loaded with $PLP_{139–151}$ was found to prevent EAE onset and modulate its course.
PLGA MPs [207]	3900	-	$MOG_{35–55}$	0.73/38	Rapamycin (loading: 0.17%/enc. eff. 42.1%)	Therapeutic: 10 days p.i.	direct intra-lymph node (LN) injection	2 mg MPs per mouse or 1 mg MPs per LN	Female C57BL/6J mice (10–11 weeks old) with EAE induced with $MOG_{35–55}$	A single intra-LN injection (at the peak of EAE) of PLGA NPs containing a MOG peptide and rapamycin was revealed to permanently reverse paralysis.
Colloidal gel based on self-assembly of PLGA-CS and PLGA-Alginate NPs [208]	PLGA-CS: 400.1, PLGA-Alginate: 208.1	PLGA-CS: 23.79 PLGA-Alginate: −38.85,	Ac-PLP-BPI-NH_2-2		-	Prophylactic: five days b.i. Preclinical/Therapeutic: four and 30 days p.i.	s.c.	300 nmol of colloidal gel per injection	Mice (6–8 weeks old) with EAE PLP139–151	A single injection of the colloidal gel containing the Ac-PLP-BPI-NH_2-2 peptide led to long-term disease suppression.

Table 5. *Cont.*

Carrier	Particle Size (nm)	Zeta Potential (mV)	Antigen	Ag Loading (wt%)/Enc. Eff. (%)	Immunomodul. Agent	Vaccination Type	Admin. Route	Dose	Animal Model	Vaccination Outcome
Soluble antigen arrays (SAgAs)										
HA-peptide conjugate [209]	HA	-	$PLP_{139–151}$	-	LABL, B7AP, CD80-CAP1, sF2 (cyclized)	Preclinical/Therapeutic: 4, 7, and 10 days p.i.	s.c.	200 nmol PLP peptide	SJL/J (H-2s) female mice (4–6 weeks old) with EAE induced with $PLP_{139–151}$	SAgAs were shown to effectively reduce EAE incidence and suppress it via co-administration of an immunodominant myelin epitope and peptides targeting the B7 signaling pathway.
SAgAs [210]	HA	-	$PLP_{139–151}$	-	LABL	Preclinical/Therapeutic: 4, 7, and 10 days p.i.	s.c.	200 nmol $PLP_{139–151}$	SJL/J female mice (4–6 weeks old) with EAE induced with $PLP_{139–151}$	Co-administration via conjugation of $PLP_{139–151}$ and LABL improved the clinical scores of EAE
cSAgAs [184]	HA	-	$PLP_{139–151}$		LABL	Preclinical/Therapeutic: 4, 7, and 10 days p.i.	s.c.	50, 133, or 200 nmol $PLP_{139–151}$	SJL/J female mice (4–6 weeks old) with EAE induced with $PLP_{139–151}$	cSAgAs was found to achieve equivalent efficiency with SAgAS regarding the suppression of EAE at a quarter of the SAgAS dose.
cSAgAs (Figure 11) [185]	HA	-	$PLP_{139–151}$	-	LABL	Preclinical/Therapeutic: 4, 7, and 10 days p.i.	s.c.	50, nmol $PLP_{139–151}$	SJL/J female mice (4–6 weeks old) with EAE induced with $PLP_{139–151}$	Low dose s.c. vaccination with cSAgAS resulted in successful suppression of EAE clinical symproms and minimization of body weight loss.
SAgAs [210]	HA	-	$PLP_{139–151}$	-	LABL	Preclinical/Therapeutic: 4, 7, and 10 days p.i.	pulmonary	65.1–74.5 mg SAgAs/mouse kg	Female SJL/J mice (four weeks old) with EAE induced with $PLP_{139–151}$	The pulmonary administration of SAgAs was found to suppress the clinical score of the disease, decrease EAE incidence and improve weight gain.

Table 5. *Cont.*

Carrier	Particle Size (nm)	Zeta Potential (mV)	Antigen	Ag Loading (wt%)/Enc. Eff. (%)	Immunomodul. Agent	Vaccination Type	Admin. Route	Dose	Animal Model	Vaccination Outcome
SAgAs [183]	HA	-	$PLP_{139–151}$	-	LABL	Preclinical/Therapeutic: 4, 7, or 10 days p.i.	i.p., upper and lower i.m., upper and lower s.c., i.v. pulmonary	200 nMol PLP per 100 μL injection volume 200 nMol PLP per 50 μL injection volume	Female SJL/J mice (6–8 weeks old) with EAE induced with $PLP_{139–151}$	i.v. administration demonstrated similar efficiency with the other routes. p.i. vaccination decreased completely clinical disease scores. Single injection-based treatment resulted in decreased efficiency compared with a triple injection treatment. Decrease of SAgAs dose and/or injection volume decreased the therapeutic efficiency.
Immune polyelectrolyte multilayers (iPEMs)										
iPEMs [186]	-	-	MOG-R3	28.4–89.7%	GpG (0.7–10.3%)	Preclinical/Therapeutic: 5 and 10 p.i.	s.c.	200 μg of (MOG-R3/GpG)3 iPEMs, per injection.	C57BL/6J mice with EAE induced with a myelin antigen	s.c. delivery of iPEMs restrained inflammation and promoted autoimmune tolerance in an EAE mouse models.
iPEMs [187]	114.9–199.2	−42.5 to 33.4	MOGR1, MOGR2	0.57–9.18 μg of MOGRx	GpG 2.18 μg–4.88 μg	Preclinical/Therapeutic: seven days or 6, 12, and 18 days p.i.	s.c.	200 μg MOGR2 (85.9 μg GpG)	Female C57BL/6J mice (10 weeks old) with EAE induced with $MOG_{35–55}$	iPEMs were shown to improve the severity, progression and incidence of EAE.
Inorganic particles and pMHC-nanoparticles (pMHC-NPs)										
Quantum dots [211]	15.0–21.0	−17.6 to −4.2	MOG	Up to 55	-	Preclinical: two days p.i.	s.c.		Female C57BL/6 mice (10–12 weeks old)	Ten-fold reduction of EAE incidence. Increased numbers of QDs with lower peptide loading were more efficient regarding the induction of immune tolerance.

Table 5. *Cont.*

Carrier	Particle Size (nm)	Zeta Potential (mV)	Antigen	Ag Loading (wt%)/Enc. Eff. (%)	Immunomodul. Agent	Vaccination Type	Admin. Route	Dose	Animal Model	Vaccination Outcome
Iron oxide NPs [212]	-	-	$MOG_{38–49}$	-	IA^b	Therapeutic: 14 or 21 days p.i.			C57BL/6 mice with EAE induced with $pMOG_{35–55}$	By administration on day 14 the NPs were found to diminish the progression of the disease, whereas when administered on day 21 they were shown to restore the motor function of paralytic mice.
Iron oxide NPs [212]	-	-	$hPLP_{175–192}$ $hMOG_{97–108}$	-	DR4-IE	Therapeutic:			*HLA-DR4-IE-* transgenic C57BL/6 *IAb*null mice	Successful EAE suppression was observed.
Pegylated gold NPs [213]	60	-	$MOG_{35–55}$ $PLP_{139–151}$ $PLP_{178–191}$		AhR ligand ITE	Prophylactic: admin. on the day of EAE induction Therapeutic: Admin. on day 17 post immunization. Weekly treatment of mice	parenteral	6 μg NPs per mouse	B6 mice with EAE induced with $MOG_{35–55}$ SJL mice with EAE induced with EAE induced with $PLP_{139–151}$	Pegylated gold NPs loaded with MOG35-55 and ITE significantly suppressed the development of EAE, whereas those loaded with PLP epitopes reduced the clinical scores of the disease and the number of relapses.
Mannan-conjugated myelin peptides										
Mannan-peptide conjugates (Figure 12) [188]	-	-	$MOG_{35–55}$, $PLP_{139–151}$, $PLP_{178–191}$, $MBP_{83–99}$	-	-	Prophylactic: 45, 30, and 15 days b.i. Preclinical/Therapeutic: Admin. on day 0 and 7 p.i.	i.d.	30 μg peptide/injection 700 μg mannan/injection	C57BL/6 mice (12–14 weeks old) with EAE induced with MOG Female SJL/J mice (6–8 weeks old) with EAE induced with PLP.	Mannan-peptide conjugates were shown to generate robust antigen-specific protection of mice from the clinical disease symptoms.
Mannan-peptide conjugates [214]	-	-	Linear and cyclic $MBP_{83–99}$ peptide analogues cyclo(83-99) [A91]MBP83-99 mutant peptide			Preclinical/Therapeutic: Admin. on day 0 and 14 p.i.	i.d.	50 μg of linear and cyclic $MBP_{83–99}$ peptide analogues	Female SJL/J mice (6–8 weeks old) with EAE induced with linear and cyclic $MBP_{83–99}$ peptide analogues	It was shown that the mutant peptide cyclo(83–99)[A91] $MBP_{83–99}$ more efficiently inhibited EAE development.

Table 5. *Cont.*

Carrier	Particle Size (nm)	Zeta Potential (mV)	Antigen	Ag Loading (wt%)/Enc. Eff. (%)	Immunomodul. Agent	Vaccination Type	Admin. Route	Dose	Animal Model	Vaccination Outcome
Liposomes										
Liposomes [190]	861.3	−36.2	$MOG_{40–55}$	-/91.5	-	Preclinical/Therapeutic: 5 and 9 days p.i.	i.p.	1.75 mg of lipid per injection	C57BL/6 female mice (8 weeks old) with EAE induced with $MOG_{40–55}$	Liposomes successfully delayed the onset, suppressed the severity and decreased the incidence of the disease.
(mannosylated) SUV [189]	~85	−7.5 to −10.5	$MBP_{46–62}$ $MBP_{124–139}$ $MBP_{147–170}$	-/90	-	Preclinical/Therapeutic: admin. on day 7 post immunization followed by five consecutive days.	s.c.		Female DA rats (8–9 weeks old) with EAE induced with a syngeneic spinal cord homogenate or with MBP_{63-81}.	It was revealed that mSUVs loaded with immunodominant epitopes of MBP could significantly suppress EAE in DA rats.
Exosomes										
mTGF-β1-EXOs [215]	50–100					Prophylactic: 8, 5, and 2 days b.i. Therapeutic: 14, 17 and 21 days p.i.	i.v.	10 μg/mouse/injection	Female C57BL/6 mice (6–8 weeks) with EAE induced with $MOG_{35–55}$ Female BALB/c mice (6–8 weeks) with EAE induced with $PLP_{180-199}$	Treatment with mTGF-β1-EXOs from C57BL/6 mice successfully inhibited the development and progression of the disease in both mice strains.

Table 5. *Cont.*

Carrier	Particle Size (nm)	Zeta Potential (mV)	Antigen	Ag Loading (wt%)/Enc. Eff. (%)	Immunomodul. Agent	Vaccination Type	Admin. Route	Dose	Animal Model	Vaccination Outcome
Antigen-presenting yeast cells										
C. utilis expressing MOG_{35-55} on its surface [216]	-	-	MOG_{35-55} pCB13 pCB10			Prophylactic: admin. on day 7 prior to immunization and for six consecutive days	Oral	1.5×10^8 *C. utilis*	Female C57BL/6 mice (eight weeks old) with EAE induced with MOG_{35-55}	*C. utilis* expressing MOG_{35-55} on its surface appeared to be a promising approach to protect myelin against autoimmunity by effectively inducing oral tolerance. Fungal viability was not found to affect the induction of tolerance.

PLGA: poly(lactide-co-glycolide); NPs: nanoparticles; MOG: myelin oligodendrocyte glycoprotein; (r) IL-10: recombinant interleukin; s.c.: subcutaneous; b.i.: before immunization; p.i.: post immunization; EAE: experimental autoimmune encephalomyelitis; PLP: proteolipid protein; TGF-β: transforming growth factor beta 1; i.v.: intravenous; MPs: microparticles; GM-CSF: granulocyte-macrophage colony-stimulating factor; PEMA: poly[ethylene-alt-maleic anhydride]; i.p.: intraperitoneal; PEG: polyethylene glycol; PLA: polylactide; PEI: polyethylene imine; Ac-PLP-BPI-NH2-2: (Ac-HSLGKWLGHPDKF-(AcpGAcpGAcp)2-ITDGEATDSG-NH2; Ac = acetyl, Acp = aminocaproic acid); CS: chitosan; SAgAs: soluble antigen arrays; HA: hyaluronic acid; LABL: ICAm-I binding peptide; cSAgAs: Click Soluble Antigen Arrays; i.p.: intraperitoneal; i.m.: intramuscular; iPEMs: immune polyelectrolyte multilayers; GpG: GpG oligonucleotide; MOGR3: MOG conjugated to tri-arginine; MOGR1 and MOGR2: MOG modified with either one or two cationic arginine residues; SUV: small unilamellar vesicles; mTGF-β1-EXOs: exosomes from dendritic cells expressing membrane-associated TGF-β1.

5. Clinical Trials

Various tolerance-inducing vaccination approaches (e.g., immunodominant myelin epitopes, APLs, DNA vaccination, attenuated autologous myelin reactive T cells, tolerogenic DCs, TCR peptide vaccination, nanocarriers loaded with encephalitogenic myelin peptides, etc.) with promising outcomes in experimental MS models have already reached the clinical development phase. Their safety, feasibility, and efficiency in inducing antigen-specific immune tolerance and reducing MRI-detected disease activity in patients with relapsing remitting and progressive MS have been preliminary demonstrated in phase I and II clinical trials [14,136,139] (Table 6).

6. Conclusions

Several exciting vaccination strategies targeting the induction of antigen-specific immune tolerance in MS have been developed during the last decades, based on a single epitope or cocktails of immunodominant epitopes of myelin proteins, altered peptide ligands, DNA vaccines, tolerogenic DCs pulsed with myelin peptides, attenuated autologous myelin reactive T cells, TCR peptide vaccines, conjugates of autoantigens with various types of cells, and different types of carriers (e.g., particles, vesicles, self-assembled structures, or molecular carriers) associated with myelin epitopes. Most of these approaches have demonstrated promising results in animal models of experimental autoimmune encephalomyelitis both in prophylactic and therapeutic vaccination protocols. They successfully prevented the disease or delayed the disease onset, reduced its clinical and pathological symptoms and decreased the number of relapses, or, in a therapeutic scheme, they reversed the clinical and histological signs of the disease. Accordingly, numerous of the abovementioned strategies reached the clinical development phase, and their safety, feasibility, and efficacy were assessed in both phase I and II clinical trials. However, the results from these trials have not indicated the same level of efficiency as in preclinical models. Even though different tolerance-inducing vaccination strategies were proven safe and well tolerated, and in some cases succeeded in inducing tolerogenic responses to patients, no major advances have been reported with respect to clinical efficiency. Consequently, despite the intensive research efforts, up to the present time, no FDA approved antigen-specific immunotherapy is available for treating MS patients. It appears that antigen-specific immunotherapies still face various major challenges such as the involvement of multiple autoantigens that can vary between patients, the epitope spreading, the vaccination of patients with inapparent infections, etc. These challenges need to be overcome in order to allow tolerogenic vaccines to play a major role in the treatment of MS patients. Progress in the scientific areas of recombinant protein expression, genome editing, and smartly designed carriers, combined with better understanding of MS immunopathogenesis and improved immunization protocols, could potentially improve these vaccination strategies in the future. Additionally, further clinical studies, such as phase II and III, including placebo groups, will be required in order to more realistically assess the clinical effectiveness of these interesting antigen-specific immunotherapies in both RRMS and SPMS patients.

Table 6. Clinical trials.

Objective	Phase	No. of Particip.	Antigen Immunotherapy	Admin. Route/Dose/Duration of Treatment	Results
To suppress disease activity in RRMS patients using CGP77116 [74]	II	24	CGP77116	s.c. injection/50 mg CGP77116 per week; 5 mg per week; 5 mg per month/9 months	Decrease of dose because of adverse effects. Trial termination due to treatment-related disease exacerbation.
Evaluation of NBI 5788 safety, and effect on RRMS patients [217]	II	144	NBI5788	s.c. injection/5, 20, or 50 mg NBI5788 per week/4 months	Trial suspension due to hypersensitivity reactions in some patients. No increase in relapses. Reduction of number and volume of enhancing lesions in patients who completed the trial receiving 5 mg of NBI5788 per week.
Assessment of safety, tolerability and clinical activity of AG284 in SPMS patients [218]	I	33	AG284	/0.6, 2, 6, 20, 60, 105, and 150 mg AG284/kg body weight; each dose was received daily for three alternate days/	No adverse events but also no significant therapeutic effect could be observed.
Assessment of the clinical efficiency of MBP_{82-98} in patients with progressive MS [219]	II	32	MBP_{82-98}	i.v./500 mg MBP_{82-98} per 6 months/24 months	Only patients with HLA haplotypes DR2 and/or DR4 appeared to have benefited from the treatment.
Evaluation of the safety and efficiency of MBP_{82-98} in SPMS patients with HLA haplotypes DR2 and/or DR4 [220]	III	612	MBP_{82-98}	i.v./500 mg MBP_{82-98} per 6 months/2 years	The administration of was safe and well tolerated. The treatment was not effective in SPMS patients with HLA $DR2^+$ or $DR4^+$
Evaluation of RTL1000 safety in MS patients [221]	I	34	RTL1000	i.v./2, 6, 20, 60, 200, and 100 mg of RTL/	RTL1000 was safe at doses ≤ 60 mg
Determination of the maximum tolerable dose and safety of RTL1000 in MS patients [222]	I	36	RTL1000	i.v./2, 6, 20, 60, 200, and 100 mg of RTL/	The maximum tolerable dose of RTL100 was 60 mg.
Examination of the effect of high dose MBP_{82-98} on the number of regulatory T cells in CPMS patients [223]		10	MBP_{82-98}	i.v./500 mg of MBP_{82-98} per 6 months/	Increase in the number of regulatory T cells in patients' PBMCs six weeks and six6 months after treatment. Renversement of the state of T cell anergy.
Assessment of safety and tolerability of autologous PBMCs coupled with 7 myelin peptides in RRMS and SPMS patients [224]	I	9	PBMCs chemically coupled with the following 7 myelin peptides: MOG_{1-20}, MOG_{35-55}, MBP_{13-32}, MBP_{83-99}, $MBP_{111-129}$, $MBP_{146-170}$, and $PLP_{139-154}$	Single infusion/1×10^3, 1×10^5, 1×10^7, 1×10^8, 1×10^9, 2.5×10^9 and 3×10^9 antigen-coupled PBMCs/3 months	The treatment was found to be safe and well-tolerated. Antigen-specific T cell responses were shown to decrease after treatment in patients who received doses $\geq 1 \times 10^9$ of antigen coupled PBMCs.
Examination of BHT-3009 safety and feasibility for immune nodulation in RRMS and SPMS patients [225]	I/II	30	BHT-3009	i.m./0.5, 1.5, and 3 mg of BHT-3009 at weeks 1, 3, 5, and 9 after patients' randomization into the clinical trial/The administration of BHT-3009 was combined or not with daily oral administration of 80 mg atorvastatin.	BHT-3009 was found to be safe and to induce antigen-specific immune tolerance in MS patients. The co-administration of atorvastatin was not considered substantially beneficial.
Assessment of the transdermal delivery of a mixture of three myelin peptides to induce immune tolerance in RRMS patients [226]		30	Mixture of the following 3 myelin peptides: MBP_{85-99}, $PLP_{139-151}$, and MOG_{35-55}	Transdermal (via an adhesive skin patch)/1 or 10 mg of each myelin peptide per week (for 4 weeks) and per month (for 11 months)/1 year	The transdermal administration of myelin peptides was proven to be tolerogenic in RRMS patients.

Table 6. *Cont.*

Objective	Phase	No. of Particip.	Antigen Immunotherapy	Admin. Route/Dose/Duration of Treatment	Results
Assessment of safety and efficiency of transdermal administration of myelin peptides in RRMS patients [227]		30	Mixture of the following three myelin peptides: $MBP_{85–99}$, $MOG_{35–55}$, and $PLP_{139–151}$	Transdermal (via an adhesive skin patch)/1 or 10 mg of each myelin peptide per week (for four weeks) and per month (for 11 months)/1 year	The transdermal delivery of myelin peptides was found to be safe, well tolerated and to reduce clinical symptoms and number of Gadolinium lesions in RRMS patients.
Evaluation of BHT-3009 regarding its safety and efficiency to induce immune tolerance in RRMS patients [228,229]	II	289	BHT-3009	i.m./ 0.5 and 1.5 mg of BHT-3009 at weeks 0, 2, 4, and every four weeks until week 44/The administration of BHT-3009 was combined or not with daily oral administration of 80 mg atorvastatin.	It was shown that treatment with the lower dose of BHT-3009 (e.g., 0.5 mg) succeeded in inducing antigen-specific immune tolerance in some patients in contrast with the higher dose (e.g., 1.5 mg) which was found to be ineffective.
Evaluation of ATX-MS-1467 safety in SPMS patients [117]	I	6	ATX-MS-1467	i.d/25, 50, 100, 400, and 800 µg of ATX-MS-1467/	The safety and tolerability of ATX-MS-1467 at a dose ≤ 800 µg, was successfully demonstrated in SPMS patients.
Evaluation of ATX-MS-1467 safety, tolerability and efficiency to induce tolerance in RRMS patients [230]	Ib, IIa	43, 37	ATX-MS-1467	Ib: i.d. (cohort 1) or s.c. (cohort 2)/25, 50, 100, 400 and 800 µg of ATXMS-1467 per two weeks (for eight weeks) and 800 µg per two weeks (for eight more weeks)/one year (including 32 weeks medication off study). IIa: i.d./50 µg of ATXMS-1467 (on day 1), 200 µg (on day 15), 800 µg (on day 29), and 800 µg per two weeks (for 16 more weeks)/one year (including 16 weeks medication off study).	Both treatment protocols were found to be safe. The relatively slow i.d. titration of ATX-MS-1467 followed by a longer high dose treatment period resulted in reduced GdE lesions which remained so even post treatment.
Tolerogenic DCs (tolDCs)					
Evaluation of the safety of myelin peptide loaded tolDCs and their ability of to induce immune tolerance in MS patients. [231]	I	8	Autologous tolDCs loaded with myelin peptides	i.v./50×10^6, 100×10^6, 150×10^6, and 300×10^6 tolDCs divided in three independent doses administered every two weeks/	Myelin peptide loaded tolDCs were proven to be safe and well tolerated, and to induce tolerogenic responses in MS patients.
Evaluation of the safety of intradermal and intranodal delivery myelin peptide loaded tolDCs and their efficacy regarding the induction of antigen-specific tolerization in MS patients [232]	I	9–15	Autologous peptide-mix loaded tolDCs	i.d. or intranodal/six repetitive doses of 5×10^6, 10×10^6 and 15×10^6 autologous peptide-mix loaded tolDCs: administration of doses 1–4 once every two weeks and of doses 5–6 once every month.	-

Table 6. *Cont.*

Objective	Phase	No. of Particip.	Antigen Immunotherapy	Admin. Route/Dose/Duration of Treatment	Results
T-cell vaccination (TCVs)					
Assessment of safety and immune efficiency of a polyclonal T cell vaccine in chronic MS patients in advanced diseases stages [233]		39	autological polyclonal TCVs	s.c./1.5–3 × 10^7 polyclonal T cells; four weekly injections followed by monthly injections.	Polyclonal TCV was proven safe and capable of inducing long-lasting, anti-inflammatory immune effects in progressive MS patients in advanced disease states.
To establish a safe and efficient dose of Tovaxin® [234]		9–15	Attenuated T cells reactive to the following myelin peptides $MBP_{83–99}$, $MBP_{151–170}$, $PLP_{30–49}$, $PLP_{180–199}$, $MOG_{1–17}$ and $MOG_{19–39}$	s.c./6–9 × 10^6, 30–45 × 10^6, and 60–90 × 10^6 administered at weeks 0, 4, 12, and 20/	The study indicated the mid-dose as optimum with respect to safety, and efficiency in reducing peripheral blood myelin reactive T cells and showing a trend to improve clinical symptoms.
Evaluation of safety and efficacy of Tovaxin in RRMS patients [235]	IIb	150	T cells reactive to different immunodominant peptides from three myelin proteins	s.c./five injections at weeks 0, 4, 8, 12, and 24	s.c. administration of Tovaxin was shown to be safe. Evidence of clinical efficiency of Tovaxin® was observed during the analysis of subgroups of patients naïve to prior disease modifying therapies.
Examination of TCV safety and efficiency in progressive MS patients [236]	II	26	T-cell lines reactive to nine different peptides of MBP, MOG and PLP.	19 patients received s.c. TCV/10–30 × 10^6 T cells, on days 1, 30, 90 and 180/7 patients received sham injections.	The clinical trial demonstrated the safety of TCV in progressive MS patients and indicated its clinical efficiency.
Assessment of TCV safety and immune modulation in RRMS and CPMS patients [237]	pilot	5	CSF derived activated CD4+T cells	3 s.c. injections; 10^6 cells at months 2, 4, and 6.	TCV was safe and well tolerated. Patients were clinically stable or exhibited reduced EDSS without relapses during and post treatment.
Examine if the depletion of T cells reactive to MBP would have a clinical benefit for RRMS and SPMS patients [238]	Preliminary	54	Irradiated autologous T cells reactive to MBP-	3 s.c. injections at 2 month intervals, 30 × 10^6–60 × 10^6 cells per injection.	A 40% decrease in the relapses rate and a minimal decrease in EDSS was observed in RRMS patients. On the other hand, a slight increase of EDSS was detected in SPMS patients. Finally, MRI scans indicated a stabilization of the lesion activity.
Assess the use of T cell lines reacting with a broad range of antigens regarding targeting and depletion of specific T cells reactive to a great number of myelin antigens in SPMS patients. [239]	Pilot	4	Peripheral blood derived T cell lines reactive to bovine myelin		TCV with T cells reactive to whole bovine myelin were shown to efficiently promote depletion of circulating T cells reactive to myelin protein.
Evaluation of the TCV efficiency in patients with aggressive RRMS non-responding to DMTs [240]		20	Autologous attenuated T cell lines reactive to MBP and MOG encephalitogenic peptides.	Three s.c. injections in six- to eight-week intervals.	TCV was proven to be safe. A decrease in the relapse rate was observed. Additionally, significant decrease in the active lesions regarding number and volume as well as in T2 lesion burden was detected.
Identification of the idiotypic determinants triggering CD81 cytotoxic anti-idiotypic responses by TCV in MS patients [241]		3	Irradiated autologous T cell clones reactive to $MBP_{83–99}$	s.c./repetitive injections of 2 × 10^7 of each cell clone every 2 months for 8 months.	CD3-specific T cells were recognized as a representative anti-idiotypic population of T cells induced by TCV.

Table 6. *Cont.*

Objective	Phase	No. of Particip.	Antigen Immunotherapy	Admin. Route/Dose/Duration of Treatment	Results
T-cell receptor (TCR)					
To examine the therapeutic potential of a trivalent TCR vaccine in MS patients [242]		23	A trivalent TCR vaccine containing the CDR2 peptides BV5S2, BV6S5 and BV13S1	12 monthly vaccinations	The therapeutic TCR vaccine induced an extended immunoregulatory network which could control complex self-reactive responses of MS.
Liposomes					
Assessment of Xemys safety and efficiency in treating RRMS and SPMS patients non-responding to DMTs [191,192]	I	20	Xemys: Liposomes loaded with MBP_{46-62}, $MBP_{124-139}$ and $MBP_{147-170}$ And targeting CD206	s.c./six weekly injections of 50, 150, 225, 450, 900, and 900 μg Xemys	The administration of Xemys was proven to be safe and well tolerated, and to normalize cytokine levels in RRMS and SPMS patients.

RRMS: relapsing remitting multiple sclerosis; CGP77116: APL of MBP_{83-99}; APL: antigen peptide ligand; MBP: myelin basic protein; s.c.: subcutaneous; NBI 5788: APL of MBP_{83-99}; AG284: solubilized complex of HLA-DR2 with MBP_{84-102}; HLA: human leucocyte antigen; SPMS: secondary progressive multiple sclerosis; i.v.: intravenous; RTL1000: recombinant T-cell receptor ligand 1000; CPMS: chronic progressive multiple sclerosis; PBMCs: peripheral blood mononuclear cells; BHT-3009: tolerizing DNA vaccine encoding MBP; i.m.: intramuscular; ATX-MS-1467: mixture of equal quantities of synthetic peptides ATX-MS1 (MBP_{30-44}), ATX-MS4 ($MBP_{131-145}$), ATX-MS6 ($MBP_{140-154}$), and ATX-MS7 (MBP_{83-99}) in PBS; PBS: phosphate-buffered saline; i.d.: intradermal; tolDCs: tolerogenic dendritic cells; Tovaxin®: autologous T-cell immunotherapy; MOG:, PLP:; CSF:; DMTs: disease modifying therapies; CDR2: complementarity determining region 2.

Author Contributions: O.K. and C.K. contributed equally to the conceptualization, writing/preparation of the original draft, and writing—review and editing of the final paper. All authors have read and agreed to the published version of the manuscript.

References

1. Harrington, E.P.; Bergles, D.E.; Calabresi, P.A. Immune cell modulation of oligodendrocyte lineage cells. *Neurosci. Lett.* **2020**, *715*, 134601. [CrossRef]
2. Baecher-Allan, C.; Kaskow, B.J.; Weiner, H.L. Multiple sclerosis: Mechanisms and immunotherapy. *Neuron* **2018**, *97*, 742–768. [CrossRef] [PubMed]
3. Dendrou, C.A.; Fugger, L.; Friese, M.A. Immunopathology of multiple sclerosis. *Nature Rev. Immunol.* **2015**, *15*, 545–558. [CrossRef] [PubMed]
4. Afshar, B.; Khalifehzadeh-Esfahani, Z.; Seyfizadeh, N.; Danbaran, G.R.; Hemmatzadeh, M.; Mohammadi, H. The role of immune regulatory molecules in multiple sclerosis. *J. Neuroimmunol.* **2019**, *337*, 577061. [CrossRef] [PubMed]
5. Greer, J.M.; Pender, M.P. Myelin proteolipid protein: An effective autoantigen and target of autoimmunity in multiple sclerosis. *J. Autoimmun.* **2008**, *31*, 281–287. [CrossRef] [PubMed]
6. Iwanowski, P.; Losy, J. Immunological differences between classical phenothypes of multiple sclerosis. *J. Neurol. Sci.* **2015**, *349*, 10–14. [CrossRef]
7. Lee, D.-H.; Linker, R.A. The role of myelin oligodendrocyte glycoprotein in autoimmune demyelination: A target for multiple sclerosis therapy? *Expert Opin. Ther. Targets* **2012**, *16*, 451–462. [CrossRef]
8. Rangachari, M.; Kuchroo, V.K. Using EAE to better understand principles of immune function and autoimmune pathology. *J. Autoimmun.* **2013**, *45*, 31–39. [CrossRef]
9. Lüssi, F.; Zipp, F.; Witsch, E. Dendritic cells as therapeutic targets in neuroinflammation. *Cell. Mol. Life Sci.* **2016**, *73*, 2425–2450. [CrossRef]
10. Ho, P.P.; Fontoura, P.; Platten, M.; Sobel, R.A.; DeVoss, J.J.; Lee, L.Y.; Kidd, B.A.; Tomooka, B.H.; Capers, J.; Agrawal, A.; et al. A Suppressive oligodeoxynucleotide enhances the efficacy of myelin cocktail/IL-4-tolerizing DNA vaccination and treats autoimmune disease. *J. Immunol.* **2005**, *175*, 6226–6234. [CrossRef]
11. Hemmer, B.; Nessler, S.; Zhou, D.; Kieseier, B.; Hartung, H.-P. Immunopathogenesis and immunotherapy of multiple sclerosis. *Nat. Clin. Prac. Neurol.* **2006**, *2*, 201–211. [CrossRef] [PubMed]
12. Hellings, N.; Raus, J.; Stinissen, P. T-cell based immunotherapy in multiple sclerosis: Induction of regulatory immune networks by T-cell vaccination. *Expert Rev. Clin. Immunol.* **2006**, *2*, 705–716. [CrossRef] [PubMed]
13. Zhou, Y.; Fang, L.; Peng, L.; Qiu, W. TLR9 and its signaling pathway in multiple sclerosis. *J. Neurol. Sci.* **2017**, *373*, 95–99. [CrossRef] [PubMed]
14. Willekens, B.; Cools, N. Beyond the magic bullet: Current progress of therapeutic vaccination in multiple sclerosis. *CNS Drugs* **2018**, *32*, 401–410. [CrossRef]
15. Skaper, S.D. Chapter 4—Oligodendrocyte precursor cells as a therapeutic target for demyelinating diseases, Prog. *Brain Res.* **2019**, *245*, 119–144. [CrossRef]
16. Gholamzad, M.; Ebtekar, M.; Ardestani, M.S.; Azimi, M.; Mahmodi, Z.; Mousavi, M.J.; Aslani, S. A comprehensive review on the treatment approaches of multiple sclerosis: Currently and in the future. *Inflamm. Res.* **2019**, *68*, 25–38. [CrossRef]
17. Derfuss, T. Personalized medicine in multiple sclerosis: Hope or reality? *BMC Medicine.* **2012**, *10*, 116. [CrossRef]
18. Lassmann, H. Pathogenic mechanisms associated with different clinical courses of multiple sclerosis. *Front. Immunol.* **2019**, *9*, 3116. [CrossRef]
19. Xie, Z.-X.; Zhang, H.-L.; Wu, X.-J.; Zhu, J.; Ma, D.-H.; Jin, T. Role of the immunogenic and tolerogenic subsets of dendritic cells in multiple sclerosis. *Mediat. Inflamm.* **2015**, *20*, 513295. [CrossRef]
20. Rostami, A.; Ciric, B. Role of Th17 cells in the pathogenesis of CNS inflammatory demyelination. *J. Neurol. Sci.* **2013**, *333*, 76–87. [CrossRef]
21. Baldassari, L.E.; Fox, R.J. Therapeutic advances and challenges in the treatment of progressive multiple sclerosis. *Drugs* **2018**, *78*, 1549–1566. [CrossRef] [PubMed]

22. Magliozzi, R.; Howell, O.; Vora, A.; Serafini, B.; Nicholas, R.; Puopolo, M.; Reynolds, R.; Aloisi, F. Meningeal B-cell follicles in secondary progressive multiple sclerosis associate with early onset of disease and severe cortical pathology. *Brain* **2007**, *130*, 1089–1104. [CrossRef] [PubMed]
23. Dolati, S.; Babaloo, Z.; Jadidi-Niaragh, F.; Ayromlou, H.; Sadreddini, S.; Yousefi, M. Multiple sclerosis: Therapeutic applications of advancing drug delivery systems. *Biomed. Pharmacother.* **2017**, *86*, 343–353. [CrossRef] [PubMed]
24. Wucherpfennig, K.W.; Strominger, J.L. Molecular mimicry in T cell-mediated autoimmunity: Viral peptides activate human T cell clones specific for myelin basic protein. *Cell* **1995**, *80*, 695–705. [CrossRef]
25. Fujinami, R.S.; von Herrath, M.G.; Christen, U.; Whitton, J.L. Molecular mimicry, bystander activation, or viral persistence: Infections and autoimmune disease. *Clin. Microbiol. Rev.* **2006**, *19*, 80–94. [CrossRef] [PubMed]
26. Kim, T.-S.; Shin, E.-C. The activation of bystander CD8+ T cells and their roles in viral infection. *Exp. Mol. Med.* **2019**, *51*, 154. [CrossRef]
27. Giacomini, P.S.; Bar-Or, A. Antigen-specific therapies in multiple sclerosis. *Expert Opin. Emerg. Drugs* **2009**, *14*, 551–560. [CrossRef]
28. Szczepanik, M. Mechanisms of immunological tolerance to the antigens of the central nervous system. Skin-induced tolerance as a new therapeutic concept. *J. Physiol. Pharmacol.* **2011**, *62*, 159–165.
29. Hellings, N.; Raus, J.; Stinissen, P. T-cell vaccination in multiple sclerosis: Update on clinical application and mode of action. *Autoimmun. Rev.* **2004**, *3*, 267–275. [CrossRef]
30. Irvine, D.J.; Hanson, M.C.; Rakhra, K.; Tokatlian, T. Synthetic nanoparticles for vaccines and immunotherapy. *Chem. Rev.* **2015**, *115*, 11109–11146. [CrossRef]
31. Selter, R.C.; Hemmer, B. Update on immunopathogenesis and immunotherapy in multiple sclerosis. *Immunotargets Ther.* **2013**, *2*, 21–30. [CrossRef]
32. Lim, E.T.; Giovannoni, G. Immunopathogenesis and immunotherapeutic approaches in multiple sclerosis. *Expert Rev. Neurother.* **2005**, *5*, 379–390. [CrossRef] [PubMed]
33. Grigoriadis, N.; van Pesch, V. A basic overview of multiple sclerosis immunopathology. *Eur. J. Neurol.* **2015**, *22*, 3–13. [CrossRef] [PubMed]
34. Sie, C.; Korn, T.; Mitsdoerffer, M. Th17 cells in central nervous system autoimmunity. *Exp. Neurol.* **2014**, *262*, 18–27. [CrossRef] [PubMed]
35. García-González, P.; Ubilla-Olguín, G.; Catalán, D.; Schinnerling, K.; Aguillón, J.C. Tolerogenic dendritic cells for reprogramming of lymphocyte responses in autoimmune diseases. *Autoimmun. Rev.* **2016**, *15*, 1071–1080. [CrossRef] [PubMed]
36. AGreenfield, L.; Hauser, S.L. B Cell therapy for multiple sclerosis: Entering an era. *Ann. Neurol.* **2018**, *83*, 13–26. [CrossRef] [PubMed]
37. Lu, L.-F.; Rudensky, A. Molecular orchestration of differentiation and function of regulatory T cells. *Genes Dev.* **2009**, *23*, 1270–1282. [CrossRef] [PubMed]
38. Gregori, S.; Goudy, K.S.; Roncarolo, M.G. The cellular and molecular mechanisms of immuno-suppression by human type 1 regulatory T cells. *Front. Immunol.* **2012**, *3*, 30. [CrossRef]
39. Lu, W.; Chen, S.; Lai, C.; Lai, M.; Fang, H.; Dao, H.; Kang, J.; Fan, J.; Guo, W.; Fu, L.; et al. Suppression of HIV replication by CD8(+) regulatory T cells in elite controllers. *Front. Immunol.* **2016**, *7*, 134. [CrossRef]
40. Vuddamalay, Y.; van Meerwijk, J.P.M. CD28- and CD28lowCD8+ regulatory T cells: Of mice and men. *Front. Immunol.* **2017**, *8*, 31. [CrossRef]
41. Milo, R. Therapeutic strategies targeting B-cells in multiple sclerosis. *Autoimmun. Rev.* **2016**, *15*, 714–718. [CrossRef]
42. Zhang, Y.; Salter, A.; Wallström, E.; Cutter, G.; Stüve, O. Evolution of clinical trials in multiple sclerosis. *Ther. Adv. Neurol. Disord.* **2019**, *12*, 1–14. [CrossRef]
43. Dargahi, N.; Katsara, M.; Tselios, T.; Androutsou, M.-E.; de Courten, M.; Matsoukas, J.; Apostolopoulos, V. Multiple sclerosis: Immunopathology and treatment update. *Brain Sci.* **2017**, *7*, 78. [CrossRef] [PubMed]
44. Gentile, A.; Musella, A.; de Vito, F.; Rizzo, F.R.; Fresegna, D.; Bullitta, S.; Vanni, V.; Guadalupi, L.; Bassi, M.S.; Buttari, F.; et al. Immunomodulatory effects of exercise in experimental multiple sclerosis. *Front. Immunol.* **2019**, *10*, 2197. [CrossRef] [PubMed]
45. Pasquier, R.A.D.; Pinschewer, D.D.; Merkler, D. Immunological mechanism of action and clinical profile of disease-modifying treatments in multiple sclerosis. *CNS Drugs* **2014**, *28*, 535–558. [CrossRef]

46. Tapeinos, C.; Battaglini, M.; Ciofani, G. Advances in the design of solid lipid nanoparticles and nanostructured lipid carriers for targeting brain diseases. *J. Control. Release* **2017**, *264*, 306–332. [CrossRef]
47. Cross, A.H.; Naismith, R.T. Established and novel disease-modifying treatments in multiple sclerosis. *J. Intern. Med.* **2014**, *275*, 350–363. [CrossRef]
48. Piehl, F. A changing treatment landscape for multiple sclerosis: Challenges and opportunities. *J. Intern. Med.* **2014**, *275*, 364–381. [CrossRef]
49. Wingerchuk, D.M.; Carter, J.L. Multiple Sclerosis: Current and Emerging Disease-Modifying Therapies and Treatment Strategies. *Mayo Clin. Proc.* **2014**, *89*, 225–240. [CrossRef]
50. Tramacere, I.; del Giovane, C.; Salanti, G.; D'Amico, R.; Pacchetti, I.; Filippini, G. Immunomodulators and immunosuppressants for relapsing-remitting multiple sclerosis: A network meta-analysis. *Cochrane Database Syst. Rev.* **2015**, *9*, CD011381. [CrossRef]
51. Wraith, D.C. The future of immunotherapy: A 20-year perspective. *Front. Immunol.* **2017**, *8*, 1668. [CrossRef] [PubMed]
52. D'Amico, E.; Patti, F.; Zanghì, A.; Zappia, M. A personalized approach in progressive multiple sclerosis: The current status of disease modifying therapies (DMTs) and future perspectives. *Int. J. Mol. Sci.* **2016**, *17*, 1725. [CrossRef] [PubMed]
53. Ciotti, J.R.; Cross, A.H. Disease-Modifying Treatment in Progressive Multiple Sclerosis. *Curr. Treat. Options Neurol.* **2018**, *20*, 12. [CrossRef] [PubMed]
54. Lassmann, H. Targets of therapy in progressive MS. *Mult. Scler.* **2017**, *23*, 1593–1599. [CrossRef]
55. Novartis Receives FDA Approval for Mayzent®(Siponimod), the First Oral Drug to Treat Secondary Progressive MS with Active Disease. Available online: https://novartis.gcs-web.com/Novartis-receives-FDA-approval-for-Mayzent-siponimod-the-first-oral-drug-to-treat-secondary-progressive-MS-with-active-disease?_ga=2.241998658.1110943223.1587297344-1758107691.1587297344 (accessed on 14 April 2020).
56. Zeposia (Ozanimod). Available online: https://multiplesclerosisnewstoday.com/zeposia-ozanimod-rpc1063-rrms/ (accessed on 14 April 2020).
57. Cladribine. Available online: https://en.wikipedia.org/wiki/Cladribine (accessed on 14 April 2020).
58. Wildner, P.; Selmaj, K.W. Multiple sclerosis: Skin-induced antigen-specific immune tolerance. *J. Neuroimmunol.* **2017**, *311*, 49–58. [CrossRef]
59. Sospedra, M.; Martin, R. Antigen-Specific Therapies in Multiple Sclerosis. *Int. Rev. Immunol.* **2005**, *24*, 393–413. [CrossRef]
60. Blanchfield, J.L. Antigen-specific tolerogenic vaccines inhibit autoimmune disease in a rodent model of multiple sclerosis. Ph.D. Thesis, The Faculty of the Department of Microbiology and Immunology Brody School of Medicine at East Carolina University, Greenville, USA, 2010.
61. Pickens, C.J.; Christopher, M.A.; Leon, M.A.; Pressnall, M.M.; Johnson, S.N.; Thati, S.; Sullivan, B.P.; Berkland, C. Antigen-drug conjugates as a novel therapeutic class for the treatment of antigen-specific autoimmune disorders. *Mol. Pharm.* **2019**, *16*, 2452–2461. [CrossRef]
62. Chunsong, Y.; Jingchao, X.; Meng, L.; Myunggi, A.; Haipeng, L. Bioconjugate strategies for the induction of antigen-specific tolerance in autoimmune diseases. *Bioconjug. Chem.* **2018**, *29*, 29719–29732. [CrossRef]
63. Mannie, M.D.; Curtis, A.D. II Tolerogenic vaccines for multiple sclerosis. *Hum. Vac. Immunother.* **2013**, *9*, 1032–1038. [CrossRef]
64. Yannakakis, M.P.; Tzoupis, H.; Michailidou, E.; Mantzourani, E.; Simal, C.; Tselios, T. Molecular dynamics at the receptor level of immunodominant myelin oligodendrocyte glycoprotein 35–55 epitope implicated in multiple sclerosis. *J. Mol. Graph. Model.* **2016**, *68*, 78–86. [CrossRef]
65. Lutterotti, A.; Martin, R. Antigen-specific tolerization approaches in multiple sclerosis. *Expert Opin. Investig. Drugs* **2014**, *23*, 9–20. [CrossRef] [PubMed]
66. Wraith, D. Antigen-specific immunotherapy. *Nature* **2016**, *530*, 422–423. [CrossRef] [PubMed]
67. Spence, A.; Klementowicz, J.E.; Bluestone, J.A.; Tang, Q. Targeting Treg signaling for the treatment of autoimmune diseases. *Curr. Opin. Immunol.* **2015**, *37*, 11–20. [CrossRef] [PubMed]
68. Sabatos-Peyton, C.A.; Verhagen, J.; Wraith, D.C. Antigen-specific immunotherapy of autoimmune and allergic diseases. *Curr. Opin. Immunol.* **2010**, *22*, 609–615. [CrossRef] [PubMed]
69. Steinman, L. The re-emergence of antigen-specific tolerance as a potential therapy for MS. *Mult. Scler. J.* **2015**, *21*, 1223–1238. [CrossRef] [PubMed]

70. Cappellano, G.; Comi, C.; Chiocchetti, A.; Dianzani, U. Exploiting PLGA-based biocompatible nanoparticles for next-generation tolerogenic vaccines against autoimmune disease. *Int. J. Mol. Sci.* **2019**, *20*, 204. [CrossRef]
71. Vanderlugt, C.L.; Miller, S.D. Epitope spreading inimmune-mediated diseases: Implications for immunotherapy. *Nat. Rev. Immunol.* **2002**, *2*, 85–95. [CrossRef]
72. Miller, S.D.; Turley, D.M.; Podojil, J.R. Antigen-specific tolerance strategies for the prevention and treatment of autoimmune disease. *Nat. Rev. Immunol.* **2007**, *7*, 665–677. [CrossRef]
73. Lutterotti, A.; Sospedra, M.; Martin, R. Antigen-specific therapies in MS—Current concepts and novel approaches. *J. Neurol. Sci.* **2008**, *274*, 18–22. [CrossRef]
74. Bielekova, B.; Goodwin, B.; Richert, N.; Cortese, I.; Kondo, T.; Afshar, G.; Grani, B.; Eaton, J.; Antel, J.; Frank, J.A.; et al. Encephalitogenic potential of the myelin basic protein peptide (amino acids 83–99) in multiple sclerosis: Results of a phase II clinical trial with an altered peptide ligand. *Nat. Med.* **2000**, *6*, 1167–1175. [CrossRef]
75. Turley, D.M.; Miller, S.D. Prospects for antigen-specific tolerance based therapies for the treatment of multiple sclerosis, Results Probl. *Cell Differ.* **2010**, *51*, 217–235. [CrossRef]
76. Constantinescu, C.S.; Farooqi, N.; O'Brien, K.; Gran, B. Experimental autoimmune encephalomyelitis (EAE) as a model for multiple sclerosis (MS). *Br. J. Pharmacol.* **2011**, *164*, 1079–1106. [CrossRef] [PubMed]
77. Fletcher, J.M.; Lalor, S.J.; Sweeney, C.M.; Tubridy, N.; Mills, K.H. T cells in multiple sclerosis and experimental autoimmune encephalomyelitis. *Clin. Exp. Immunol.* **2010**, *162*, 1–11. [CrossRef] [PubMed]
78. Libbey, J.E.; Fujinami, R.S. Experimental autoimmune encephalomyelitis as a testing paradigm for adjuvants and vaccines. *Vaccine* **2011**, *29*, 3356–3362. [CrossRef] [PubMed]
79. Tabansky, I.; Keskin, D.B.; Watts, D.; Petzold, C.; Funaro, M.; Sands, W.; Wright, P.; Yunis, E.J.; Najjar, S.; Diamond, B.; et al. Targeting DEC-205–DCIR2+ dendritic cells promotes immunological tolerance in proteolipid protein-induced experimental autoimmune encephalomyelitis. *Mol. Med.* **2018**, *24*, 17. [CrossRef]
80. Huang, X.; Lu, H.W.Q. The mechanisms and applications of T cell vaccination for autoimmune diseases: A comprehensive review. *Clinic. Rev. Allerg. Immunol.* **2014**, *47*, 219–233. [CrossRef] [PubMed]
81. Grau-López, L.; Raïch, D.; Ramo-Tello, C.; Naranjo-Gómez, M.; Dàvalos, A.; Pujol-Borrell, R.; Borràs, F.E.; Martínez-Cáceres, E. Myelin peptides in multiple sclerosis. *Autoimmun. Rev.* **2009**, *8*, 650–653. [CrossRef]
82. Kuchroo, V.K.; Anderson, A.C.; Waldner, H.; Munder, M.; Bettelli, E.; Nicholson, L.B. T cell response in experimental autoimmune encephalomyelitis (EAE): Role of Self and Cross-Reactive Antigens in Shaping, Tuning, and Regulating the Autopathogenic T Cell Repertoire. *Annu. Rev. Immunol.* **2002**, *20*, 101–123. [CrossRef]
83. Matsoukas, J.; Apostolopoulos, V.; Kalbacher, H.; Papini, A.-M.; Tselios, T.; Chatzantoni, K.; Biagioli, T.; Lolli, F.; Deraos, S.; Papathanassopoulos, P.; et al. Design and synthesis of a novel potent myelin basic protein epitope 87-99 cyclic analogue: Enhanced stability and biological properties of mimics render them a potentially new class of immunomodulators. *J. Med. Chem.* **2005**, *48*, 1470–1480. [CrossRef]
84. Reindl, M.; Waters, P. Myelin oligodendrocyte glycoprotein antibodies in neurological disease. *Nat. Rev. Neurol.* **2019**, *15*, 89–102. [CrossRef]
85. Kaushansky, N.; Eisenstein, M.; Zilkha-Falb, R.; Ben-Nun, A. The myelin-associated oligodendrocytic basic protein (MOBP) as a relevant primary target autoantigen in multiple sclerosis. *Autoimmun. Rev.* **2010**, *9*, 233–236. [CrossRef] [PubMed]
86. Androutsou, M.E.; Tapeinou, A.; Vlamis-Gardikas, A.; Tselios, T. Myelin oligodendrocyte glycoprotein and multiple sclerosis. *Med. Chem.* **2018**, *14*, 120–128. [CrossRef] [PubMed]
87. Tselios, T.; Aggelidakis, M.; Tapeinou, A.; Tseveleki, V.; Kanistras, I.; Gatos, D.; Matsoukas, J. Rational design and synthesis of altered peptide ligands based on human myelin oligodendrocyte glycoprotein 35–55 epitope: Inhibition of chronic experimental autoimmune encephalomyelitis in mice. *Molecules* **2014**, *19*, 17968–17984. [CrossRef] [PubMed]
88. Deraos, G.; Kritsi, E.; Matsoukas, M.-T.; Christopoulou, K.; Kalbacher, H.; Zoumpoulakis, P.; Apostolopoulos, V.; Matsoukas, J. Design of linear and cyclic mutant analogues of dirucotide peptide (MBP82–98) against multiple sclerosis: Conformational and binding studies to MHC Class II. *Brain Sci.* **2018**, *8*, 213. [CrossRef] [PubMed]

89. Tapeinou, A.; Giannopoulou, E.; Hansen, C.S.B.E.; Kalofonos, H.; Apostolopoulosd, V.; Vlamis-Gardikas, A.; Tselios, T. Design, synthesis and evaluation of an anthraquinone derivative conjugated to myelin basic protein immunodominant (MBP85-99) epitope: Towards selective immunosuppression. *Eur. J. Med. Chem.* **2018**, *143*, 621–631. [CrossRef]
90. Yannakakis, M.-P.; Simal, C.; Tzoupis, H.; Rodi, M.; Dargahi, N.; Prakash, M.; Mouzaki, A.; Platts, J.A.; Apostolopoulos, V.; Tselios, T.V. Design and synthesis of non-peptide mimetics mapping the immunodominant myelin basic protein (MBP83–96) epitope to function as T-cell receptor antagonists. *Int. J. Mol. Sci.* **2017**, *18*, 1215. [CrossRef]
91. Correale, J.; Farez, M.; Gilmore, W. Vaccines for multiple sclerosis: Progress to date. *CNS Drugs* **2008**, *22*, 175–198. [CrossRef]
92. Mantzourani, E.D.; Platts, J.A.; Brancale, A.; Mavromoustakos, T.M.; Tselios, T.V. Molecular dynamics at the receptor level of immunodominant myelin basic protein epitope 87–99 implicated in multiple sclerosis and its antagonists altered peptide ligands: Triggering of immune response. *J. Mol. Graph. Model.* **2007**, *26*, 471–481. [CrossRef]
93. Kaushansky, N.; de Rosbo, N.K.; Zilkha-Falb, R.; Yosef-Hemo, R.; Cohen, L.; Ben-Nun, A. 'Multi-epitope-targeted' immune-specific therapy for a multiple sclerosis-like disease via engineered multi-epitope protein is superior to peptides. *PLoS ONE* **2011**, *6*, e27860. [CrossRef]
94. Kaushansky, N.; Kaminitz, A.; Allouche-Arnon, H.; Ben-Nun, A. Modulation of MS-like disease by a multi epitope protein is mediated by induction of CD11c+ CD11b+ Gr1+ myeloid-derived dendritic cells. *J. Neuroimmunol.* **2019**, *333*, 476953. [CrossRef]
95. Moorman, C.D.; Curtis, A.D., 2nd; Bastian, A.G.; Elliott, S.E.; Mannie, M.D. A GMCSF-Neuroantigen Tolerogenic Vaccine Elicits Systemic Lymphocytosis of CD4+ CD25high FOXP3+ Regulatory T Cells in Myelin-Specific TCR Transgenic Mice Contingent Upon Low-Efficiency T Cell Antigen Receptor Recognition. *Front. Immunol.* **2019**, *9*, 3119. [CrossRef] [PubMed]
96. Mannie, M.D.; Blanchfield, J.L.; Islam, S.M.T.; Abbott, D.J. Cytokine-neuroantigen fusion proteins as a new class of tolerogenic, therapeutic vaccines for treatment of inflammatory demyelinating disease in rodent models of multiple sclerosis. *Front. Immunol.* **2012**, *3*, 255. [CrossRef] [PubMed]
97. Abbott, D.J.; Blanchfield, J.L.; Martinson, D.A.; Russell, S.C.; Taslim, N.; Curtis, A.D.; Mannie, M.D. Neuroantigen-specific, tolerogenic vaccines: GMCSF is a fusion partner that facilitates tolerance rather than immunity to dominant self-epitopes of myelin in murine models of experimental autoimmune encephalomyelitis (EAE). *BMC Immunol.* **2011**, *12*, 72. [CrossRef] [PubMed]
98. Blanchfield, J.L.; Mannie, M.D. A GMCSF-neuroantigen fusion protein is a potent tolerogen in experimental autoimmune encephalomyelitis (EAE) that is associated with efficient targeting of neuroantigen to APC. *J. Leukoc. Biol.* **2010**, *87*, 509–521. [CrossRef]
99. Petzold, C.; Schallenberg, S.; Stern, J.N.H.; Kretschmer, K. Targeted antigen delivery to DEC-205+ dendritic cells for tolerogenic vaccination. *Rev. Diabet. Stud.* **2012**, *9*, 305–318. [CrossRef]
100. Idoyaga, J.; Fiorese, C.; Zbytnuik, L.; Lubkin, A.; Miller, J.; Malissen, B.; Mucida, D.; Merad, M.; Steinman, R.M. Specialized role of migratory dendritic cells in peripheral tolerance induction. *J. Clin. Investig.* **2013**, *123*, 844–854. [CrossRef]
101. Stern, J.N.H.; Keskin, D.B.; Kato, Z.; Waldner, H.; Schallenberg, S.; Anderson, A.; von Boehmer, H.; Kretschmer, K.; Strominger, J.L. Promoting tolerance to proteolipid protein-induced experimental autoimmune encephalomyelitis through targeting dendritic cells. *Proc. Natl. Acad. Sci. USA* **2010**, *107*, 17280–17285. [CrossRef]
102. Ring, S.; Maas, M.; Nettelbeck, D.M.; Enk, A.H.; Mahnke, K. Targeting of autoantigens to DEC205+ dendritic cells in vivo suppresses experimental allergic encephalomyelitis in mice. *J. Immunol.* **2013**, *191*, 2938–2947. [CrossRef]
103. Kasagi, S.; Wang, D.; Zhang, P.; Zanvit, P.; Chen, H.; Zhang, D.; Li, J.; Che, L.; Maruyama, T.; Nakatsukasa, H.; et al. Combination of apoptotic T cell induction and self-peptide administration for therapy of experimental autoimmune encephalomyelitis. *EBioMedicine* **2019**, *44*, 50–59. [CrossRef]
104. Clemente-Casares, X.; Tsai, S.; Yang, Y.; Santamaria, P. Peptide-MHC-based nanovaccines for the treatment of autoimmunity: A "one size fits all" approach? *J. Mol. Med.* **2011**, *89*, 733–742. [CrossRef]

105. Offner, H.; Sinha, S.; Wang, C.; Burrows, G.G.; Vandenbark, A.A. Recombinant T-cell receptor ligands: Immunomodulatory, neuroprotective and neuroregenerative effects suggest application as therapy for multiple sclerosis. *Rev. Neurosci.* **2008**, *19*, 327–339. [CrossRef] [PubMed]
106. Sinha, S.; Subramanian, S.; Emerson-Webber, A.; Lindner, M.; Burrows, G.G.; Grafe, M.; Linington, C.; Vandenbark, A.A.; Bernard, C.C.A.; Offner, H. Recombinant TCR ligand reverses clinical signs and CNS damage of EAE induced by recombinant human MOG. *J. Neuroimmune Pharmacol.* **2010**, *5*, 231–239. [CrossRef] [PubMed]
107. Gong, Y.; Wang, Z.; Liang, Z.; Duan, H.; Ouyang, L.; Yu, Q.; Xu, Z.; Shen, G.; Weng, X.; Wu, X. Soluble MOG35-55/I-Ab Dimers Ameliorate Experimental Autoimmune Encephalomyelitis by Reducing Encephalitogenic T Cells. *PLoS ONE* **2012**, *7*, e47435. [CrossRef] [PubMed]
108. Vandenbark, A.A.; Rich, C.; Mooney, J.; Zamora, A.; Wang, C.; Huan, J.; Fugger, L.; Offner, H.; Jones, R.; Burrows, G.G. Recombinant TCR ligand induces tolerance to myelin oligodendrocyte glycoprotein 35-55 peptide and reverses clinical and histological signs of chronic experimental autoimmune encephalomyelitis in HLA-DR2 transgenic mice. *J. Immunol.* **2003**, *171*, 127–133. [CrossRef]
109. White, D.R.; Khedri, Z.; Kiptoo, P.; Siahaan, T.J.; Tolbert, T.J. Synthesis of a bifunctional peptide inhibitor–IgG1 Fc fusion that suppresses experimental autoimmune encephalomyelitis. *Bioconjug. Chem.* **2017**, *28*, 1867–1877. [CrossRef]
110. Ridwan, R.; Kiptoo, P.; Kobayashi, N.; Weir, S.; Hughes, M.; Williams, T.; Soegianto, R.; Siahaan, T.J. Antigen-specific suppression of experimental autoimmune encephalomyelitis by a novel bifunctional peptide inhibitor: Structure optimization and pharmacokinetics. *JPET* **2010**, *332*, 1136–1145. [CrossRef]
111. Badawi, A.H.; Siahaan, T.J. Suppression of MOG- and PLP-induced experimental autoimmune encephalomyelitis using a novel multivalent bifunctional peptide inhibitor. *J. Neuroimmunol.* **2013**, *263*, 20–27. [CrossRef]
112. Majewska, M.; Zając, K.; Srebro, Z.; Sura, P.; Książek, L.; Zemelka, M.; Szczepanik, M. Epicutaneous immunization with myelin basic protein protects from the experimental autoimmune encephalomyelitis. *Pharmacol. Rep.* **2007**, *59*, 74–79.
113. Szczepanik, M.; Tutaj, M.; Bryniarski, K.; Dittel, B.N. Epicutaneously induced TGF-h-dependent tolerance inhibits experimental autoimmune encephalomyelitis. *J. Neuroimmunol.* **2005**, *164*, 105–114. [CrossRef]
114. Tutaj, M.; Szczepanik, M. Epicutaneous (EC) immunization with myelin basic protein (MBP) induces TCRabþ CD4þ CD8þ double positive suppressor cells that protect from experimental autoimmune encephalomyelitis (EAE). *J. Autoimmun.* **2007**, *28*, 208–215. [CrossRef]
115. Li, H.; Zhang, G.-X.; Chen, Y.; Xu, H.; Fitzgerald, D.C.; Zhao, Z.; Rostami, A. CD11c+CD11b+ Dendritic cells play an important role in intravenous tolerance and the suppression of experimental autoimmune encephalomyelitis. *J. Immunol.* **2008**, *181*, 2483–2493. [CrossRef] [PubMed]
116. Lourbopoulos, A.; Deraos, G.; Matsoukas, M.-T.; Touloumi, O.; Giannakopoulou, A.; Kalbacher, H.; Grigoriadis, N.; Apostolopoulos, V.; Matsoukas, J. Cyclic MOG35–55 ameliorates clinical and neuropathological features of experimental autoimmune encephalomyelitis, Bioorgan. *Med. Chem.* **2017**, *25*, 4163–4174. [CrossRef] [PubMed]
117. Streeter, H.B.; Rigden, R.; Martin, K.F.; Scolding, N.J.; Wraith, D.C. Preclinical development and first-in-human study of ATX-MS-1467 for immunotherapy of MS. *Neurol. Neuroimmunol. Neuroinflamm.* **2015**, *2*, e93. [CrossRef] [PubMed]
118. Billetta, R.; Ghahramani, N.; Morrow, O.; Prakken, B.; de Jong, H.; Meschter, C.; Lanza, P.; Albani, S. Epitope-specific immune tolerization ameliorates experimental autoimmune encephalomyelitis. *Clin. Immunol.* **2012**, *145*, 94–101. [CrossRef]
119. Peron, J.P.S.; Yang, K.; Chen, M.-L.; Brandao, W.N.; Basso, A.S.; Commodaro, A.G.; Weiner, H.L.; Rizzo, L.V. Oral tolerance reduces Th17 cells as well as the overall inflammation in the central nervous system of EAE mice. *J. Neuroimmunol.* **2010**, *227*, 10–17. [CrossRef]
120. Song, F.; Guan, Z.; Gienapp, I.E.; Shawler, T.; Benson, J.; Whitacre, C.C. The thymus plays a role in oral tolerance in experimental autoimmune encephalomyelitis. *J. Immunol.* **2006**, *177*, 1500–1509. [CrossRef]
121. Deraos, G.; Rodi, M.; Kalbacher, H.; Chatzantoni, K.; Karagiannis, F.; Synodinos, L.; Plotas, P.; Papalois, A.; Dimisianos, N.; Papathanasopoulos, P.; et al. Properties of myelin altered peptide ligand cyclo(8–99)(Ala91,Ala96) MBP87-99 render it a promising drug lead for immunotherapy of multiple sclerosis. *Eur. J. Med.Chem.* **2015**, *101*, 13–23. [CrossRef]

122. Islam, S.M.T.; Curtis, A.D., 2nd; Taslim, N.; Wilkinson, D.S.; Mannie, M.D. GM-CSF-neuroantigen fusion proteins reverse experimental autoimmune encephalomyelitis and mediate tolerogenic activity in adjuvant-primed environments: Association with inflammation-dependent, inhibitory antigen presentation. *J. Immunol.* **2014**, *193*, 2317–2329. [CrossRef]
123. Mannie, M.D.; Clayson, B.A.; Buskirk, E.J.; DeVine, J.L.; Hernandez, J.J.; Abbott, D.J. IL-2/Neuroantigen fusion proteins as antigen-specific tolerogens in experimental autoimmune encephalomyelitis (EAE): Correlation of T cell-mediated antigen presentation and tolerance induction. *J. Immunol.* **2007**, *178*, 2835–2843. [CrossRef]
124. Link, J.M.; Rich, C.M.; Korat, M.; Burrows, G.G.; Offner, H.; Vandenbark, A.A. Monomeric DR2/MOG-35–55 recombinant TCR ligand treats relapses of experimental encephalomyelitis in DR2 transgenic mice. *Clin. Immunol.* **2007**, *123*, 95–104. [CrossRef]
125. Huan, J.; Subramanian, S.; Jones, R.; Rich, C.; Link, J.; Mooney, J.; Bourdette, D.N.; Vandenbark, A.A.; Burrows, G.G.; Offner, H. Monomeric recombinant TCR ligand reduces relapse rate and severity of experimental autoimmune encephalomyelitis in SJL/J mice through cytokine switch. *J. Immunol.* **2004**, *172*, 4556–4566. [CrossRef] [PubMed]
126. Offner, H.; Subramanian, S.; Wang, C.; Afentoulis, M.; Vandenbark, A.A.; Huan, J.; Burrows, G.G. Treatment of passive experimental autoimmune encephalomyelitis in SJL mice with a recombinant TCR ligand induces IL-13 and prevents axonal injury. *J. Immunol.* **2005**, *175*, 4103–4111. [CrossRef] [PubMed]
127. Sinha, S.; Subramanian, S.; Proctor, T.M.; Kaler, L.J.; Grafe, M.; Dahan, R.; Huan, J.; Vandenbark, A.A.; Burrows, G.G.; Offner, H. A promising therapeutic approach for multiple sclerosis: Recombinant T-cell receptor ligands modulate experimental autoimmune encephalomyelitis by reducing interleukin-17 production and inhibiting migration of encephalitogenic cells into the CNS. *J. Neurosci.* **2007**, *27*, 12531–12539. [CrossRef] [PubMed]
128. Sinha, S.; Subramanian, S.; Miller, L.; Proctor, T.M.; Roberts, C.; Burrows, G.G.; Vandenbark, A.A.; Offner, H. Cytokine switch and bystander suppression of autoimmune responses to multiple antigens in experimental autoimmune encephalomyelitis by a single recombinant T-Cell receptor ligand. *J. Neurosci.* **2009**, *29*, 3816–3823. [CrossRef] [PubMed]
129. Sinha, S.; Miller, L.; Subramanian, S.; McCarty, O.; Proctor, T.; Meza-Romero, R.; Burrows, G.G.; Vandenbark, A.A.; Offner, H. Binding of recombinant T cell receptor ligands (RTL) to antigen presenting cells prevents upregulation of CD11b and inhibits T cell activation and transfer of experimental autoimmune encephalomyelitis. *J. Neuroimmunol.* **2010**, *225*, 52–61. [CrossRef] [PubMed]
130. Wang, C.; Gold, B.G.; Kaler, L.J.; Yu, X.; Afentoulis, M.E.; Burrows, G.G.; Vandenbark, A.A.; Bourdette, D.N.; Offner, H. Antigen-specific therapy promotes repair of myelin and axonal damage in established EAE. *J. Neurochem.* **2006**, *98*, 1817–1827. [CrossRef] [PubMed]
131. Badawi, A.H.; Kiptoo, P.; Siahaan, T.J. Immune tolerance induction against experimental Autoimmune Encephalomyelitis (EAE) Using A New PLP-B7AP Conjugate that simultaneously targets B7/CD28 costimulatory signal and TCR/MHC-II signal. *J. Mult. Scler. (Foster City)* **2015**, *2*, 1000131.
132. Badawi, A.H.; Kiptoo, P.; Wang, W.-T.; Choi, I.-Y.; Lee, P.; Vines, C.M.; Siahaan, T.J. Suppression of EAE and prevention of blood-brain barrier breakdown after vaccination with novel bifunctional peptide inhibitor. *Neuropharmacology* **2012**, *62*, 1874–1881. [CrossRef]
133. Kobayashi, N.; Kobayashi, H.; Gu, L.; Malefyt, T.; Siahaan, T.J. Antigen-specific suppression of experimental autoimmune encephalomyelitis by a novel bifunctional peptide inhibitor. *JPET* **2007**, *322*, 879–886. [CrossRef]
134. Kobayashi, N.; Kiptoo, P.; Kobayashi, H.; Ridwan, R.; Brocke, S.; Siahaan, T.J. Prophylactic and therapeutic suppression of experimental autoimmune encephalomyelitis by a novel bifunctional peptide inhibitor. *Clin. Immunol.* **2008**, *129*, 69–79. [CrossRef]
135. Kiptoo, P.; Büyüktimkin, B.; Badawi, A.H.; Stewart, J.; Ridwan, R.; Siahaan, T.J. Controlling immune response and demyelination using highly potent bifunctional peptide inhibitors in the suppression of experimental autoimmune encephalomyelitis. *Clin. Exp. Immunol.* **2012**, *172*, 23–36. [CrossRef] [PubMed]
136. Fissolo, N.; Montalban, X.; Comabella, M. DNA vaccination techniques. *Methods Mol. Biol.* **2016**, *1304*, 39–50. [CrossRef] [PubMed]
137. Garren, H. DNA vaccines for autoimmune diseases. *Expert Rev. Vaccines* **2009**, *8*, 1195–1203. [CrossRef] [PubMed]
138. Fontoura, P.; Garren, H.; Steinman, L. Antigen-specific therapies in multiple sclerosis: Going beyond proteins and peptides. *Int. Rev. Immunol.* **2005**, *24*, 415–446. [CrossRef] [PubMed]

139. Fissolo, N.; Montalban, X.; Comabella, M. DNA-based vaccines for multiple sclerosis: Current status and future directions. *Clin. Immunol.* **2012**, *142*, 76–83. [CrossRef]
140. Stuve, O.; Cravens, P.; Eagar, T.N. DNA-based vaccines: The future of multiple sclerosis therapy? *Expert Rev. Neurother.* **2008**, *8*, 351–360. [CrossRef] [PubMed]
141. Jakimovski, D.; Weinstock-Guttman, B.; Ramanathan, M.; Dwyer, M.G.; Zivadinov, R. Infections, vaccines and autoimmunity: A multiple sclerosis perspective. *Vaccines* **2020**, *8*, 50. [CrossRef]
142. Garren, H.; Ruiz, P.J.; Watkins, T.A.; Fontoura, P.; Nguyen, L.-V.T.; Estline, E.R.; Hirschberg, D.L.; Steinman, L. Combination of gene delivery and DNA vaccination to protect from and reverse Th1 autoimmune disease via deviation to the Th2 pathway. *Immunity* **2001**, *15*, 15–22. [CrossRef]
143. Wefer, J.; Harris, R.A.; Lobell, A. Protective DNA vaccination against experimental autoimmune encephalomyelitis is associated with induction of IFNh. *J. Neuroimmunol.* **2004**, *149*, 66–76. [CrossRef]
144. Schif-Zuck, S.; Wildbaum, G.; Karin, N. Coadministration of plasmid DNA constructs encoding an encephalitogenic determinant and IL-10 elicits regulatory T cell-mediated protective immunity in the central nervous system. *J. Immunol.* **2006**, *177*, 8241–8247. [CrossRef]
145. Lobell, A.; Weissert, R.; Eltayeb, S.; de Graaf, K.L.; Wefer, J.; Storch, M.K.; Lassmann, H.; Wigzell, H.; Olsson, T. Suppressive DNA vaccination in myelin oligodendrocyte glycoprotein peptide-induced experimental autoimmune encephalomyelitis involves a T1-biased immune response. *J. Immunol.* **2003**, *170*, 1806–1813. [CrossRef] [PubMed]
146. Andersson, A.; Isaksson, M.; Wefer, J.; Norling, A.; Flores-Morales, A.; Rorsman, F.; Kämpe, O.; Harris, R.A.; Lobell, A. Impaired autoimmune T helper 17 cell responses following DNA vaccination against rat experimental autoimmune encephalomyelitis. *PLoS ONE* **2008**, *3*, e3682. [CrossRef] [PubMed]
147. Kang, Y.; Sun, Y.; Zhang, J.; Gao, W.; Kang, J.; Wang, Y.; Wang, B.; Xia, G. Treg cell resistance to apoptosis in DNA vaccination for experimental autoimmune encephalomyelitis treatment. *PLoS ONE* **2012**, *7*, e49994. [CrossRef] [PubMed]
148. Walczak, A.; Szymanska, B.; Selmaj, K. Differential prevention of experimental autoimmune encephalomyelitis with antigen-specific DNA vaccination. *Clin. Neurol. Neurosurg.* **2004**, *106*, 241–245. [CrossRef] [PubMed]
149. Liu, J.; Cao, X. Regulatory dendritic cells in autoimmunity: A comprehensive review. *J. Autoimmun.* **2015**, *63*, 1–12. [CrossRef] [PubMed]
150. Domogalla, M.P.; Rostan, P.V.; Raker, V.K.; Steinbrink, K. Tolerance through education: How tolerogenic dendritic cells shape immunity. *Front. Immunol.* **2017**, *8*, 1764. [CrossRef]
151. Van Brussel, I.; Lee, W.P.; Rombouts, M.; Nuyts, A.H.; Heylen, M.; DeWinter, B.Y.; Cools, N.; Schrijvers, D.M. Tolerogenic dendritic cell vaccines to treat autoimmune diseases: Can the unattainable dream turn into reality? *Autoimmun. Rev.* **2014**, *13*, 138–150. [CrossRef]
152. Flórez-Grau, G.; Zubizarreta, I.; Cabezón, R.; Villoslada, P.; Benitez-Ribas, D. Tolerogenic dendritic cells as a promising antigen-specific therapy in the treatment of multiple sclerosis and neuromyelitis optica from preclinical to clinical trials. *Front. Immunol.* **2018**, *9*, 1169. [CrossRef]
153. Obregon, C.; Kumar, R.; Pascual, M.A.; Vassalli, G.; Golshayan, D. Update on dendritic cell-induced immunological and clinical tolerance. *Front. Immunol.* **2017**, *8*, 1514. [CrossRef]
154. Derdelinckx, J.; Mansilla, M.J.; de Laere, M.; Lee, W.-P.; Navarro-Barriuso, J.; Wens, I.; Nkansah, I.; Daans, J.; de Reu, H.; Keliris, A.J.; et al. Clinical and immunological control of experimental autoimmune encephalomyelitis by tolerogenic dendritic cells loaded with MOG-encoding RNA. *J. Neuroinflam.* **2019**, *16*, 167. [CrossRef]
155. Iberg, C.A.; Hawiger, D. Natural and induced tolerogenic dendritic cells. *J. Immunol.* **2020**, *204*, 733–744. [CrossRef] [PubMed]
156. Vandenbark, A.A.; Abulafia-Lapid, R. Autologous T-cell vaccination for multiple sclerosis: A perspective on progress. *BioDrugs* **2008**, *22*, 265–273. [CrossRef] [PubMed]
157. Volovitz, I.; Marmora, Y.; Mor, F.; Flügel, A.; Odoardi, F.; Eisenbach, L.; Cohen, I.R. T cell vaccination induces the elimination of EAE effector T cells: Analysis using GFP-transduced, encephalitogenic T cells. *J. Autoimmun.* **2010**, *35*, 135–144. [CrossRef] [PubMed]
158. Turley, D.M.; Miller, S.D. Peripheral tolerance induction using ethylenecarbodiimide-fixed APCs uses both direct and indirect mechanisms of antigen presentation for prevention of experimental autoimmune encephalomyelitis. *J. Immunol.* **2007**, *178*, 2212–2220. [CrossRef] [PubMed]

159. Getts, D.R.; Turley, D.M.; Smith, C.E.; Harp, C.T.; McCarthy, D.; Feeney, E.M.; Getts, M.T.; Martin, A.J.; Luo, X.; Terry, R.R.; et al. Tolerance Induced by Apoptotic Antigen-Coupled Leukocytes is Induced by PD-L1+, IL-10-Producing Splenic Macrophages and Maintained by Tregs. *J. Immunol.* **2011**, *187*, 2405–2417. [CrossRef] [PubMed]
160. Pishesha, N.; Bilate, A.M.; Wibowo, M.C.; Huang, N.-J.; Lia, Z.; Deshycka, R.; Bousbaine, D.; Lia, H.; Pattersona, H.C.; Dougana, S.K.; et al. Engineered erythrocytes covalently linked to antigenic peptides can protect against autoimmune disease. *Proc. Natl. Acad. Sci. USA* **2017**, *114*, 3157–3162. [CrossRef]
161. Chen, Z.; Yang, D.; Peng, X.; Lin, J.; Suc, Z.; Lia, J.; Zhang, X.; Weng, Y. Beneficial effect of atorvastatin-modified dendritic cells pulsed with myelin oligodendrocyte glycoprotein autoantigen on experimental autoimmune encephalomyelitis. *Neuroreport* **2018**, *29*, 317–327. [CrossRef]
162. Wang, X.; Zhang, J.; Baylink, D.J.; Li1, C.-H.; Watts, D.M.; Xu, Y.; Qin, X.; Walter, M.H.; Tang, X. Targeting non-classical myelin epitopes to treat experimental autoimmune encephalomyelitis. *Sci. Rep.* **2016**, *6*, 36064. [CrossRef]
163. Kalantari, T.; Karimi, M.H.; Ciric, B.; Yan, Y.; Rostami, A.; Kamali-Sarvestani, E. Tolerogenic dendritic cells produced by lentiviral-mediated CD40- and interleukin-23p19-specific shRNA can ameliorate experimental autoimmune encephalomyelitis by suppressing T helper type 17 cells. *Clin. Exp. Immunol.* **2014**, *176*, 180–189. [CrossRef]
164. Mansilla, M.J.; Sellès-Moreno, C.; Fàbregas-Puig, S.; Amoedo, J.; Navarro-Barriuso, J.; Teniente-Serra, A.; Grau-López, L.; Ramo-Tello, C.; Martínez-Cáceres, E.M. Beneficial effect of tolerogenic dendritic cells pulsed with MOG autoantigen in experimental autoimmune encephalomyelitis. *CNS Neurosci. Ther.* **2015**, *21*, 222–230. [CrossRef]
165. Mansilla, M.J.; Contreras-Cardone, R.; Navarro-Barriuso, J.; Cools, N.; Berneman, Z.; Ramo-Tello, C.; Martínez-Cáceres, E.M. Cryopreserved vitamin D3-tolerogenic dendritic cells pulsed with autoantigens as a potential therapy for multiple sclerosis patients. *J. Neuroinflamm.* **2016**, *13*, 113. [CrossRef] [PubMed]
166. Zhou, Y.; Leng, X.; Luo, S.; Su, Z.; Luo, X.; Guo, H.; Mo, C.; Zou, Q.; Liu, Y.; Wang, Y. Tolerogenic dendritic cells generated with tofacitinib ameliorate experimental autoimmune encephalomyelitis through modulation of Th17/Treg balance. *J. Immunol. Res.* **2016**, *2016*, 5021537. [CrossRef] [PubMed]
167. Xie, Z.; Chen, J.; Zheng, C.; Wu, J.; Cheng, Y.; Zhu, S.; Lin, C.; Cao, Q.; Zhu, J.; Jin, T. 1,25-dihydroxyvitamin D3-induced dendritic cells suppress experimental autoimmune encephalomyelitis by increasing proportions of the regulatory lymphocytes and reducing T helper type 1 and type 17 cells. *Immunology* **2017**, *152*, 414–424. [CrossRef] [PubMed]
168. Papenfuss, T.L.; Powell, N.D.; McClain, M.A.; Bedarf, A.; Singh, A.; Gienapp, I.E.; Shawler, T.; Whitacre, C.C. Estriol generates tolerogenic dendritic cells in vivo that protect against autoimmunity. *J. Immunol.* **2011**, *15*, 186–3346. [CrossRef] [PubMed]
169. Menges, M.; Rößner, S.; Voigtländer, C.; Schindler, H.; Kukutsch, N.A.; Bogdan, C.; Erb, K.; Schuler, G.; Lutz, M.B. Repetitive injections of dendritic cells matured with tumor necrosis factor α induce antigen-specific protection of mice from autoimmunity. *J. Exp. Med.* **2002**, *195*, 15–21. [CrossRef] [PubMed]
170. Xiao, B.-G.; Huang, Y.-M.; Yang, J.-S.; Xu, L.-Y.; Link, H. Bone marrow-derived dendritic cells from experimental allergic encephalomyelitis induce immune tolerance to EAE in Lewis rats. *Clin. Exp. Immunol.* **2001**, *125*, 300–309. [CrossRef] [PubMed]
171. Kim, Y.C.; Zhang, A.-H.; Yoon, J.; Culp, W.E.; Leesa, J.R.; Wucherpfennig, K.W.; Scott, D.W. Engineered MBP-specific human Tregs ameliorate MOG-induced EAE through IL-2-triggered inhibition of effector T cells. *J. Autoimmun.* **2018**, *92*, 77–86. [CrossRef]
172. Pereira, B.d.; Fraefel, C.; Hilbe, M.; Ackermann, M.; Dresch, C. Transcriptional targeting of DCs with lentiviral vectors induces antigen-specific tolerance in a mouse model of multiple sclerosis. *Gene Ther.* **2013**, *20*, 556–566. [CrossRef]
173. Eixarch, H.; Espejo, C.; Gómez, A.; Mansilla, M.J.; Castillo, M.; Mildner, A.; Vidal, F.; Gimeno, R.; Prinz, M.; Montalban, X.; et al. Tolerance induction in experimental autoimmune encephalomyelitis using non-myeloablative hematopoietic gene therapy with autoantigen. *Mol. Ther.* **2009**, *17*, 897–905. [CrossRef]
174. Casacuberta-Serra, S.; Costa, C.; Eixarch, H.; Mansilla, M.J.; López-Estévez, S.; Martorell, L.; Parés, M.; Montalban, X.; Espejo, C.; Barquinero, J. Myeloid-derived suppressor cells expressing a self-antigen ameliorate experimental autoimmune encephalomyelitis. *Exp. Neurol.* **2016**, *286*, 50–60. [CrossRef]

175. Tabansky, I.; Messina, M.D.; Bangeranye, C.; Goldstein, J.; Blitz-Shabbir, K.M.; Machado, S.; Jeganathan, V.; Wright, P.; Najjar, S.; Cao, Y.; et al. Advancing drug delivery systems for the treatment of multiple sclerosis. *Immunol. Res.* **2015**, *63*, 58–69. [CrossRef] [PubMed]
176. Ballerini, C.; Baldi, G.; Aldinucci, A.; Maggi, P. Nanomaterial applications in multiple sclerosis inflamed Brain. *J. Neuroimmune Pharmacol.* **2015**, *10*, 1–13. [CrossRef] [PubMed]
177. Gharagozloo, M.; Majewski, S.; Foldvari, M. Therapeutic applications of nanomedicine in autoimmune diseases: From immunosuppression to tolerance induction. *Nanomed. Nanotechnol.* **2015**, *11*, 1003–1018. [CrossRef] [PubMed]
178. Pires, L.R.; Marques, F.; Sousa, J.C.; Cerqueira, J.; Pinto, I.M. Nano- and micro-based systems for immunotolerance induction in multiple sclerosis. *Hum. Vaccines Immunother.* **2016**, *12*, 1886–1890. [CrossRef] [PubMed]
179. Veld, R.H.I.; da Silva, C.G.; Kaijzel, E.L.; Chan, A.B.; Cruz, L.J. The Potential of nano-vehicle mediated therapy in vasculitis and multiple sclerosis. *Curr. Pharm. Des.* **2017**, *23*, 1985–1992. [CrossRef]
180. Gammon, J.M.; Jewell, C.M. Engineering immune tolerance with biomaterials. *Adv. Healthc. Mater.* **2019**, *8*, e1801419. [CrossRef]
181. Pei, W.; Wan, X.; Shahzad, K.A.; Zhang, L.; Song, S.; Jin, X.; Wang, L.; Zhao, C.; Shen, C. Direct modulation of myelin-autoreactive CD4+ and CD8+ T cells in EAE mice by a tolerogenic nanoparticle co-carrying myelin peptide-loaded major histocompatibility complexes, CD47 and multiple regulatory molecules. *Int. J. Nanomed.* **2018**, *13*, 3731–3750. [CrossRef]
182. Sestak, J.O.; Sullivan, B.P.; Thati, S.; Northrup, L.; Hartwell, B.; Antunez, L.; Forrest, M.L.; Vines, C.M.; Siahaan, T.J.; Berkland, C. Codelivery of antigen and an immune cell adhesion inhibitor is necessary for efficacy of soluble antigen arrays in experimental autoimmune encephalomyelitis. *Mol. Ther. Methods Clin. Dev.* **2014**, *1*, 14008. [CrossRef]
183. Thati, S.; Kuehl, C.; Hartwell, B.; Sestak, J.; Siahaan, T.; Forrest, M.L.; Berkland, C. Routes of Administration and dose optimization of soluble antigen arrays in mice with experimental autoimmune encephalomyelitis. *J. Pharm. Sci.* **2015**, *104*, 714–721. [CrossRef]
184. Hartwell, B.L.; Pickens, C.J.; Leon, M.; Berkland, C. Multivalent antigen arrays exhibit high avidity binding and modulation of B cell receptor-mediated signaling to drive efficacy against experimental autoimmune encephalomyelitis. *Biomacromolecules* **2017**, *18*, 1893–1907. [CrossRef]
185. Hartwell, B.L.; Pickens, C.J.; Leon, M.; Northrup, L.; Christopher, M.; Griffin, J.D.; Martinez-Becerra, F.; Berkland, C. Soluble antigen arrays disarm antigen-specific B cells to promote lasting immune tolerance in experimental autoimmune encephalomyelitis. *J. Autoimmun.* **2018**, *93*, 76–88. [CrossRef] [PubMed]
186. Tostanoski, L.H.; Chiu, Y.-C.; Andorko, J.I.; Guo, M.; Zeng, X.; Zhang, P.; Royal, W., III; Jewell, C.M. Design of polyelectrolyte multilayers to promote immunological tolerance. *ACS Nano* **2016**, *10*, 9334–9345. [CrossRef] [PubMed]
187. Hess, K.L.; Andorko, J.I.; Tostanoski, L.H.; Jewell, C.M. Polyplexes assembled from self-peptides and regulatory nucleic acids blunt toll-like receptor signaling to combat autoimmunity. *Biomaterials* **2017**, *118*, 51–62. [CrossRef] [PubMed]
188. Tseveleki, V.; Tselios, T.; Kanistras, I.; Koutsoni, O.; Karamita, M.; Vamvakas, S.-S.; Apostolopoulos, V.; Dotsika, E.; Matsoukas, J.; Lassmann, H.; et al. Mannan-conjugated myelin peptides prime non-pathogenic Th1 and Th17 cells and ameliorate experimental autoimmune encephalomyelitis. *Exp. Neurol.* **2015**, *267*, 254–267. [CrossRef] [PubMed]
189. Belogurov, A.A., Jr.; Stepanov, A.V.; Smirnov, I.V.; Melamed, D.; Bacon, A.; Mamedov, A.E.; Boitsov, V.M.; Sashchenko, L.P.; Ponomarenko, N.A.; Sharanova, S.N.; et al. Liposome-encapsulated peptides protect against experimental allergic encephalitis. *FASEB J.* **2013**, *27*, 222–231. [CrossRef] [PubMed]
190. Pujol-Autonell, I.; Mansilla, M.-J.; Rodriguez-Fernandez, S.; Cano-Sarabia, M.; Navarro-Barriuso1, J.; Ampudia, R.-M.; Rius, A.; Garcia-Jimeno, S.; Perna-Barrull, D.; Martinez-Caceres, E.; et al. Liposome-based immunotherapy against autoimmune diseases: Therapeutic effect on multiple sclerosis. *Nanomedicine* **2017**, *12*, 1231–1242. [CrossRef]
191. Belogurov, A.; Zakharov, K.; Lomakin, Y.; Surkov, K.; Avtushenko, S.; Kruglyakov, P.; Smirnov, I.; Makshakov, G.; Lockshin, C.; Gregoriadis, G.; et al. CD206-targeted liposomal myelin basic protein peptides in patients with multiple sclerosis resistant to first-line disease-modifying therapies: A first-in-human, proof-of-concept dose-escalation study. *Neurotherapeutics* **2016**, *13*, 895–904. [CrossRef]

192. Lomakin, Y.; Belogurov, A., Jr.; Glagoleva, I.; Stepanov, A.; Zakharov, K.; Okunola, J.; Smirnov, I.; Genkin, D.; Gabibov, A. Administration of myelin basic protein peptides encapsulated in mannosylated liposomes normalizes level of serum TNF-α and IL-2 and chemoattractants CCL2 and CCL4 in multiple sclerosis patients. *Mediat. Inflamm.* **2016**, *2016*, 2847232. [CrossRef]
193. Cappellano, G.; Woldetsadik, A.D.; Orilieri, E.; Shivakumar, Y.; Rizzi, M.; Carniato, F.; Gigliotti, C.L.; Boggio, E.; Clemente, N.; Comi, C.; et al. Subcutaneous inverse vaccination with PLGA particles loaded with aMOG peptide and IL-10 decreases the severity of experimental autoimmune encephalomyelitis. *Vaccine* **2014**, *32*, 5681–5689. [CrossRef]
194. Casey, L.M.; Pearson, R.M.; Hughes, K.R.; Liu, J.M.H.; Rose, J.A.; North, M.G.; Wang, L.Z.; Lei, M.; Miller, S.D.; Shea, L.D. Conjugation of transforming growth factor Beta to antigen-loaded Poly(lactide-co-glycolide) nanoparticles enhances efficiency of antigen-specific tolerance. *Bioconjug. Chem.* **2018**, *29*, 813–823. [CrossRef]
195. Cho, J.J.; Stewart, J.M.; Drashansky, T.T.; Brusko, M.A.; Zuniga, A.N.; Lorentsen, K.J.; Keselowsky, B.G.; Avram, D. An antigen-specific semi-therapeutic treatment with local delivery of tolerogenic factors through a dual-sized microparticle system blocks experimental autoimmune encephalomyelitis. *Biomaterials* **2017**, *143*, 79–92. [CrossRef] [PubMed]
196. Gholamzad, M.; Ebtekar, M.; Ardestani, M.S. Intravenous injection of myelin oligodendrocyte glycoprotein-coated PLGA microparticles have tolerogenic effects in experimental autoimmune encephalomyelitis. *Iran J. Allergy Asthma Immunol.* **2017**, *16*, 27–281.
197. Hunter, Z.; McCarthy, D.P.; Yap, W.T.; Harp, C.T.; Getts, D.R.; Shea, L.D.; Miller, S.D. A biodegradable nanoparticle platform for the induction of antigen-specific immune tolerance for treatment of autoimmune disease. *ACS Nano* **2014**, *8*, 2148–2160. [CrossRef] [PubMed]
198. Maldonado, R.A.; LaMothe, R.A.; Ferrari, J.D.; Zhang, A.-H.; Rossi, R.J.; Kolte, P.N.; Griset, A.P.; O'Neil, C.; Altreuter, D.H.; Browning, E.; et al. Polymeric synthetic nanoparticles for the induction of antigen-specific immunological tolerance. *Proc. Natl. Acad. Sci. USA* **2014**, *112*, E156–E165. [CrossRef]
199. McCarthy, D.P.; Yap, J.W.-T.; Harp, C.T.; Song, W.K.; Chen, J.; Pearson, R.M.; Miller, S.D.; Shea, L.D. An antigen-encapsulating nanoparticle platform for TH1/17 immune tolerance therapy. *Nanomedicine* **2017**, *13*, 191–200. [CrossRef]
200. Saito, E.; Kuo, R.; Kramer, K.R.; Gohel, N.; Giles, D.A.; Moore, B.B.; Miller, S.D.; Shea, L.D. Design of biodegradable nanoparticles to modulate phenotypes of antigen presenting cells for antigen-specific treatment of autoimmune disease. *Biomaterials* **2019**, *222*, 119432. [CrossRef]
201. Wan, X.; Pei, W.; Shahzad, K.A.; Zhang, L.; Song, S.; Jin, X.; Wang, L.; Zhao, C.; Shen, C. A Tolerogenic artificial APC durably ameliorates experimental autoimmune encephalomyelitis by directly and selectively modulating myelin peptide–autoreactive $CD4^+$ and $CD8^+$ T cell. *J. Immunol.* **2018**, *201*, 1194–1210. [CrossRef]
202. Zhao, H.; Kiptoo, P.; Williams, T.D.; Siahaan, T.J.; Topp, E.M. Immune response to controlled release of immunomodulating peptides in a murine experimental autoimmune encephalomyelitis (EAE) model. *J. Control. Release* **2010**, *141*, 145–152. [CrossRef]
203. Pearson, R.M.; Casey, L.M.; Hughes, K.R.; Wang, L.Z.; North, M.G.; Getts, D.R.; Miller, S.D.; Shea, L.D. Controlled delivery of single or multiple antigens in tolerogenic nanoparticles using peptide-polymer bioconjugates. *Mol. Ther.* **2017**, *25*, 1655–1664. [CrossRef]
204. Sestak, J.O.; Fakhari, A.; Badawi, A.H.; Siahaan, T.J.; Berkland, C. Structure, size, and solubility of antigen arrays determines efficacy in experimental autoimmune encephalomyelitis. *AAPS J.* **2014**, *16*, 1185–1193. [CrossRef]
205. Kuo, R.; Saito, E.; Miller, S.D.; Shea, L.D. Peptide-conjugated nanoparticles reduce positive co-stimulatory expression and T cell activity to induce tolerance. *Mol. Ther.* **2017**, *25*, 1676–1685. [CrossRef] [PubMed]
206. Getts, D.R.; Martin, A.J.; McCarthy, D.P.; Terry, R.L.; Hunter, Z.N.; Yap, W.T.; Getts, M.T.; Pleiss, M.; Luo, X.; King, N.J.C.; et al. Microparticles bearing encephalitogenic peptides induce T-cell tolerance and ameliorate experimental autoimmune encephalomyelitis. *Nat. Biotechnol.* **2012**, *30*, 1217–1224. [CrossRef] [PubMed]
207. Tostanoski, L.H.; Chiu, Y.-C.; Gammon, J.M.; Simon, T.; Andorko, J.I.; Bromberg, J.S.; Jewell, C.M. Reprogramming the local lymph node microenvironment promotes tolerance that is systemic and antigen-specific. *Cell Rep.* **2016**, *16*, 2940–2952. [CrossRef] [PubMed]
208. Büyüktimkin, B.; Wang, Q.; Kiptoo, P.; Stewart, J.M.; Berkland, C.; Siahaan, T.J. Vaccine-like controlled-release delivery of an immunomodulating peptide to treat experimental autoimmune encephalomyelitis. *Mol. Pharm.* **2012**, *9*, 979–985. [CrossRef]

209. Northrup, L.; Sestak, J.O.; Sullivan, B.P.; Thati, S.; Hartwell, B.L.; Siahaan, T.J.; Vines, C.M.; Berkland, C. Co-delivery of autoantigen and B7 pathway modulators suppresses experimental autoimmune encephalomyelitis. *AAPS J.* **2014**, *16*, 1204–1213. [CrossRef]
210. Kuehl, C.; Thati, S.; Sullivan, B.; Sestak, J.; Thompson, M.; Siahaan, T.; Berkland, C. Pulmonary administration of soluble antigen arrays is superior to antigen in treatment of experimental autoimmune encephalomyelitis. *J. Pharm. Sci.* **2017**, *106*, 3293–3302. [CrossRef]
211. Hess, K.L.; Oh, E.; Tostanoski, L.H.; Andorko, J.I.; Susumu, K.; Deschamps, J.R.; Medintz, I.L.; Jewell, C.M. Engineering immunological tolerance using quantum dots to tune the density of self-antigen display. *Adv. Funct. Mater.* **2017**, *27*. [CrossRef]
212. Clemente-Casares, X.; Blanco, J.; Ambalavanan, P.; Yamanouchi, J.; Singha, S.; Fandos, C.; Tsai, S.; Wang, J.; Garabatos, N.; Izquierdo, C.; et al. Expanding antigen-specific regulatory networks to treat autoimmunity. *Nature* **2016**, *530*, 434–440. [CrossRef]
213. Yeste, A.; Nadeau, M.; Burns, E.J.; Weiner, H.L.; Qu, F.J. Nanoparticle-mediated codelivery of myelin antigen and a tolerogenic small molecule suppresses experimental autoimmune encephalomyelitis. *Proc. Natl. Acad. Sci. USA* **2012**, *109*, 11270–11275. [CrossRef]
214. Katsara, M.; Deraos, G.; Tselios, T.; Matsoukas, J.; Apostolopoulos, V. Design of novel cyclic altered peptide ligands of myelin basic protein MBP83–99 that modulate immune responses in SJL/J mice. *J. Med. Chem.* **2008**, *51*, 3971–3978. [CrossRef]
215. Yu, L.; Yang, F.; Jiang, L.; Chen, Y.; Wang, K.; Xu, F.; Wei, Y.; Cao, X.; Wang, J.; Cai, Z. Exosomes with membrane-associated TGF-β1 from gene-modified dendritic cells inhibit murine EAE independently of MHC restriction. *Eur. J. Immunol.* **2013**, *43*, 2461–2472. [CrossRef] [PubMed]
216. Buerth, C.; Mausberg, A.K.; Heininger, M.K.; Hartung, H.-P.; Kieseier, B.C.; Ernst, J.F. Oral tolerance induction in experimental autoimmune encephalomyelitis with Candida utilis expressing the immunogenic MOG35-55 peptide. *PLoS ONE* **2016**, *11*, e0155082. [CrossRef] [PubMed]
217. Kappos, L.; Comi, G.; Panitch, H.; Oger, J.; Antel, J.; Conlon, P.; Steinman, L. The Altered peptide ligand in relapsing MS study group, Induction of a non-encephalitogenic type 2 T helper-cell autoimmune response in multiple sclerosis after administration of an altered peptide ligand in a placebo-controlled, randomized phase II trial. *Nat. Med.* **2000**, *6*, 1176–1182. [CrossRef] [PubMed]
218. Goodkin, D.E.; Shulman, M.; Winkelhake, J.; Waubant, E.; Andersson, P.; Stewart, T.; Nelson, S.; Fischbein, N.; Coyle, P.K.; Frohman, E.; et al. A phase I trial of solubilized DR2:MBP84-102 (AG284) in multiple sclerosis. *Neurology* **2000**, *54*, 1414–1420. [CrossRef] [PubMed]
219. Warren, K.G.; Catz, I.; Ferenczi, L.Z.; Krantz, M.J. Intravenous synthetic peptide MBP8298 delayed disease progression in an HLA Class II-defined cohort of patients with progressive multiple sclerosis: Results of a 24-month double-blind placebo-controlled clinical trial and 5 years of follow-up treatment. *Eur. J. Neurol.* **2006**, *13*, 887–895. [CrossRef]
220. Freedman, M.S.; Bar-Or, A.; Oger, J.; Traboulsee, A.; Patry, D.; Young, C.; Olsson, T.; Li, D.; Hartung, H.-P.; Krantz, M.; et al. A phase III study evaluating the efficacy and safety of MBP8298 in secondary progressive MS. *Neurology* **2011**, *77*, 1551–1560. [CrossRef]
221. Offner, H.; Burrows, G.G.; Ferro, A.J.; Vandenbark, A.A. RTL therapy for multiple sclerosis: A Phase I clinical study. *J. Neuroimmunol.* **2011**, *231*, 7–14. [CrossRef]
222. Yadav, V.; Bourdette, D.N.; Bowen, J.D.; Lynch, S.G.; Mattson, D.; Preiningerova, J.; Bever, C.T.; Simon, J.; Goldstein, A.; Burrows, G.G.; et al. Recombinant T-cell receptor ligand (RTL) for treatment of multiple sclerosis: A double-blind, placebo-controlled, Phase 1, dose-escalation study. *Autoimmune Dis.* **2012**, *2012*, 954739. [CrossRef]
223. Loo, E.W.; Krantz, M.J.; Agrawal, B. High dose antigen treatment with a peptide epitope of myelin basic protein modulates T cells in multiple sclerosis patients. *Cell. Immunol.* **2012**, *280*, 10–15. [CrossRef]
224. Lutterotti, A.; Yousef, S.; Sputtek, A.; Stürner, K.H.; Stellmann, J.-P.; Breiden, P.; Reinhardt, S.; Schulze, C.; Bester, M.; Heesen, C.; et al. Antigen-specific tolerance by autologous myelin peptide–coupled cells: A Phase 1 trial in multiple sclerosis. *Sci. Transl. Med.* **2013**, *5*, 188ra75. [CrossRef]
225. Bar-Or, A.; Vollmer, T.; Antel, J.; Arnold, D.L.; Bodner, C.A.; Campagnolo, D.; Gianettoni, J.; Jalili, F.; Kachuck, N.; Lapierre, Y.; et al. Induction of antigen-specific tolerance in multiple sclerosis after immunization with a DNA encoding myelin basic protein in a randomized, placebo-controlled Phase I/II trial. *Arch. Neurol.* **2007**, *64*, 1407–1415. [CrossRef] [PubMed]

226. Juryńczyk, M.; Walczak, A.; Jurewicz, A.; Jesionek-Kupnicka, D.; Szczepanik, M.; Selmaj, K. Immune regulation of multiple sclerosis by transdermally applied myelin peptides. *Ann. Neurol.* **2010**, *68*, 593–601. [CrossRef] [PubMed]
227. Walczak, A.; Siger, M.; Ciach, A.; Szczepanik, M.; Selmaj, K. Transdermal application of myelin peptides in multiple sclerosis treatment. *JAMA Neurol.* **2013**, *70*, 1105–1109. [CrossRef] [PubMed]
228. Garren, H.; Robinson, W.H.; Krasulova´, E.; Havrdova´, E.; Nadj, C.; Selmaj, K.; Losy, J.; Nadj, I.; Radue, E.-W.; Kidd, B.A.; et al. Steinman, and the BHT-3009 Study Group, Phase 2 trial of a DNA vaccine encoding myelin basic protein for multiple sclerosis. *Ann. Neurol.* **2008**, *63*, 611–620. [CrossRef]
229. Papadopoulou, A.; von Felten, S.; Traud, S.; Rahman, A.; Quan, J.; King, R.; Garren, H.; Steinman, L.; Cutter, G.; Kappos, L.; et al. Evolution of MS lesions to black holes under DNA vaccine treatment. *J. Neurol.* **2012**, *259*, 1375–1382. [CrossRef]
230. Chataway, J.; Martin, K.; Barrell, K.; Sharrack, B.; Stolt, P.; Wraith, D.C. Effects of ATX-MS-1467 immunotherapy over 16 weeks in relapsing multiple sclerosis. *Neurology* **2018**, *90*, e955–e962. [CrossRef]
231. Zubizarreta, I.; Flórez-Graub, G.; Vila, G.; Cabezón, R.; España, C.; Andorra, M.; Saiza, A.; Llufriu, S.; Sepulveda, M.; Sola-Valls, N.; et al. Immune tolerance in multiple sclerosis and neuromyelitis optica with peptide-loaded tolerogenic dendritic cells in a phase 1b trial. *Proc. Natl. Acad. Sci. USA* **2019**, *116*, 8463–8470. [CrossRef]
232. Willekens, B.; Presas-Rodríguez, S.; Mansilla, M.J.; Derdelinckx, J.; Lee, W.-P.; Nijs, G.; de Laere, M.; Wens, I.; Cras, P.; Parizel, P.; et al. On behalf of the RESTORE consortium, Tolerogenic dendritic cell-based treatment for multiple sclerosis (MS): A harmonized study protocol for two phase I clinical trials comparing intradermal and intranodal cell administration. *BMJ Open* **2019**, *9*, e030309. [CrossRef]
233. Seledtsova, G.V.; Ivanova, I.P.; Shishkov, A.A.; Seledtsov, V.I. Immune responses to polyclonal T-cell vaccination in patients with progressive multiple sclerosis. *J. Immunotoxicol.* **2016**, *13*, 879–884. [CrossRef]
234. Loftus, B.; Newsom, B.; Montgomery, M.; von Gynz-Rekowski, K.; Riser, M.; Inman, S.; Garces, P.; Rill, D.; Zhang, J.; Williams, J.C. Autologous attenuated T-cell vaccine (Tovaxin®) dose escalation in multiple sclerosis relapsing–remitting and secondary progressive patients nonresponsive to approved immunomodulatory therapies. *Clin. Immunol.* **2009**, *131*, 202–215. [CrossRef]
235. Fox, E.; Wynn, D.; Cohan, S.; Rill, D.; McGuire, D.; Markowitz, C. A randomized clinical trial of autologous T-cell therapy in multiple sclerosis: Subset analysis and implications for trial design. *Mult. Scler. J.* **2012**, *18*, 843–852. [CrossRef] [PubMed]
236. Karussis, D.; Shor, H.; Yachnin, J.; Lanxner, N.; Amiel, M.; Baruch, K.; Keren-Zur, Y.; Haviv, O.; Filippi, M.; Petrou, P.; et al. T Cell vaccination benefits relapsing progressive multiple sclerosis patients: A randomized, double-blind clinical trial. *PLoS ONE* **2012**, *7*, e50478. [CrossRef] [PubMed]
237. Van der, A.A.; Hellings, N.; Medaer, R.; Gelin, G.; Palmers, Y.; Rauss, J.; Stinissen, P. T cell vaccination in multiple sclerosis patients with autologous CSF-derived activated T cells: Results from a pilot study. *Clin. Exp. Immunol.* **2003**, *131*, 155–168. [CrossRef] [PubMed]
238. Zhang, J.Z.; Rivera, V.M.; Tejada-Simon, M.V.; Yang, D.; Hong, J.; Li, S.; Haykal, H.; Killian, J.; Zang, Y.C.Q. T cell vaccination in multiple sclerosis: Results of a preliminary study. *J. Neurol.* **2002**, *249*, 212–218. [CrossRef] [PubMed]
239. Correale, J.; Lunda, B.; McMillan, M.; Koa, D.Y.; McCarthy, K.; Weiner, L.P. T cell vaccination in secondary progressive multiple sclerosis. *J. Neuroimmunol.* **2000**, *107*, 130–139. [CrossRef]
240. Achiron, A.; Lavie, G.; Kishner, I.; Stern, Y.; Sarova-Pinhas, I.; Ben-Aharon, T.; Barak, Y.; Raz, H.; Lavie, M.; Barliya, T.; et al. T cell vaccination in multiple sclerosis relapsing–remitting nonresponders patients. *Clin. Immunol.* **2004**, *113*, 155–160. [CrossRef]
241. Zang, Y.C.Q.; Hong, J.; Rivera, V.M.; Killian, J.; Zhang, J.Z. Preferential recognition of TCR hypervariable regions by human anti-idiotypic T cells induced by T cell vaccination. *J. Immunol.* **2000**, *164*, 4011–4017. [CrossRef]
242. Vandenbark, A.A.; Culbertson, N.E.; Bartholomew, R.M.; Huan, J.; Agotsch, M.; LaTocha, D.; Yadav, V.; Mass, M.; Whitham, R.; Lovera, J.; et al. Therapeutic vaccination with a trivalent T-cell receptor (TCR) peptide vaccine restores deficient FoxP3 expression and TCR recognition in subjects with multiple sclerosis. *Immunology* **2007**, *123*, 66–78. [CrossRef]

9

Lost in Classification: Lower Cognitive Functioning in Apparently Cognitive Normal Newly Diagnosed RRMS Patients

Marco Pitteri *, Stefano Ziccardi, Caterina Dapor, Maddalena Guandalini and Massimiliano Calabrese *

Neurology section, Department of Neurosciences, Biomedicine and Movement Sciences, University of Verona, 37134 Verona, Italy; stefano.ziccardi@univr.it (S.Z.); caterina.dapor@univr.it (C.D.); maddalena.guandalini@univr.it (M.G.)

* Correspondence: marco.pitteri@univr.it (M.P.); massimiliano.calabrese@univr.it (M.C.);

Abstract: Cognitive functioning in multiple sclerosis (MS) patients is usually related to the classic, dichotomic classification of impaired vs. unimpaired cognition. However, this approach is far from mirroring the real efficiency of cognitive functioning. Applying a different approach in which cognitive functioning is considered as a continuous variable, we aimed at showing that even newly diagnosed relapsing–remitting MS (RRMS) patients might suffer from reduced cognitive functioning with respect to a matched group of neurologically healthy controls (HCs), even if they were classified as having no cognitive impairment (CI). Fifty newly diagnosed RRMS patients and 36 HCs were tested with an extensive battery of neuropsychological tests. By using Z-scores applied to the whole group of RRMS and HCs together, a measure of cognitive functioning (Z-score index) was calculated. Among the 50 RRMS patients tested, 36 were classified as cognitively normal (CN). Even though classified as CN, RRMS patients performed worse than HCs at a global level ($p = 0.004$) and, more specifically, in the domains of memory ($p = 0.005$) and executive functioning ($p = 0.006$). These results highlight that reduced cognitive functioning can be present early in the disease course, even in patients without an evident CI. The current classification criteria of CI in MS should be considered with caution.

Keywords: multiple sclerosis; cognitive impairment; diagnosis; neuropsychological assessment

1. Introduction

Multiple Sclerosis (MS) is one of the most common inflammatory neurodegenerative disorders of the human central nervous system (CNS), characterized histologically by multifocal areas of inflammation, demyelination, and neurodegeneration [1] within the white matter (WM) [2] as well as within cortical and deep gray matter (GM) [3].

In addition to physical disability, cognitive impairment (CI) is common in MS patients, with frequencies ranging from 43% to 70% [4] depending on the studied population, the tests used, and the applied cut-off scores [5,6]. CI can occur early in the disease course [7] and has been strongly associated with both focal and diffuse GM damage [8,9] and WM lesion measures [10,11]. The mainly affected cognitive domains are verbal learning and memory, attention, information processing speed, and executive functions [12]. CI can alter MS patients' behavior and quality of life [13,14], leading to social and personal difficulties, despite minimal physical disability [15]. Longitudinal studies have shown that CI detected at the time of diagnosis can predict the conversion from clinically isolated syndrome to definite MS [16], the progression of physical disability [17], the transition to the secondary progressive (SP) phase [18], and the worsening of physical disability and GM atrophy in the long term [19]. These studies suggest that assessing cognitive functioning since the early phases of the disease is of paramount importance [20,21].

Despite the different batteries of neuropsychological tests used to assess cognitive functioning, the classification of CI is undoubtedly affected by the chosen cut-off applied [6,22] and by the number of neuropsychological tests used. Usually, MS patients are classified as having either "normal cognition" or "impaired cognition" in a perspective of dichotomous classification (unimpaired vs. impaired). This approach, however, is far from being meaningful considering the real life [5], in which measures of functional aspects, such as cognitive functioning, resemble continuous variables, as also underlined in other neurological populations (e.g., see [23,24]).

Dichotomizing continuous variables, such as cognitive functions, carries the risk of losing information that might increase the number of false positive results, as well as of underestimating the extent of variation in patients' performance [25], rendering difficult the diagnosis and the subsequent clinical decisions. For this reason, it would be more appropriate to use different psychometric methods, switching from a "cognitive impairment-based" to a "cognitive functioning-based" approach, considering cognitive functioning as a continuum variable as it is in real life, ranging from a minimum to a maximum level of performance. This is of particular interest given that cognitive decline may develop as a result of gradual progression, related to neurodegeneration and brain atrophy, or of acute disease activity, for which decline in cognitive performance can be often followed by incomplete recovery, thus contributing to the burden of CI in the long term [11].

In order to investigate the usefulness of this approach, with the present study we aimed at investigating the cognitive performance of a group of newly diagnosed MS patients with relapsing–remitting (RR) course as compared to a group of healthy controls (HCs). We expected that also the newly diagnosed MS patients, even if classified as being "cognitively normal" when referring to the classic, dichotomous approach, would rather show reduced cognitive functioning with respect to HCs.

2. Materials and Methods

2.1. Participants

Fifty consecutive newly diagnosed RRMS patients (37 females, mean ± SD age = 38.2 ± 11.6 years; mean ± SD education = 14.2 ± 2.7 years; mean ± SD disease duration from onset = 3.5 ± 5.2 years; median [range] effects of disability (EDSS) = 1.5 (0–4)) were tested with an extensive battery of neuropsychological tests near the time of MS diagnosis (average: 6 months). At the time of neuropsychological testing, 31 RRMS patients were still untreated, whereas 14 were treated with dymethilfumarate, 1 with fingolimod, 1 with natalizumab, 1 with interferon beta1-a, 1 with peg-interferon beta1-a, and 1 with azathioprine. Inclusion criteria for RRMS patients comprised diagnosis of RRMS [26], no relapse or steroid treatment in the 30 days before neuropsychological assessment, no concomitant neurological or other pathological health conditions, no substance abuse or other MS concomitant medication (as benzodiazepines or antidepressant drugs), and no visual impairment.

A group of 36 HCs, matched with RRMS patients for age, education, and gender, was recruited and tested with the same battery of neuropsychological tests used to assess RRMS patients. Inclusion criteria for HCs comprised no cognitive deficits measured with the Montreal Cognitive Assessment (MoCA) test [27], a test of global cognitive functioning; no neurologic, psychiatric, or other concomitant pathologies; normal or corrected to normal vision; no substance abuse or other prior or concomitant medications.

All participants were recruited at the MS Center of the Verona University Hospital (Verona, Italy). The study was approved by the local Ethics Committee, and written informed consent was collected from all participants. Demographic and clinical characteristics of RRMS and HCs are listed in Table 1.

Table 1. Demographic and clinical characteristics of relapsing–remitting multiple sclerosis (RRMS) patients and healthy controls (HCs).

	CI ($n = 14$)	CN ($n = 36$)	HCs ($n = 36$)	p
Gender (M/F)	3/11	10/26	13/23	0.547
Age (years)	39.3 ± 14.0	37.8 ± 10.8	33.6 ± 10.4	0.170
Education (years)	13.8 ± 4.0	14.4 ± 2.0	15.1 ± 2.6	0.229
EDSS [1]	2.0 (0–4)	1.0 (0–3)	/	/
Disease duration (years)	4.4 ± 8.2	3.1 ± 3.6	/	/
Time between diagnosis and neuropsychological assessment (months)	6 (±3)	6 (±2)	/	/

[1] Means ± SDs were provided for continuous variables. Median (range) was provided for effects of disability (EDSS). EDSS = Expanded Disability Status Scale; CI = cognitive impairment; CN = cognitive normal.

2.2. *Neuropsychological Assessment*

RRMS patients and HCs were tested with an extensive battery of neuropsychological tests, which included the Brief Repeatable Battery (BRB) of neuropsychological tests [28]; the Stroop Test, ST [29]; the Phonological, Semantic, and Alternate Verbal Fluency test, (VF [30]); and the Modified Five Point Test (MFPT; [31]). The BRB is composed of tests of verbal learning and delayed memory recall (Selective Reminding Test, SRT); visuospatial learning and delayed memory recall (10/36 Spatial Recall Test, SPART); visual information processing speed and attention (Symbol Digit Modalities Test, SDMT); auditory information processing speed, attention, and calculation (Paced Auditory Serial Addition Task, PASAT); and semantic verbal fluency (Word List Generation, WLG). The ST is a test of attention and of automatic response inhibition; the VF test is a test of verbal fluency (phonemic, semantic, and alternate); the MFPT is a test of figurative fluency and use of strategies.

Depression, anxiety, and stress were evaluated with the 21-item Depression Anxiety Stress Scale (DASS-21; [32]) and subjective fatigue with the Fatigue Severity Scale (FSS; [33]). According to the most used method [6], RRMS patients were classified as "cognitive normal" (CN) if they scored below the cut-off (5° percentile; z-score = −1.65) on zero, one, or two neuropsychological tests administered; otherwise, if RRMS patients obtained a score below the cut-off on three or more neuropsychological tests, they were classified as having CI.

For each neuropsychological test and for each RRMS patient and HC, we calculated the Z-score index (for details see [34]), in which we did not use the normative data of the Italian validation of each test but, rather, the mean and standard deviation (SD) of scores of the RRMS patients and the HCs together. Considering the mean and SD of both groups together, in which MS patients and HCs compose the same population, allows to normalize the dependent variable (Z-score index) in a unique gaussian distribution with overlapped curves, mimicking a more real-life condition. Following this procedure, we calculated: (1) a global cognitive functioning index (Z-global) considering the average of the Z-scores of each neuropsychological test; and (2) three domain-specific Z-score indexes: memory (Z-MEM), attention/information processing speed (Z-ATT/IPS), and executive functions (Z-EF). For the detailed classification of each cognitive domain, see Table 2.

Table 2. Neuropsychological tests considered for each Z-score domain index.

Z-MEM	Z-ATT/IPS	Z-EF
SRT-LTS	SDMT	ST (average EIT and EIE)
SRT-CLTR	PASAT-3	Phonemic VF
SRT-D	PASAT-2	Alternate VF
SPART-I		MFPT-UDs
SPART-D		MFPT-CSs

Z-MEM = Z-score–Memory; Z-ATT/IPS = Z-score–Attention/Information Processing Speed; Z-EF = Z-score–Executive Functions; SRT-LTS = Selective Reminding Test-Long-Term Storage; SRT-CLTR = Selective Reminding Test-Consistent Long-Term Retrieval; SRT-D = Selective Reminding Test-Delayed; SPART-I = Spatial Recall Test-Immediate; SPART-D = Spatial Recall Test-Delayed; SDMT = Symbol Digit Modalities Test; PASAT = Paced Auditory Serial Addition Test; ST-EIT = Stroop Test-Effect Interference Time; ST-EIE = Stroop Test-Effect Interference Error; VF = Verbal Fluency; MFPT-UDs = Modified Five Point Test-Unique Designs; MFPT-CSs = Modified Five Point Test-Cumulative Strategies.

2.3. *Statistical Analyses*

ANOVA models with Tukey post-hoc analysis and chi-square test were applied to compare demographic, clinical, and Z-index scores among CI, CN, and HCs. Effects of EDSS, disease duration, emotional state (DASS-21), and fatigue (FSS) on the global cognitive functioning index (Z-score global index) and on the three cognitive domains (Z-MEM, Z-ATT/IPS, Z-EF) were controlled for RRMS patients' by using a stepwise multiple regression analysis.

3. Results

Among the 50 RRMS patients tested, 14 were classified as having CI, and 36 as being CN. The majority (12/14: 86%) of the CI patients were impaired in the domains of ATT/IPS (64%) and EF (71%).

Group comparison results between CI ($n = 14$), CN ($n = 36$), and HCs ($n = 36$) showed no significant difference between the three groups in terms of age ($p = 0.170$), education ($p = 0.229$), and gender ($p = 0.547$).

The Z-score global index was significantly different among the three groups ($p < 0.001$). Post-hoc comparisons showed a significant difference between CI and HCs ($p < 0.001$), between CI and CN ($p < 0.001$), and also between CN and HCs ($p = 0.004$) (Figure 1).

Significant difference was found among the three groups also for Z-MEM ($p < 0.001$), Z-ATT/IPS ($p < 0.001$), and Z-EFs ($p < 0.001$). Post-hoc analysis showed a significant difference between CI and HCs for Z- MEM ($p < 0.001$), Z-ATT/IPS ($p < 0.001$), and Z-EF ($p < 0.001$); between CI and CN for Z-MEM ($p = 0.009$), Z-ATT/IPS ($p < 0.001$), and Z-EF ($p < 0.001$); and between CN and HCs for Z-MEM ($p = 0.005$) and Z-EF ($p = 0.006$). No significant difference was found between CN and HCs for Z-ATT/IPS ($p = 0.087$), as shown in Figure 1.

Considering CI and CN patients together, the results of the multiple regression analysis (final model $R^2 = 0.254$, $p = 0.170$) showed no significant effects of age ($\beta = -0.255$, $p = 0.155$), education ($\beta = 0.196$, $p = 0.240$), gender ($\beta = 0.224$, $p = 0.185$), disability ($\beta = -0.125$, $p = 0.437$), disease duration ($\beta = 0.085$, $p = 0.591$), emotional state ($\beta = -0.197$, $p = 0.288$), and fatigue ($\beta = -0.145$, $p = 0.477$) on the Z-global index. No significant effect of these variables was also found on Z-MEM ($R^2 = 0.289$, $p = 0.099$), Z-ATT/IPS ($R^2 = 0.208$, $p = 0.311$), and Z-EF ($R^2 = 0.252$, $p = 0.173$).

Considering each single neuropsychological test, we found a significant difference among the three groups (CI, CN, and HCs) in all the neuropsychological tests (all $p < 0.05$), except for the WLG test ($p = 0.180$). Post-hoc analysis showed a significant difference between CI and HCs in all neuropsychological tests (all $p < 0.05$). Moreover, we found a significant difference between CI and CN for the SRT-CLTR ($p = 0.013$), SRT-D ($p = 0.026$), SDMT ($p = 0.040$), PASAT-3 ($p = 0.001$), PASAT-2 ($p = 0.043$), ST-Effect Interference Time (EIT) ($p = 0.049$), ST-Effect Interference Error (EIE) ($p < 0.001$), Phonemic Verbal Fluency ($p = 0.023$), Semantic Verbal Fluency ($p = 0.042$), MFPT-Unique Designs (UDs)

(p = 0.001), and MFPT-Error Index (p = 0.020), as shown in Table 3. Finally, comparing CN and HCs, we found significant difference for the SRT-LTS (p = 0.012), SRT–CLTR (p = 0.016), SRT-D (p = 0.007), SDMT (p = 0.014), Phonemic Verbal Fluency (p = 0.034), MFPT-UDs (p = 0.003), and MFPT-Cumulative Strategies (CSs) (p = 0.019), as shown in Table 3.

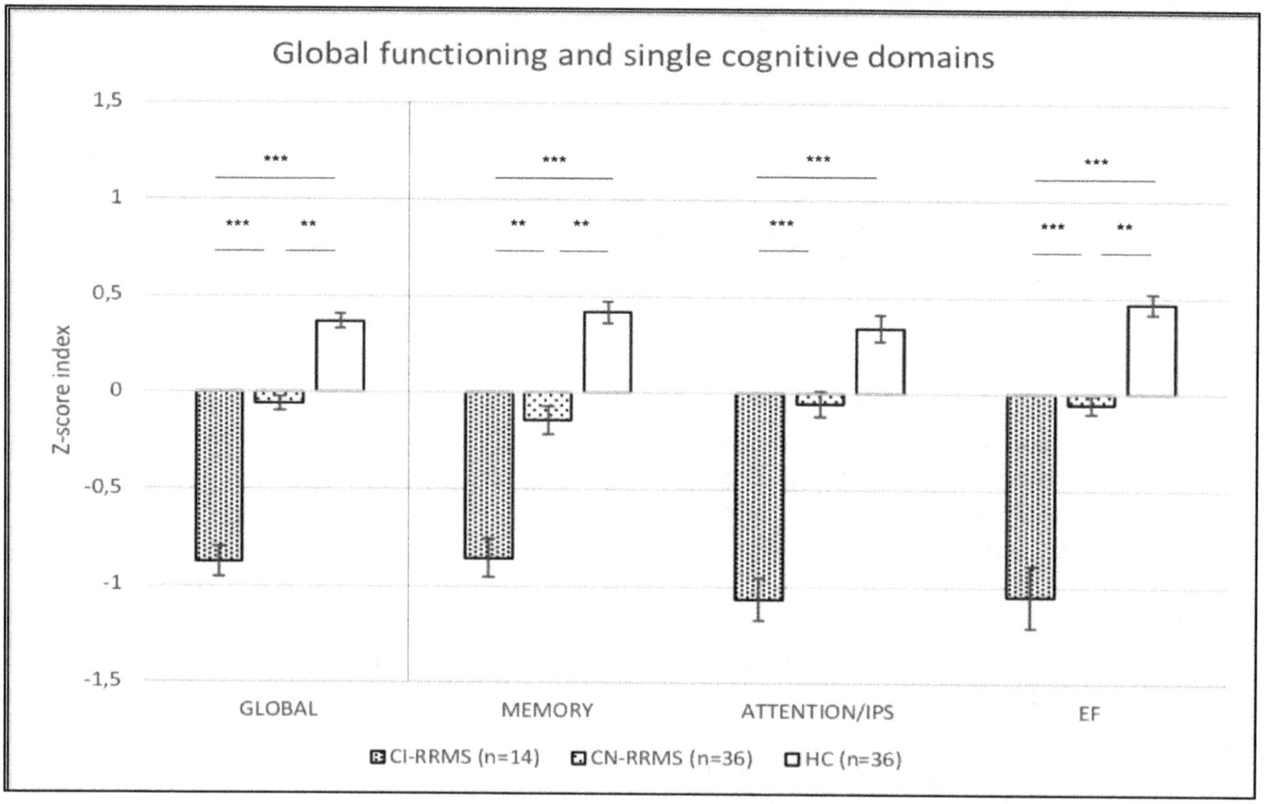

Figure 1. Functioning at a global level and on single cognitive domains of patients with cognitive impairment (CI), cognitive normal (CN) patients and healthy controls (HCs). ** = $p < 0.01$, *** = $p < 0.001$.

Table 3. Neuropsychological performance of RRMS patients and HCs and results of the comparison between the Z-score indexes of each subtest. Means ± SDs are provided.

		CI (n = 14)		CN (n = 36)		HCs (n = 36)			
NP Battery/NP Test	Subtest	Raw Scores	Z-score Index	Raw Scores	Z-score Index	Raw Scores	Z-score Index	p CI vs. CN	p CN vs. HCs
BRB (Brief Repeatable Battery)	SRT-LTS	38.5 ± 15.7	−0.8 ± 1.2	47.3 ± 12.8	−0.2 ± 0.9	55.7 ± 10.2	0.5 ± 0.8	0.076	0.012 *
	SRT-CLTR	26.2 ± 13.1	−1.0 ± 0.8	39.9 ± 15.2	−0.1 ± 0.9	49.7 ± 14.3	0.5 ± 0.9	0.013 *	0.016 *
	SRT-D	6.8 ± 2.5	−0.9 ± 1	8.7 ± 2.5	−0.2 ± 1	10.3 ± 1.7	0.5 ± 0.7	0.026 *	0.007 *
	SPART	20.3 ± 4.4	−0.7 ± 1	22.7 ± 4.4	−0.1 ± 1	25 ± 4.1	0.4 ± 0.9	0.211	0.054
	SPART-D	6.9 ± 1.7	−0.6 ± 0.9	7.9 ± 2	−0.1 ± 1	8.8 ± 1.8	0.3 ± 0.9	0.246	0.145
	SDMT	45.1 ± 11.3	−0.8 ± 0.9	53.9 ± 9.7	−0.1 ± 0.8	61.7 ± 12.9	0.5 ± 1	0.04 *	0.014 *
	PASAT-3	31.2 ± 11.5	−1.1 ± 1	43.6 ± 10.6	0.009 ± 0.9	47.8 ± 9.6	0.4 ± 0.8	0.001*	0.198
	PASAT-2	26.1 ± 10.8	−0.9 ± 1.1	35.3 ± 9.9	0.009 ± 0.1	37.1 ± 8.7	0.2 ± 0.9	0.043 *	0.689
	WLG	23.8 ± 7	−0.5 ± 1.1	27.2 ± 6.6	0.06 ± 1	27.5 ± 6	0.1 ± 0.9	0.231	0.974
Stroop Test (ST)	ST-EIT	17.3 ± 7.8	−0.7 ± 1.4	13.4 ± 5.4	−0.04 ± 1	11.3 ± 3.5	0.3 ± 0.6	0.049 *	0.202
	ST-EIE	1.6 ± 2.3	−1.1 ± 2.1	0.2 ± 0.5	0.2 ± 0.4	0.1 ± 0.4	0.3 ± 0.3	0.000 *	0.882
Verbal Fluency Test (VF)	Phonemic	34.1 ± 11.9	−0.8 ± 0.9	44.7 ± 12.7	−0.01 ± 0.9	53.9 ± 10.6	0.7 ± 0.8	0.023 *	0.034 *
	Semantic	47.5 ± 11.5	−0.7 ± 1	56.2 ± 11.3	−0.005 ± 0.9	63.5 ± 9.1	0.6 ± 0.8	0.042 *	0.071
	Alternate	37.8 ± 12.3	−0.6 ± 1.1	43.2 ± 10.8	−0.09 ± 0.9	50.5 ± 9.9	0.5 ± 0.9	0.350	0.073
	Shifting Index	0.9 ± 0.3	0.06 ± 1.5	0.9 ± 0.1	−0.06 ± 0.9	0.9 ± 0.1	−0.02 ± 0.9	0.944	0.993
Modified Five Point Test (MFPT)	MFPT-UDs	23.2 ± 12.7	−1.1 ± 1.2	34.3 ± 7.7	−0.07 ± 0.7	41.9 ± 7.5	0.6 ± 0.7	0.001 *	0.003 *
	MFPT-CSs	8.7 ± 11.9	−0.7 ± 1	14.9 ± 10.6	−0.1 ± 0.9	22.8 ± 11.1	0.5 ± 0.9	0.193	0.019 *
	MFPT-Error Index	15.3 ± 16.8	−0.7 ± 1.7	6.7 ± 6.9	0.2 ± 0.7	7.1 ± 8.4	0.1 ± 0.8	0.02 *	0.985

* = significant result.

4. Discussion

With the present study, we aimed at investigating the cognitive performance of a group of newly diagnosed RRMS patients as compared to a matched group of HCs by using a cognitive "functioning-based" approach instead of the classic "impairment-based" approach, in order to obtain a better real-life picture of RRMS patients' effective cognitive functioning.

Considering a functioning-based approach (i.e., Z-score index), the results of the present study showed that newly diagnosed RRMS patients can differ significantly from a group of HCs both on a global level and with reference to the cognitive domains of attention/processing speed, memory, and executive functioning. However, the most interesting finding is related to the fact that this significant difference between RRMS patients and HCs persists even after isolating those patients classified as CN, considering the classic categorization criterion [6]. Specifically, the group of CN patients showed a significant decrease in cognitive performance as compared to HCs at the global level as well as in the domains of memory and executive functions. The grading scores assigned on the basis of this cognitive "functioning-based" approach, as opposed to the classic "impairment-based" approach, highlight that also newly diagnosed CN RRMS patients can show worse cognitive performance as compared to HCs since the early stages of the disease, independently of the effect of other clinical and demographical variables like age, education, physical disability, disease duration, fatigue, or emotional state. The classic cognitive "impairment-based" approach is undoubtedly affected by different cut-offs threshold and by the different number of neuropsychological tests used, which can render the diagnosis of CI uncertain. Given that cognitive decline can occur as a result of gradual progression related to neurodegeneration or of more transient changes related to inflammatory (i.e., relapses) disease activity, by using a functioning-based approach (i.e., Z-score index) we expected that also newly diagnosed RRMS patients would perform worse with respect to HCs. In fact, it has been found that brain alterations due to GM and WM lesions and inflammatory phenomena can be observed since the time of diagnosis and are related to differences in the inflammatory profile [35,36]. Considering previous studies that showed that early neurodegeneration phenomena affect mainly the frontal and the temporal lobes since the early stage of the disease [8], it is remarkable that a significant difference between newly diagnosed CN patients and HCs was found specifically in the domains of memory and executive functions, that are mainly related to the activity of frontal and temporal brain areas, respectively. We would like to strongly highlight the alterations in executive functioning, since this domain is often neglected and not included in the most used batteries of neuropsychological tests in MS (i.e., the BRB and the Brief International Cognitive Assessment for MS, BICAMS).

The Z-score index, in which cognitive performance is considered as a continuum, seemed to effectively reflect the accumulation of cognitive alterations even in those RRMS patients that would be classified as "cognitively normal". As recently highlighted [37], if we accept that cognitive deficits in MS patients, or cognitive decline from baseline, reflect mainly cerebral dysfunctions related to MS disease, after excluding other confounding factors such as physical disability, fatigue, and emotional state, then cognitive functioning merits clinical attention as would any other indication of disease activity.

With this perspective, the classic impairment-based approach, usually limited by outdated and less representative normative data, can be overcome, optimizing the identification of slight alterations in cognitive performance already evident in newly diagnosed RRMS patients classified as being "cognitively normal" according to the traditional classification method. As underlined in previous studies, the early detection and monitoring of cognitive dysfunction may be crucial to identify MS patients with a probable worse prognosis and more severe disease progression [18,19], enabling early pharmacological and non-pharmacological interventions aimed at preventing further cognitive decline and disability in the long term [38]. According to this, a complete neuropsychological assessment in terms of level of performance, not just prone to classification criteria, seems of paramount importance not only in patients that show evident cognitive impairment [20], but also in apparently "cognitively normal" patients, as highlighted in the present study.

As recently underlined by Weber et al. [39], neuropsychological tests have shown a significant predictive value also regarding everyday-life activity and can be used in the clinical setting as one of several measures to help the clinician understand the impact of MS disease on the patients and their families. This view of considering patients' "cognitive performance" instead of patients' "cognitive impairment" might be an invaluable window on the real-life performance of MS patients since the time of diagnosis, given that early cognitive alterations can be considered as a signal of increased risk of disease progression [20].

We are aware that this study has some limitations. First, considering the variability of the MS population, further studies should include a larger number of both MS patients and matched HCs to substantiate the results of the present study. Second, the study is limited by the lack of a longitudinal neuropsychological assessment; this functioning-based approach should be tested more extensively with follow-up measures. Third, this study focused only on patients with RR course; future studies should extend this approach by investigating different MS populations. However, this is a proof-of-concept study, with which we aimed at highlighting the limitation of using the dichotomic approach derived from the classic neuropsychological assessment, frequently used for MS patients.

5. Conclusions

The results of the present study suggest that cognitive dysfunction in RRMS is a phenomenon that can be detected also in newly diagnosed patients. Extensive cognitive assessment since the early phase of the disease would be then of critical importance. This would support an accurate judgement of decline in cognitive functioning and would be clinically meaningful to determine a baseline cognitive profile to be monitored in the follow-up. We suggest approaching with extreme caution the traditional classification method of cognitive impairment: this classification criterion might fail in measuring the actual cognitive performance and should be interpreted with caution. In this regard, preferring an approach based on the evaluation of cognitive functioning as a continuous variable should be therefore recommended, also considering computerized devices [40,41].

Author Contributions: Conceptualization, M.P.; methodology, M.P. and S.Z.; formal analysis, S.Z.; investigation, M.P., S.Z., M.G., C.D., and M.C.; data curation, M.P., S.Z., M.G., C.D., and M.C.; writing—original draft preparation, S.Z.; writing—review and editing, M.P., S.Z., M.G., C.D., and M.C.; supervision, M.P. and M.C.; project administration, M.P.

References

1. Kutzelnigg, A.; Lassmann, H. *Pathology of Multiple Sclerosis and Related Inflammatory Demyelinating Diseases*, 1st ed.; Elsevier: Amsterdam, The Netherlands, 2014; Volume 122, ISBN 9780444520012.
2. Noseworthy, J.; Lucchinetti, C.; Rodriguez, M.; Weinshenker, B. Multiple Sclerosis. *N. Engl. J. Med.* **2000**, *343*, 938–952. [CrossRef] [PubMed]
3. Calabrese, M.; Magliozzi, R.; Ciccarelli, O.; Geurts, J.J.G.; Reynolds, R.; Martin, R. Exploring the origins of grey matter damage in multiple sclerosis. *Nat. Rev. Neurosci.* **2015**, *16*, 147–158. [CrossRef] [PubMed]
4. Chiaravalloti, N.D.; DeLuca, J. Cognitive impairment in multiple sclerosis. *Lancet Neurol.* **2008**, *7*, 1139–1151. [CrossRef]
5. Amato, M.P.; Morra, V.B.; Falautano, M.; Ghezzi, A.; Goretti, B.; Patti, F.; Riccardi, A.; Mattioli, F.; Amato, M.P. Cognitive assessment in multiple sclerosis—An Italian consensus. *Neurol. Sci.* **2018**, *39*, 1317–1324. [CrossRef]
6. Fischer, M.; Kunkel, A.; Bublak, P.; Faiss, J.H.; Hoffmann, F.; Sailer, M.; Schwab, M.; Zettl, U.K.; Köhler, W. How reliable is the classification of cognitive impairment across different criteria in early and late stages of multiple sclerosis? *J. Neurol. Sci.* **2014**, *343*, 91–99. [CrossRef]
7. Amato, M.P.; Portaccio, E.; Goretti, B.; Zipoli, V.; Hakiki, B.; Giannini, M.; Pastò, L.; Razzolini, L.; Pia, M.; Portaccio, A.E. Cognitive impairment in early stages of multiple sclerosis. *Neurol. Sci.* **2010**, *31*, 211–214. [CrossRef]

8. Calabrese, M.; Agosta, F.; Rinaldi, F.; Mattisi, I.; Grossi, P.; Favaretto, A.; Atzori, M.; Bernardi, V.; Barachino, L.; Rinaldi, L.; et al. Cortical lesions and atrophy associated with cognitive impairment in relapsing-remitting multiple sclerosis. *Arch. Neurol.* **2009**, *66*, 1144–1150. [CrossRef]
9. Eijlers, A.J.C.; van Geest, Q.; Dekker, I.; Steenwijk, M.D.; Meijer, K.A.; Hulst, H.E.; Barkhof, F.; Uitdehaag, B.M.J.; Schoonheim, M.M.; Geurts, J.J.G. Predicting cognitive decline in multiple sclerosis: A 5-year follow-up study. *Brain* **2018**, *141*, 2605–2618. [CrossRef]
10. Preziosa, P.; Rocca, M.A.; Pagani, E.; Stromillo, M.L.; Enzinger, C.; Gallo, A.; Hulst, H.E.; Atzori, M.; Pareto, D.; Riccitelli, G.C.; et al. Structural MRI correlates of cognitive impairment in patients with multiple sclerosis. *Hum. Brain Mapp.* **2016**, *37*, 1627–1644. [CrossRef]
11. Rocca, M.A.; Amato, M.P.; De Stefano, N.; Enzinger, C.; Geurts, J.J.; Penner, I.-K.; Rovira, A.; Sumowski, J.F.; Valsasina, P.; Filippi, M. Clinical and imaging assessment of cognitive dysfunction in multiple sclerosis. *Lancet Neurol.* **2015**, *14*, 302–317. [CrossRef]
12. Benedict, R.H.B.; Cookfair, D.; Gavett, R.; Gunther, M.; Munschauer, F.; Garg, N.; Weinstock-Guttman, B. Validity of the minimal assessment of cognitive function in multiple sclerosis (MACFIMS). *J. Int. Neuropsychol. Soc.* **2006**, *12*, 549–558. [CrossRef]
13. Amato, M.P.; Zipoli, V.; Portaccio, E. Multiple sclerosis-related cognitive changes: A review of cross-sectional and longitudinal studies. *J. Neurol. Sci.* **2006**, *245*, 41–46. [CrossRef] [PubMed]
14. Rao, S.M. Cognitive function in patients with multiple sclerosis: Impairment and treatment. *Int. J. MS Care* **2004**, *6*, 9–22. [CrossRef]
15. Benedict, R.H.B.; Zivadinov, R. Risk factors for and management of cognitive dysfunction in multiple sclerosis. *Nat. Rev. Neurol.* **2011**, *7*, 332–342. [CrossRef] [PubMed]
16. Zipoli, V.; Goretti, B.; Hakiki, B.; Siracusa, G.; Sorbi, S.; Portaccio, E.; Amato, M.P. Cognitive impairment predicts conversion to multiple sclerosis in clinically isolated syndromes. *Mult. Scler.* **2010**, *16*, 62–67. [CrossRef] [PubMed]
17. Deloire, M.; Ruet, A.; Hamel, D.; Bonnet, M.; Brochet, B. Early cognitive impairment in multiple sclerosis predicts disability outcome several years later. *Mult. Scler.* **2010**, *16*, 581–587. [CrossRef]
18. Moccia, M.; Lanzillo, R.; Palladino, R.; Chang, K.C.-M.M.C.-M.; Costabile, T.; Russo, C.; De Rosa, A.; Carotenuto, A.; Sacca, F.; Maniscalco, G.T.; et al. Cognitive impairment at diagnosis predicts 10-year multiple sclerosis progression. *Mult. Scler.* **2016**, *22*, 659–667. [CrossRef]
19. Pitteri, M.; Romualdi, C.; Magliozzi, R.; Monaco, S.; Calabrese, M. Cognitive impairment predicts disability progression and cortical thinning in MS: An 8-year study. *Mult. Scler.* **2017**, *23*, 848–854. [CrossRef]
20. Kalb, R.; Beier, M.; Benedict, R.H.; Charvet, L.; Costello, K.; Feinstein, A.; Gingold, J.; Goverover, Y.; Halper, J.; Harris, C.; et al. Recommendations for cognitive screening and management in multiple sclerosis care. *Mult. Scler. J.* **2018**, *24*, 1665–1680. [CrossRef]
21. Sumowski, J.F.; Benedict, R.; Enzinger, C.; Filippi, M.; Geurts, J.J.; Hamalainen, P.; Hulst, H.; Inglese, M.; Leavitt, V.M.; Rocca, M.A.; et al. Cognition in multiple sclerosis. *Neurology* **2018**, *90*, 278–288. [CrossRef]
22. Binder, L.M.; Iverson, G.L.; Brooks, B.L. To err is human: "abnormal" Neuropsychological scores and variability are common in healthy adults. *Arch. Clin. Neuropsychol.* **2009**, *24*, 31–46. [CrossRef] [PubMed]
23. Azouvi, P. The ecological assessment of unilateral neglect. *Ann. Phys. Rehabil. Med.* **2017**, *60*, 186–190. [CrossRef] [PubMed]
24. Pitteri, M.; Chen, P.; Passarini, L.; Albanese, S.; Meneghello, F.; Barrett, A.M. Conventional and functional assessment of spatial neglect: Clinical practice suggestions. *Neuropsychology* **2018**, *32*, 835. [CrossRef] [PubMed]
25. Altman, D.G.; Royston, P. The cost of dichotomising continuous variables. *BMJ* **2006**, *332*, 1080. [CrossRef] [PubMed]
26. Polman, C.H.; Reingold, S.C.; Banwell, B.; Clanet, M.; Cohen, J.A.; Filippi, M.; Fujihara, K.; Havrdova, E.; Hutchinson, M.; Kappos, L.; et al. Diagnostic criteria for multiple sclerosis: 2010 revisions to the McDonald criteria. *Ann. Neurol.* **2011**, *69*, 292–302. [CrossRef] [PubMed]
27. Santangelo, G.; Siciliano, M.; Pedone, R.; Vitale, C.; Falco, F.; Bisogno, R.; Siano, P.; Barone, P.; Grossi, D.; Santangelo, F.; et al. Normative data for the Montreal Cognitive Assessment in an Italian population sample. *Neurol. Sci.* **2015**, *36*, 585–591. [CrossRef]

28. Amato, M.P.; Portaccio, E.; Goretti, B.; Zipoli, V.; Ricchiuti, L.; De Caro, M.F.; Patti, F.; Vecchio, R.; Sorbi, S.; Trojano, M.; et al. The Rao's Brief Repeatable Battery and Stroop test: Normative values with age, education and gender corrections in an Italian population. *Mult. Scler.* **2006**, *12*, 787–793. [CrossRef]
29. Caffarra, P.; Vezzadini, G.; Dieci, F.; Zonato, F.; Venneri, A. Una versione abbreviata del test di Stroop: Dati normativi nella popolazione italiana. *Riv. Neurol.* **2002**, *12*, 111–115.
30. Costa, A.; Bagoj, E.; Monaco, M.; Zabberoni, S.; De Rosa, S.; Papantonio, A.M.; Mundi, C.; Caltagirone, C.; Carlesimo, G.A. Standardization and normative data obtained in the Italian population for a new verbal fluency instrument, the phonemic/semantic alternate fluency test. *Neurol. Sci.* **2014**, *35*, 365–372. [CrossRef]
31. Cattelani, R.; Dal Sasso, F.; Corsini, D.; Posteraro, L. The Modified Five-Point Test: Normative data for a sample of Italian healthy adults aged 16–60. *Neurol. Sci.* **2011**, *32*, 595–601. [CrossRef]
32. Bottesi, G.; Ghisi, M.; Altoè, G.; Conforti, E.; Melli, G.; Sica, C. The Italian version of the Depression Anxiety Stress Scales-21: Factor structure and psychometric properties on community and clinical samples. *Compr. Psychiatry* **2015**, *60*, 170–181. [CrossRef] [PubMed]
33. Krupp, L.B.; Larocca, N.G.; Muir Nash, J.; Steinberg, A.D. The fatigue severity scale: Application to patients with multiple sclerosis and systemic lupus erythematosus. *Arch. Neurol.* **1989**, *46*, 1121–1123. [CrossRef] [PubMed]
34. Strauss, E.; Sherman, E.M.S.; Spreen, O. *A Compendium of Neuropsychological Tests: Administration, Norms and Commentary*, 3rd ed.; Oxford University Press: New York, NY, USA, 2006.
35. Frischer, J.M.; Bramow, S.; Dal-bianco, A.; Lucchinetti, C.F.; Rauschka, H.; Schmidbauer, M.; Laursen, H.; Sorensen, P.S.; Lassmann, H. Neurodegeneration in multiple sclerosis brains. *Brain* **2009**, *132*, 1175–1189. [CrossRef]
36. Magliozzi, R.; Howell, O.W.; Nicholas, R.; Cruciani, C.; Castellaro, M.; Romualdi, C.; Rossi, S.; Pitteri, M.; Benedetti, M.D.; Gajofatto, A.; et al. Inflammatory intrathecal profiles and cortical damage in multiple sclerosis. *Ann. Neurol.* **2018**, *83*, 739–755. [CrossRef]
37. Weinstock-Guttman, B.; Eckert, S.; Benedict, R.H.B. A decline in cognitive function should lead to a change in disease-modifying therapy—Yes. *Mult. Scler. J.* **2018**, *24*, 1681–1682. [CrossRef]
38. Forn, C.; Rocca, M.A.; Valsasina, P.; Boscá, I.; Casanova, B.; Sanjuan, A.; Ávila, C.; Filippi, M. Functional magnetic resonance imaging correlates of cognitive performance in patients with a clinically isolated syndrome suggestive of multiple sclerosis at presentation: An activation and connectivity study. *Mult. Scler. J.* **2012**, *18*, 153–163. [CrossRef]
39. Weber, E.; Goverover, Y.; DeLuca, J. Beyond cognitive dysfunction: Relevance of ecological validity of neuropsychological tests in multiple sclerosis. *Mult. Scler. J.* **2019**, *25*, 1412–1419. [CrossRef]
40. Golan, D.; Wilken, J.; Doniger, G.M.; Fratto, T.; Kane, R.; Srinivasan, J.; Zarif, M.; Bumstead, B.; Buhse, M.; Fafard, L.; et al. Validity of a Multi-Domain Computerized Cognitive Assessment battery for Patients with Multiple Sclerosis. *Mult. Scler. Relat. Disord.* **2019**, *30*, 154–162. [CrossRef]
41. De Meijer, L.; Merlo, D.; Skibina, O.; Grobbee, E.J.; Gale, J.; Haartsen, J.; Maruff, P.; Darby, D.; Butzkueven, H.; Van der Walt, A. Monitoring cognitive change in multiple sclerosis using a computerized cognitive battery. *Mult. Scler. J. Exp. Transl. Clin.* **2018**, *4*, 205521731881551. [CrossRef]

10

*HLA-DPB1*03* as Risk Allele and *HLA-DPB1*04* as Protective Allele for Both Early- and Adult-Onset Multiple Sclerosis in a Hellenic Cohort

Maria Anagnostouli [1,2,*], Artemios Artemiadis [2,3], Maria Gontika [2], Charalampos Skarlis [2], Nikolaos Markoglou [2], Serafeim Katsavos [2], Konstantinos Kilindireas [4], Ilias Doxiadis [5] and Leonidas Stefanis [6]

1 Faculty of Neurology in Demyelinating Disease Unit & Director of Immunogenetics Laboratory, 1st Department of Neurology, Medical School, National and Kapodistrian University of Athens, NKUA, Aeginition Hospital, 115 28 Athens, Greece

2 Immunogenetics Laboratory, 1st Department of Neurology, Medical School, National and Kapodistrian University of Athens, NKUA, Aeginition Hospital, 115 28 Athens, Greece; kmwartem@yahoo.com (A.A.); mary212009@windowslive.com (M.G.); charskarlis@med.uoa.gr (C.S.); nmarkoglou@yahoo.gr (N.M.); serafkatsavos@gmail.com (S.K.)

3 Medical School, University of Cyprus, Nicosia 1678, Cyprus

4 Demyelinating Diseases Unit, 1st Department of Neurology, Medical School, National and Kapodistrian University of Athens, NKUA, Aeginition Hospital, 115 28 Athens, Greece; kildrcost@med.uoa.gr

5 Transplantation Immunological Laboratory, Institute of Transfusion Medicine, University Hospital Leipzig, 04103 Leipzig, Germany; ilidox@planet.nl

6 1st Department of Neurology, Medical School, National and Kapodistrian University of Athens, NKUA, Aeginition Hospital, 115 28 Athens, Greece; lstefanis@med.uoa.gr

* Correspondence: managnost@med.uoa.gr

Abstract: Background: Human Leucocyte Antigens (HLA) represent the genetic loci most strongly linked to Multiple Sclerosis (MS). Apart from *HLA-DR* and *HLA–DQ*, *HLA-DP* alleles have been previously studied regarding their role in MS pathogenesis, but to a much lesser extent. Our objective was to investigate the risk/resistance influence of *HLA-DPB1* alleles in Hellenic patients with early- and adult-onset MS (EOMS/AOMS), and possible associations with the *HLA-DRB1*15:01* risk allele. **Methods**: One hundred MS-patients (28 EOMS, 72 AOMS) fulfilling the McDonald-2010 criteria were enrolled. HLA genotyping was performed with standard low-resolution Sequence-Specific Oligonucleotide techniques. Demographics, clinical and laboratory data were statistically processed using well-defined parametric and nonparametric methods and the SPSSv22.0 software. **Results**: No significant *HLA-DPB1* differences were found between EOMS and AOMS patients for 23 distinct *HLA-DPB1* and 12 *HLA-DRB1* alleles. The *HLA-DPB1*03* allele frequency was found to be significantly increased, and the *HLA-DPB1*02* allele frequency significantly decreased, in AOMS patients compared to controls. The *HLA-DPB1*04* allele was to be found significantly decreased in AOMS and EOMS patients compared to controls. **Conclusions**: Our study supports the previously reported risk susceptibility role of the *HLA-DPB1*03* allele in AOMS among Caucasians. Additionally, we report for the first time a protective role of the *HLA-DPB1*04* allele among Hellenic patients with both EOMS and AOMS.

Keywords: Multiple Sclerosis; early-onset; adult-onset; Human Leucocyte Antigens; immunogenetics; clinical phenotype; clinical outcome; therapeutics

1. Introduction

Multiple sclerosis (MS) is considered a complex, multifactorial disease entity, as both environmental and genetic factors have been implicated in its pathogenesis [1]. The Major Histocompatibility Complex (MHC) represents a cluster of highly polymorphic genes, including mainly the Human Leukocyte Antigens (HLA) system, namely Class I (A, B, C) and II (DR, DQ, DP) genes, and genes encoding for some other immune factors, like complement components, Bf, C2, C4 and TNF, in Class III and IV loci [2]. HLA molecules mediate antigen presentation to T-lymphocytes, playing a crucial role in immune response and affecting all clinical and neuroimaging characteristics and response to treatment in MS [3,4]. Linkage studies in various populations have consistently demonstrated that the MHC and its polymorphisms represent the genetic locus most strongly linked to MS [3–5], and that the MHC class II (*HLA-DR, HLA-DQ, HLA-DP*) region is the susceptibility complex that accounts for the majority of familial clustering in MS [6].

The MHC class II linkage to MS differs in various populations, with the highest association conferred by the *HLA-DRB1*15:01/HLA-DQB1*06:02* haplotype, present in Caucasians [5]. In 2011, in a collaborative European study, the *HLA-DRB1*15:01* allele exhibited the strongest association with MS, along with the *HLA-DRB1* 03:01* and *HLA-DRB1*13:01* alleles [7], although *DRB1*15:01* was recently found to be hypomethylated and predominantly expressed in monocytes among carriers of *DRB1*15:01*, suggesting putative therapeutic strategies targeting methylation-mediated regulation of this major risk gene [8].

Recent studies have further established the role of *HLA-DRB1*15:01* in early-onset (pediatric and adolescent) MS (EOMS), which accounts for 3–5% of all MS cases, while the role of *HLA-DRB1*04* and *HLA-DRB1*03* remains to be clarified [9–11].

Apart from the well examined *HLA-DR* and *HLA-DQ* genes, other class II genes and their products, *HLA-DP* alleles, have been previously studied regarding their role in MS pathogenesis. One of the earliest studies regarding *HLA-DP* genotyping was performed three decades ago using a small sample of 45 Swedish patients with MS in comparison with 166 Danish controls [12]. Since then, few studies have been published on the role of the *HLA- DPB1* locus concerning genetic risk in adult-onset MS (AOMS), either in Asian [13–16] or European populations [17–21], and no such studies have been performed on EOMS. In 2013, Patsopoulos et al. used single nucleotide polymorphisms (SNP) data from genome-wide studies and tested classical alleles and polymorphisms in eight classical HLA genes in 5091 AOMS cases and 9595 controls [22]. Among a total of 11 identified statistically independent effects, they confirmed a possible association of *HLA-DPB1*03:01*, and also highlighted a more statistically significant effect at amino acid position 65 in the peptide binding groove of *HLA-DPB1** [22]. So far, *HLA-DPB1** alleles have been mainly correlated with neuromyelitis optica spectrum disorders (NMOSD) in Asian but not Caucasian populations [23], while a series of studies suggest a possible role in other autoimmune disorders as well, including juvenile idiopathic arthritis [24], type I diabetes [25] and atopic myelitis in Japanese [26].

The present study attempts to expand the existing data on HLA and MS by investigating the influence of *HLA-DPB1** alleles on disease risk and resistance in a Hellenic sample of 100 patients of both EOMS and AOMS, using healthy controls (HC) for comparisons, given the pre-existing difference in *HLA-DRB1* allele frequencies in EOMS and AOMS in our ethnic group [11] and the total absence of information on *HLA-DPB1* genotyping in the Hellenic MS population.

Additionally, we examined, the putative positive or negative association between the well-defined *HLA-DRB1*15:01* allele and the various *HLA-DPB1** alleles, given the extensive epistatic mechanisms that exist in HLA loci, as clearly illustrated in previous reports [12,19,27,28].

2. Materials and Methods

2.1. Patients

One hundred patients with MS (62 females, 38 males, mean age 36.9 ± 11.4 years old) were selected, fulfilling the McDonald criteria for MS diagnosis [29]. These patients were enrolled from the outpatient clinic at the Neurology Department of the Aeginition University Hospital (Athens, Greece) after providing written informed consent. The study received ethical approval by the Hospital's Ethics Committee (ethic approval code number: 117/2-4-13), as it was found consistent with the Declaration of Helsinki. At the time this study, 42 patients had the relapsing-remitting type of the disease (RRMS), and 10 patients were identified with primary progressive MS (PPMS), while the rest had the secondary progressive type (SPMS). For all patients, the mean age of disease onset was 27.8 ± 10.8 years old, the mean disease duration was 100.9 ± 80.4 months and the median Expanded Disability Status Scale (EDSS) was 3.0 (range:1.0–8.0) [30]. There were two MS onset groups; 28 in the ≤19 years old or early onset MS (EOMS) group and 72 in the >19 years old or adult onset MS (AOMS) group. Valid Magnetic Resonance Imaging (MRI) and cerebrospinal fluid (CSF) (i.e., presence of oligoclonal bands and IgG index calculation) assessments were available 60 (60%) of the patients. Missing data for MRIs were attributed to the lack of recent MRI scans. With regards to CSF, some but not all patients had been subjected to CSF analysis, since this was not a prerequisite for the MS diagnosis, according to the revised 2010 McDonald criteria [29]. All patients provided informed consent for participation and publication.

2.2. *HLA-DPB1** and *HLA-DRB1** Genotyping

HLA genotyping was performed at the Immunogenetics Laboratory of the 1st Department of Neurology, in Aeginition Hospital. High molecular weight DNA was extracted from peripheral blood samples (8 mL peripheral blood in sodium citrate, ACD Vacutainer® tube) using the DNA extraction, Maxi Kit (QIAGEN, Venlo, the Netherlands) as per manufacturer's guidelines in the commercial kit. HLA class II (*HLA-DRB1* and *HLA-DPB1*) frequencies were determined by molecular techniques for all the specificities included in the HLA Nomenclature of 2012 (we present only the first two or four digits of each allele, for low or high resolution respectively) [31]. *HLA-DRB1* genotyping had been previously performed, using a PCR-SSO (Polymerase-Chain-Reaction, PCR, Sequence-Specific Oligonucleotide, SSO) technique (Elpha Bio-Rad, High resolution), as described elsewhere [11]. *HLA-DPB1* genotyping was performed using a different PCR-SSO technique, based on a method that depends on reverse hybridization (Line Probe Assay, INNO-LiPA, Low Resolution, Innogenetics, Fujirebio, Europe) according to the manufacturer's protocol.

2.3. Statistical Analyses

The Hardy-Weinberg proportions (HWP) and linkage disequilibrium for *HLA-DPB1*, *HLA-DRB1* haplotypes were ascertained using the PyPoP software [32]. An Ewens-Watterson (EW) homozygosity test for neutrality was also performed. Calculation of the normalized deviate of the homozygosity (i.e., Fnd) was done, with positive and negative values implying directional and balancing selection, respectively. *HLA-DPB1** genotype frequency in patients with MS was compared with that reported in a previous study of Hellenic HC by using multiple binomial tests [33].

Separate analyses were performed in the EOMS and AOMS groups using the same expected genotype frequencies of the healthy controls [33]. A Fisher's exact test for categorical and Mann-Whitney U test for numerical variables were performed to allow us to make group comparisons. Mantel-Haenszel statistics were used to ascertain the role of MS groups in the association between *HLA-DPB1* genotypes and categorical clinical parameters. In *HLA-DPB1* genotype-related tests (except those for clinical parameters), p value correction was made according to the Benjamini–Yekutieli method (or B–Y) based on the following formula: p (B–Y) = a/(Σ1/i), where i denotes the number of comparisons and a = 0.05 [34,35]. Statistical analyses were performed using the SPSS v22.0 software (Armonk, NY, USA: IBM Corp).

3. Results

3.1. HWP and Linkage Disequilibrium of the Study's Sample

Twenty-three distinct *HLA-DPB1* alleles were identified (total alleles: 200). There were 28 homozygote and 72 heterozygote patients with MS. There were no deviations from the HWP (homozygotes: 29.71 expected, F(1) = 0.1, $p = 0.754$, heterozygotes: 70.29 expected, F(1) = 0.04, $p = 0.838$). The most common haplotypes were *HLA-DPB1*04/DPB1*04* (27%), followed by *HLA-DPB1*02/DPB1*04* (13%), *HLA-DPB1*03/DPB1*04* (11%) and *HLA-DPB1*10/DPB1*04* (6%). The EW homozygosity test of neutrality was found to be significantly positive (i.e., Fnd = 3.79, $p = 0.992$, i.e., over the limit 0.975), denoting a directional selection of the *HLA-DPB1*04* allele.

Twelve distinct *HLA-DRB1* alleles were identified (total alleles: 174) in 87 out of the 100 patients. There were 11 (12.6%) homozygote and 76 (87.3%) heterozygote patients. There were no deviations from the HWP (homozygotes: 10.84 expected, F(1) = 0, $p = 0.962$, heterozygotes: 76.16 expected, F(1) = 0, $p = 0.986$). The most common allele was *HLA-DRB1*11* (20.1%), followed by *HLA-DRB1*16* (15.5%), *HLA-DRB1*15* (13.2%), *HLA-DRB1*04* (12.1%) and *HLA-DRB1*13* (10.4%). The most common, but still of low frequency (4.6%), genotype was *HLA-DRB1*11/DRB1*16*. The EW homozygosity test of neutrality was found to be significantly negative (i.e., Fnd = −1.41, $p = 0.0033$, i.e., lower the limit 0.05), indicating a balancing selection.

The delta distance for the *HLA-DPB1* and *HLA-DRB1* haplotypes was 0.00938 ($p = 0.303$), denoting linkage equilibrium. This did not change when age of MS onset was taken into account (EOMS: delta 0.0128, $p = 0.954$, AOMS: delta 0.0133, $p = 0.351$). The most common (i.e., over 5%) *HLA-DPB1/HLA-DRB1* haplotypes were *HLA-DPB1*04/HLA-DRB1*11* (10.8%), *HLA-DPB1*04/HLA-DRB1*16* (7.7%), *HLA-DPB1*04/HLA-DRB1*04* (7%), *HLA-DPB1*02/HLA-DRB1*11* (6.6%) and *HLA-DPB1*04/HLA-DRB1*03* (5.5%).

3.2. Nongenetic Comparisons between Age of Onset Groups

Table 1 presents the main characteristics of the two MS groups. Patients with EOMS were significantly younger and had longer disease duration compared to AOMS, which primarily reflects the blood sampling timing, and has no specific clinical significance. Of most importance, patients with EOMS had significantly higher IgG indexes compared to AOMS. It should be noted that this difference reflects 60 out of the 100 patients with MS of this study, since, as mentioned in the methods section, no CSF testing was available for 40 patients.

Table 1. Nongenetic Comparisons Between Age of Multiple Sclerosis (MS) Onset Groups.

Characteristics	EOMS	AOMS	Sig [1]
Females	19/28 (67.9%)	43/72 (59.7%)	0.499
Age (years old)	29.9 ± 9.8	39.8 ± 10.8	0.001 *
Duration of MS (months)	148.1 ± 105.4	81.3 ± 69.1	0.011 *
EDSS	3.1 ± 1.7	3.3 ± 1.6	0.414
Primary Progressive	3/28 (10.7%)	7/72 (9.7%)	0.917
Relapses since onset	5.2 ± 6.1	3.7 ± 2.5	0.393
IgG index [2]	1.3 ± 0.7	0.8 ± 0.4	0.004 *
Presence of OCBs [2]	13/15 (86.7%)	31/45 (68.9%)	0.312
Subcortical lesions [2]	12/17 (70.6%)	27/43 (62.8%)	0.765
Periventricular lesions [2]	16/17 (94.1%)	42/43 (97.7%)	0.49
Infratentorial lesions [2]	12/17 (70.6%)	30/43 (69.8%)	1.000
Spinal cord lesions [2]	12/14 (85.7%)	29/31 (93.5%)	0.578

Numbers represent means ± standard deviation and absolute (%) frequencies; 1 Fisher exact test for categorical and Mann-Whitney U test for numerical characteristics. OCBs: Oligoclonal Bands, Sig.: significance. 2 Valid MRI and cerebrospinal fluid assessments were available for 60 (66%) and 60 (60%) patients, respectively. * $p \leq 0.05$.

3.3. HLA-DPB1 Allele Comparisons between the Age of Onset Groups

No significant *HLA-DPB1* allele differences were found between patients with EOMS and AOMS (Table 2). However, there were significantly fewer *HLA-DPB1*04*-positive patients in the EOMS group compared to HC (64.3% vs. 92.7%). The *HLA-DPB1*03* allele was found to be significantly increased in patients with AOMS compared to HC (23.6% vs. 13.4%). On the other hand, *HLA-DPB1*02* and *HLA-DPB1*04* were found to be significantly decreased ($p < 0.001$) in patients with AOMS compared to HC (22.2% vs. 36.6% and 79.2% vs.92.7%).

A total of 21 out of 87 patients (24.1%) were positive for the *HLA-DRB1*15* allele, which is significantly higher than the expected 11.4% allele frequency in HC ($p < 0.001$), confirming the well-established role of this allele in MS pathogenesis [33]. *HLA-DRB1*15* allele positivity was 20.8% (5/24) for EOMS and 25.4% (16/63) for AOMS ($p = 0.783$).

Table 3 presents the *HLA-DRB1*15* allele frequency among the different *HLA-DPB1** alleles. Only statistically significant associations are presented. The *HLA-DRB1*15* allele was statistically significantly absent among *HLA-DPB1*03* positive patients ($p = 0.001$) and among *HLA-DPB1*03* positive AOMS ($p = 0.003$), whereas it was significantly increased among *HLA-DPB1*04* ($p = 0.048$), *HLA-DPB1*14* ($p = 0.008$) -positive genotype patients. Finally, the *HLA-DRB1*15* allele was positive in the two *HLA-DPB1*14* positive patients with EOMS ($p = 0.036$).

In the 60 patients with available CSF examination, those with the *HLA-DPB1*02* allele had significantly higher IgG indexes than those who were negative for *HLA-DPB1*02* (mean 1.22 ± 0.70 vs. 0.75 ± 0.39, respectively, $p = 0.02$), irrespective of age of MS onset. There were no other significant associations between the *HLA-DPB1* or *HLA-DRB1* alleles (i.e., presence or not of each *HLA-DPB1** allele and *HLA-DRB1*15* allele) and gender, type of MS, MRI or CSF assessments (data not shown). Patients with AOMS who were positive for *HLA-DPB1*02* had significantly fewer relapses since onset than *HLA-DPB1*02* negative patients with AOMS (2.7 ± 2.5 vs. 3.9 ± 2.4, $p = 0.033$), corroborating the protective role of *HLA-DPB1*02* phenotype, as reported above (Figure 1). No other MS group effects on the HLA and clinical parameter associations were found.

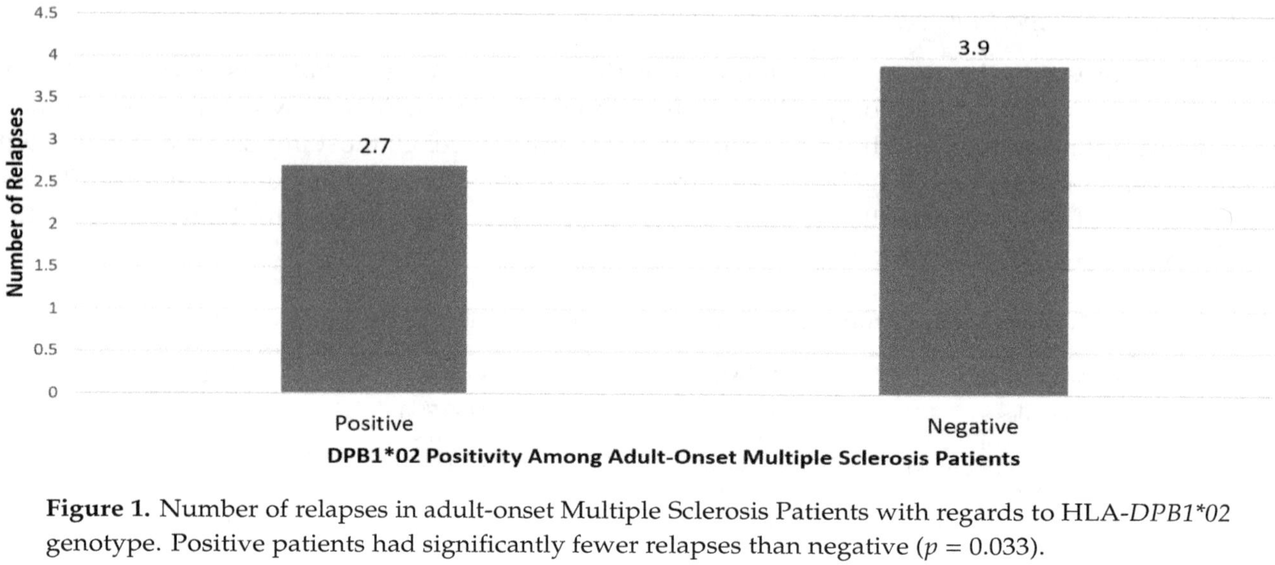

Figure 1. Number of relapses in adult-onset Multiple Sclerosis Patients with regards to HLA-*DPB1*02* genotype. Positive patients had significantly fewer relapses than negative ($p = 0.033$).

Table 2. *HLA-DPB1* Allele Frequencies Among Different Age of Multiple Sclerosis (MS) Onset Groups of Patients.

Early MS		Adult MS	HCs	Early vs. Adult MS	Early MS vs. HCs	Adult MS vs. HCs
	(N = 28)	(N = 72)	(N = 246)	Sig [1]	Sig [2]	Sig [2]
*HLA-DPB1*01*	3.6	4.2	4.5	0.85 (0.09–8.55) 1.000	0.79 (0.1–6.37) 0.500	0.92 (0.25–3.42) 0.500
*HLA-DPB1*02*	39.3	22.2	36.6	2.27 (0.89–5.80) 0.131	1.12 (0.5–2.5) 0.461	0.5 (0.23–0.91) 0.008 **
*HLA-DPB1*03*	17.9	23.6	13.4	0.7 (0.23–2.13) 0.602	1.4 (0.50–3.95) 0.339	2.0 (1.04–3.84) 0.009 **
*HLA-DPB1*04*	64.3	79.2	92.7	0.47 (0.18–1.24) 0.132	0.14 (0.06–0.35) <0.001 **	0.3 (0.14–0.63) <0.001 **
*HLA-DPB1*05*	3.6	2.8	2.4	1.3 (0.11–14.89) 1.000	1.48 (0.17–12.77) 0.500	1.14 (0.23–5.79) 0.500
*HLA-DPB1*06*	0	1.4	0.8	- 1.000	- 0.500	1.72 (0.15–19.23) 0.500
*HLA-DPB1*09*	0	1.4	2.8	- 1.000	- 0.372	0.48 (0.06-3.97) 0.356
*HLA-DPB1*10*	10.7	9.7	4.9	1.11 (0.27–4.65) 1.000	2.34 (0.62–8.85) 0.162	2.1 (0.8–5.55) 0.052
*HLA-DPB1*11*	0	1.4	-	- 1.000	-	-
*HLA-DPB1*13*	3.6	2.8	6.1	1.3 (0.11–14.89) 1.000	0.57 (0.07–4.49) 0.435	0.44 (0.1–1.97) 0.176
*HLA-DPB1*14*	7.1	6.9	3.7	1 (0.18–5.48) 1.000	2.03 (0.42–9.88) 0.321	1.97 (0.64–6.06) 0.126
*HLA-DPB1*15*	0	4.2	2.0	- 0.557	- 0.468	2.1 (0.49–8.99) 0.186
*HLA-DPB1*19*	0	1.4	0.4	- 1.000	- 0.500	3.45 (0.21–55.87) 0.346
*HLA-DPB1*22*	3.6	0	-	- 0.280	-	-
*HLA-DPB1*23*	3.6	0	2.4	- 0.280	1.48 (0.17–12.77) 0.500	- 0.172

Table 2. *Cont.*

Early MS		Adult MS	HCs	Early vs. Adult MS	Early MS vs. HCs	Adult MS vs. HCs
	(N = 28)	(N = 72)	(N = 246)	Sig [1]	Sig [2]	Sig [2]
*HLA-DPB1*32*	3.6	0	0.8	- 0.280	4.52 (0.4–51.49) 0.279	- 0.460
*HLA-DPB1*33*	3.6	2.8	0.4	1.3 (0.11–14.89) 1.000	9.07 (0.55–149.24) 0.123	7.0 (0.63–78.34) 0.130
*HLA-DPB1*34*	0	1.4	-	- 1.000	-	-
*HLA-DPB1*35*	0	4.2	0.8	- 0.557	- 0.500	10.65 (1.09–104.03) 0.005 **
*HLA-DPB1*38*	3.6	0	-	- 0.280	-	-
*HLA-DPB1*46*	3.6	0	-	- 0.280	-	-
*HLA-DPB1*50*	0	1.4	0.4	- 1.000	- 0.500	3.45 (0.21–55.87) 0.346
*HLA-DPB1*56*	0	1.4	-	- 1.000	-	-

Numbers represent frequencies (%). 1 Fishers's exact test (23 comparisons) 2 Binomial tests (17 comparisons). ** $p \leq 0.015$ (17 comparisons) or $p \leq 0.013$ (23 comparisons), according to the Benjamini–Yekutieli method for 17 comparisons, HCs: Healthy Control

Table 3. Significant DRB1*15 Positivity Differences among *HLA-DPB1* Alleles and Age of Onset Groups in Multiple Sclerosis (MS) Patients.

	Total Sample of MS Patients	
*HLA-DPB1** Genotype	*HLA-DRB1*15* Positive	Sig [1]
*HLA-DPB1*03*	0/22 (0%)	0.001 *
*HLA-DPB1*04*	19/63 (30.2%)	0.048 *
*HLA-DPB1*14*	5/7 (71.4%)	0.008 *
	Adult-Onset MS	
*HLA-DPB1** Genotype	*HLA-DRB1*15* Positive	Sig [1]
*HLA-DPB1*03*	0/17 (0%)	0.003 *
	Early-Onset MS	
*HLA-DPB1** Genotype	*HLA-DRB1*15* Positive	Sig [1]
*HLA-DPB1*14*	2/2 (100%)	0.036 *

Values represent observed frequencies (%) of *HLA-DRB1*15* allele positivity among the different *HLA-DPB1* genotypes. 1 Fisher exact tests. * $p \leq 0.05$.

4. Discussion

HLA-immunogenetics is an old but still rapidly expanding field in MS pathogenesis. In order to keep abreast of rapid developments in this field, we investigated the role of the *HLA-DP* locus in MS pathophysiology. We genotyped 100 Hellenic patients with MS for *HLA-DR* and *HLA-DP* alleles, as described above, which is a rather small sample and the main limitation of this study. *HLA-DPB1* genotyping was performed for the first time on a Hellenic MS population and in patients with EOMS, which is the core novelty of our research, albeit on a small sample (28 patients); however, we highlight again that EOMS is a rare disease entity and represents only the 3–5% of all MS patients in Caucasian populations.

In our study, we replicated the well-established predominance of the *HLA-DRB1*15* genotype in Hellenic patients with MS compared to HC, independently of age at disease onset [11].

No statistically significant *HLA-DPB1* allele differences were found between patients with EOMS and AOMS. All statistically significant differences were investigated in the AOMS group, except for the *HLA-DPB1*04* allele, which is lower in EOMS and AOMS, compared to the HC group at a high statistical level ($p < 0.001$, Table 2), suggesting a possible protective role in the Hellenic population. This is in contrast with an early study in 1988 [12] where the frequencies of DPw4 were 93.3% in patients with MS and 72.3% in controls (relative risk, $R^2 = 5.4$, $p = 0.0014$). Nevertheless, we have to mention that in this early study, the HLA-DNA typing was carried out on a small sample of 45 patients with MS and 63 controls of different ethnic European groups (Swedish and Danish), using the Restriction Fragment Length Polymorphism (RFLP) technique for *HLA-DP* and *HLA-DR* genes. In this same study, the *HLA-DR2* antigen was present in 75.5% of patients and in 33.7% of the controls ($R^2 = 6.1$, p less than 10(-6)). *HLA-DPw4* was not associated (i.e., was not in linkage disequilibrium) with *HLA-DR2* in patients or controls. Thus, the researchers concluded that in MS, the associations with *HLA-DP* and *HLA-DR* are independent of each other, but the combined presence of *HLA-DPw4* (cellularly defined) and *HLA-DR2* represented a significantly higher risk than either antigen alone, indicating that synergism between *HLA-DP* and *HLA-DR* gene products may play a role in the genetic susceptibility to MS. On the other hand, a recent study on celiac disease showed that the *HLA-DPB1*04:01* allele protects genetically-susceptible children from celiac disease [36], a fact that is in line with our results, concerning children and adults with MS, while in another study in 2015, another *HLA-DPB1*04* allele, namely *HLA-DPB1*04:02*, conferred a strong protective effect against narcolepsy [37]. Finally, the worldwide risk *HLA-DRB1*15* allele in MS, in Caucasians, was found to be significantly increased among *HLA-DPB1*04* positive patients with MS ($p = 0.048$) in our sample.

In another early study in France in 1991, it was found that the distribution of *HLA-DPB1* alleles was not significantly different in patients with MS and controls [20]. Nowadays, it is perfectly clear that the *HLA-DP*03* allele is associated with MS and epitope spreading in MS [17,22], and in this study, we observed the risk susceptibility of this allele in our Hellenic MS sample, at a highly significant level ($p < 0.009$, Table 2).

Regarding AOMS, the *HLA-DPB1*03* allele could be a risk factor for the disease, as it was found to be significantly increased in patients with AOMS compared to HC. The percentage of *HLA-DPB1*03* positive patients with EOMS was higher than HC (17.9% vs. 13.4%), although at a nonstatistically significant level. The *HLA-DRB1*15* allele was absent among *HLA-DPB1*03* positive patients. This cannot be attributed to linkage disequilibrium, as this was tested. Linkage disequilibrium for the *HLA-DR* and *HLA-DP* genes was excluded in previous studies as well [12]. Since *HLA-DPB1*03* was found to be increased in AOMS, it may constitute a risk factor; this genotype may exert its risk factor effect only in the absence of *HLA-DRB1*15*, at least in AOMS. Moreover, the *HLA-DRB1*15* allele was found to be significantly increased among *HLA-DPB1*04*-positive patients, suggesting that *HLA-DPB1*04* exerts a protective effect only in the absence of *HLA-DRB1*15*. Despite the relatively small sample size in our study, these findings suggest that epistatic mechanisms between Class II *HLA-DR* and *HLA-DP* alleles may play a role in disease pathogenesis and risk of disease occurrence. This conclusion is in line with the results of Dekker et al. [19] who observed that in patients with MS who lacked *HLA-DQB1*06:02* allele, the *HLA-DPB1*03:01* allele frequency was significantly ($p = 0.006$) increased (50.0%) compared with *HLA-DQB1*06:02*-negative controls (9.1%). In parallel, in 2009, Lincoln et al. highlighted the role of epistasis between *HLA-DRB1*15* and *HLA-DQA1*01:02* alleles. More specifically, they proved that *HLA-DQA1*01:02*, which shows no primary MS association, increases disease risk when combined with *HLA-DRB1*15:01*, through transepistatic interactions [27]. Of note is the fact that the presented slight *HLA-DPB1* allele differences between AOMS and EOMS could also reflect the different clinical course of these two groups, given that patients with older age at onset are known to be more at risk of having secondary-progressive disease. For instance, predicting the onset of secondary-progressive multiple sclerosis is accomplished using genetic and nongenetic factors, with the *HLA-A*02:01* allele conferring a decreased risk for MS and also contributing to decreased hazards for SPMS [38].

Another finding in our study that is worthy of mention is the possible protective role of the *HLA-DPB1*02* allele in AOMS. *HLA-DPB1*02* was found to be significantly decreased in AOMS, while those who were *HLA-DPB1*02* positive had, in general, fewer relapses since onset compared to *HLA-DPB1*02*-negative patients with AOMS, corroborating the protective role of the *HLA-DPB1*02* allele reported above (Figure 1).

The *HLA-DPB1*35* allele was found to be significantly increased in patients with AOMS compared to HC, while increased prevalence of the *HLA- DRB1*15* allele in *HLA-DPB1*14*-positive patients with MS and patients with EOMS was also noted. Nevertheless, their possible genetic risk should be interpreted with caution, due to the very low frequency of these alleles.

At this point, we have to mention that the *HLA-DPB1*04* allele is the most frequent in the Hellenic population (92.7%), followed by *HLA-DP*02* (36.6%) and *HLA-DP*03* (13.4%) [30]. Additionally, according to our results, the most common *HLA-DPB1*-haplotypes in Hellenic patients with MS were *HLA-DPB1*04/DPB1*04* (27%), followed by *HLA-DPB1*02/DPB1*04* (13%), *HLA-DPB1*03/DPB1*04* (11%) and *HLA-DPB1*10/DPB1*04* (6%). Thus, the emerging protective role of the *HLA-DP*04* allele is in parallel with the *HLA-DR*11* allele, which is the most common in the Hellenic population, and the protective *HLA-DRB1* allele in Hellenic patients with MS [11].

The role of *HLA-DPB1* alleles has been studied in a range of other autoimmune diseases, especially NMOSD [23]. More specifically, *HLA-DPB1*05:01*, which is extremely rare in Caucasian populations, has the strongest association with opticospinal MS and anti-AQP4 seropositivity in Asian populations, while *HLA-DPB1*03* possibly offers genetic protection against the disease [23]. Moreover, *HLA-DPB1*02:01* has been associated with oligoarticular and rheumatoid factor-negative polyarticular juvenile idiopathic arthritis and childhood-onset diabetes type I in the Japanese population [24,25].

Therapeutic interventions in MS are sometimes difficult, because the patient's symptoms at the initial stages are not clearly suggestive of a definite demyelinating syndrome, especially in children. Furthermore, sometimes the neuroradiological (MRI) aspects and blood antibody tests are not helpful. In these situations, having a marker or a combination of markers that supports the differential diagnosis is of crucial importance, and has a direct impact on therapeutic decision making. The *HLA-DR* alleles, and especially the *HLA-DR*15* allele, are the most robust genetic markers for almost every clinical or paraclinical aspect of the disease [4] in Caucasians and for the therapeutic response to different Disease Modified Treatments (DMTs) [4]. Nowadays, the expansion and overlap of various demyelinating diseases, namely MS, NMOSD, ADEM (Acute Disseminating Encephalomyelitis), MOG-Demyelinating (Myelin Oligodendrocyte Glycoprotein-Demyelinating) disease, Optic Neuritis, etc., make the need for specific biomarkers more urgent than ever before, as noted in our previous critical review [39] and in this works of other researchers [40].

Apart from a genetic association with MS and other demyelinating diseases, *HLA-DP* molecules play a key role in MS pathogenesis and progression, as described many years ago [17,41].

Additionally, in our Hellenic cohort, the *HLA-DP* alleles seemed to play an independent role in patients with MS (risk/protective), apart from the *HLA-DR* alleles, a fact that has to be confirmed in larger cohorts in the future. This could pave the way for the usage of these alleles in patient stratification (carriers and noncarriers)—as already happens with various HLA-DRB1 alleles and especially with the *HLA-DRB1*15* allele [4,42]—for many MS characteristics and therapy responses in different DMTs in Caucasian populations [4,42].

Altogether, clarification of *HLA-DP* allele associations with both EOMS and AOMS is needed in every ethnic group to get a better idea of clinical features and MS phenotypes and disease progression, and as a form of future putative data for better therapeutics.

5. Conclusions-Limitations

In conclusion, our study supports the previously reported risk susceptibility role of the *HLA-DPB1*03* allele in AOMS in many Caucasian populations. Additionally, we report, for the first time in the international literature, the protective role of the *HLA-DPB1*04* allele for patients with both EOMS and AOMS, and the putative protective role of the *HLA-DPB1*02* allele in patients with AOMS in our sample. Another finding that is worthy of mention is the total absence of the well-established *HLA-DRB1*15* allele among patients having the most statistically frequent *HLA-DPB1*03* allele in our cohort.

A limitation of our study was the relatively small sample size (28 patients with EOMS and 72 patients with AOMS). Indeed, observed small effect sizes for DPB1 alleles from the different group comparisons were the following: EOMS vs. AOMS 7%, EOMS vs. HCs 21.9% and AOMS vs. HCs 25.8%. However, this is a first attempt towards clarifying the role of the *HLA-DPB1* alleles in MS in a Hellenic AOMS and EOMS cohort. Moreover, the small study sample did not allow us to conduct multivariable analyses, which would more readily reveal confounding effects in our analyses.

These novel data could also contribute to personalized MS-therapeutics in the near future, taking into account the rapid expansion of our knowledge of multiple sclerosis and other distinct demyelinating diseases in many ethnic groups.

Author Contributions: Conceptualization, methodology, patients' curating, manuscript's drafting, manuscript's proofreading, M.A., statistical analyses, manuscript's drafting, manuscript's proofreading, A.A., patients' curating, bibliography manuscript's drafting, M.G., project administration, bibliography, C.S., data curating, N.M., S.K., critical review of the manuscript, K.K., L.S., statistical suggestions, validation, critical review of the manuscript, I.D. All authors have read and agreed to the published version of the manuscript

Acknowledgments: We want to gratefully thank the patients and their families for their valuable contribution in our research.

References

1. Ramagopalan, S.V.; Dyment, D.A.; Ebers, G.C. Genetic epidemiology: The use of old and new tools for multiple sclerosis. *Trends Neurosci.* **2008**, *31*, 645–652. [CrossRef]
2. Gruen, J.R.; Weissman, S.M. Human MHC Class III and IV Genes and Disease Associations. *Front. Biosci.* **2001**, *6*, D960–D972. [CrossRef] [PubMed]
3. Katsavos, S.; Anagnostouli, M. Biomarkers in Multiple Sclerosis: An Up-to-Date Overview. *Mult. Scler. Int.* **2013**, *2013*, 340508. [CrossRef] [PubMed]
4. Stamatelos, P.; Anagnostouli, M. HLA-Genotype in Multiple Sclerosis: The Role in Disease onset, Clinical Course, Cognitive Status and Response to Treatment: A Clear Step Towards Personalized Therapeutics. *Immunogenet* **2017**, *2*, 116.
5. Goodin, D.; Khankhanian, P.; Gourraud, P.A.; Vince, N. Highly conserved extended haplotypes of the major histocompatibility complex and their relationship to multiple sclerosis susceptibility. *PLoS ONE* **2018**, *13*, e0190043. [CrossRef] [PubMed]
6. Bozikas, V.P.; Anagnostouli, M.C.; Petrikis, P.; Sitzoglou, C.; Phokas, C.; Tsakanikas, C.; Karavatos, A. Familial bipolar disorder and multiple sclerosis: A three-generation HLA family study. *Prog. Neuropsychopharmacol. Biol. Psychiatry* **2003**, *27*, 835–839. [CrossRef]
7. International Multiple Sclerosis Genetics Consortium; Wellcome Trust Case Control Consortium 2; Sawcer, S.; Hellenthal, G.; Pirinen, M.; Spencer, C.C.; Patsopoulos, N.A.; Moutsianas, L.; Dilthey, A.; Su, Z.; et al. Genetic risk and a primary role for cell-mediated immune mechanisms in multiple sclerosis. *Nature* **2011**, *476*, 214–219.
8. Kular, L.; Liu, Y.; Ruhrmann, S.; Zheleznyakova, G.; Marabita, F.; Gomez-Cabrero, D.; James, T.; Ewing, E.; Lindén, M.; Górnikiewicz, B.; et al. DNA Methylation as a Mediator of HLA-DRB1*15:01 and a Protective Variant in Multiple Sclerosis. *Nat. Commun.* **2018**, *9*, 2397. [CrossRef]
9. Gianfrancesco, M.; Stridh, P.; Shao, X.; Rhead, B.; Graves, J.S.; Chitnis, T.; Waldman, A.; Lotze, T.; Schreiner, T.; Belman, A.; et al. Genetic risk factors for pediatric–onset multiple sclerosis. *Mult. Scler.* **2018**, *24*, 1825–1834. [CrossRef]
10. Venkateswaran, S.; Banwell, B. Pediatric multiple sclerosis. *Neurologist* **2010**, *16*, 92–105. [CrossRef]
11. Anagnostouli, M.C.; Manouseli, A.; Artemiadis, A.; Katsavos, S.; Fillipopoulou, C.; Youroukos, S.; Efthimiopoulos, S.; Doxiadis, I. HLA-DRB1* Allele Frequencies in Pediatric, Adolescent and Adult-Onset Multiple Sclerosis Patients, in a Hellenic Sample. Evidence for New and Established Associations. *J. Mult. Scler.* **2014**, *1*, 104. [CrossRef]
12. Odum, N.; Hyldic-Nielsenn, J.J.; Morling, N.; Sandberg-Wollheim, M.; Platz, P.; Svejgaard, A. HLA-DP antigens are involved in the susceptibility to multiple sclerosis. *Tissue Antigens* **1988**, *31*, 235–237. [CrossRef] [PubMed]
13. Wu, X.M.; Wang, C.; Zhang, K.N.; Lin, A.Y.; Kira, J.; Hu, G.Z.; Qu, X.H.; Xiong, Y.Q.; Cao, W.F.; Gong, L.Y. Association of susceptibility to multiple sclerosis in Southern Han Chinese with HLA-DRB1, -DPB1 alleles and DRB1-DPB1 haplotypes: Distinct from other populations. *Mult. Scler.* **2009**, *15*, 1422–1430. [CrossRef]
14. Fukazawa, T.; Yamasaki, K.; Ito, H.; Kikuchi, S.; Minohara, M.; Horiuchi, I.; Tsukishima, E.; Sasaki, H.; Hamada, T.; Nishimura, Y.; et al. Both the HLA-DPB1 and -DRB1 alleles correlate with risk for multiple sclerosis in Japanese: Clinical phenotypes and gender as important factors. *Tissue Antigens* **2000**, *55*, 199–205. [CrossRef] [PubMed]
15. Fukazawa, T.; Kikuchi, S.; Miyagishi, R.; Miyazaki, Y.; Yabe, I.; Hamada, T.; Sasaki, H. HLA-DPB1*0501 is not uniquely associated with opticospinal multiple sclerosis in Japanese patients. Important role of DPB1*0301. *Mult. Scler.* **2006**, *12*, 19–23. [CrossRef] [PubMed]
16. Yoshimura, S.; Isobe, N.; Yonekawa, T.; Matsushita, T.; Masaki, K.; Sato, S.; Kawano, Y.; Yamamoto, K.; Kira, J.; South Japan Multiple Sclerosis Genetics Consortium. Genetic and infectious profiles of Japanese multiple sclerosis patients. *PLoS ONE* **2012**, *7*, e48592. [CrossRef]
17. Yu, M.; Kinkel, R.P.; Weinstock-Guttman, B.; Cook, D.J.; Tuohy, V.K. HLADP: A class II restriction molecule involved in epitope spreading during the development of multiple sclerosis. *Hum. Immunol.* **1998**, *59*, 15–24. [CrossRef]

18. Field, J.; Browning, S.R.; Johnson, L.J.; Danoy, P.; Varney, M.D.; Tait, B.D.; Gandhi, K.S.; Charlesworth, J.C.; Heard, R.N.; Australia and New Zealand Multiple Sclerosis Genetics Consortium; et al. A polymorphism in the HLA-DPB1 gene is associated with susceptibility to multiple sclerosis. *PLoS ONE* **2010**, *5*, e13454. [CrossRef]
19. Dekker, J.W.; Easteal, S.; Jakobsen, I.B.; Gao, X.; Stewart, G.J.; Buhler, M.M.; Hawkins, B.R.; Higgins, D.A.; Yu, Y.L.; Serjeantson, S.W. HLA-DPB1 alleles correlate with risk for multiple sclerosis in Caucasoid and Cantonese patients lacking the high-risk DQB1*0602 allele. *Tissue Antigens* **1993**, *41*, 31–36. [CrossRef]
20. Roth, M.P.; Coppin, H.; Descoins, P.; Ruidavets, J.B.; Cambon-Thomsen, A.; Clanet, M. HLA-DPB1 gene polymorphism and multiple sclerosis: A large case-control study in the southwest of France. *J. Neuroimmunol.* **1991**, *34*, 215–222. [CrossRef]
21. Marrosu, M.G.; Cocco, E.; Costa, G.; Murru, M.R.; Mancosu, C.; Murru, R.; Lai, M.; Sardu, C.; Contu, P. Interaction of loci within the HLA region influences multiple sclerosis course in the Sardinian population. *J. Neurol.* **2006**, *253*, 208–213. [CrossRef] [PubMed]
22. Patsopoulos, N.A.; Barcellos, L.F.; Hintzen, R.Q.; Schaefer, C.; van Duijn, C.M.; Noble, J.A.; Raj, T.; IMSGC; ANZgene; Gourraud, P.A.; et al. Fine-mapping the genetic association of the major histocompatibility complex in multiple sclerosis: HLA and non-HLA effects. *PLoS Genet.* **2013**, *9*, e1003926.
23. Gontika, M.P.; Anagnostouli, M.C. Human leukocyte antigens immunogenetics of neuromyelitis optica or Devic's disease and the impact on the immunopathogenesis, diagnosis and treatment: A critical review. *Neuroimmunol. Neuroinflamm.* **2014**, *1*, 44–50. [CrossRef]
24. Hersh, A.O.; Prahalad, S. Immunogenetics of juvenile idiopathic arthritis: A comprehensive review. *J. Autoimmun.* **2015**, *64*, 113–124. [CrossRef] [PubMed]
25. Nishimaki, K.; Kawamura, T.; Inada, H.; Yagawa, K.; Nose, Y.; Nabeya, N.; Isshiki, G.; Tatsumi, N.; Niihira, S. HLA DPB1*0201 gene confers disease susceptibility in Japanese with childhood onset type I diabetes, independent of HLA-DR and DQ genotypes. *Diabetes Res. Clin. Pract.* **2000**, *47*, 49–55. [CrossRef]
26. Sato, S.; Isobe, N.; Yoshimura, S.; Kanamori, Y.; Masaki, K.; Matsushita, T.; Kira, J. HLA-DPB1*0201 is associated with susceptibility to atopic myelitis in Japanese. *J. Neuroimmunol.* **2012**, *251*, 110–113. [CrossRef] [PubMed]
27. Lincoln, M.R.; Ramagopalan, S.V.; Chao, M.J.; Herrera, B.M.; Deluca, G.C.; Orton, S.M.; Dyment, D.A.; Sadovnick, A.D.; Ebers, G.C. Epistasis among HLA-DRB1, HLA-DQA1, and HLA-DQB1 loci determines multiple sclerosis susceptibility. *Proc. Natl. Acad. Sci. USA* **2009**, *106*, 7542–7547. [CrossRef] [PubMed]
28. Moutsianas, L.; Jostins, L.; Beecham, A.H.; Dilthey, A.T.; Xifara, D.K.; Ban, M.; Shah, T.S.; Patsopoulos, N.A.; Alfredsson, L.; Anderson, C.A.; et al. Class II HLA interactions modulate genetic risk for multiple sclerosis. *Nat. Genet.* **2015**, *47*, 1107–1113.
29. Polman, C.H.; Reingold, S.C.; Banwell, B.; Clanet, M.; Cohen, J.A.; Filippi, M.; Fujihara, K.; Havrdova, E.; Hutchinson, M.; Kappos, L.; et al. Diagnostic criteria for multiple sclerosis: 2010 revisions to the McDonald criteria. *Ann. Neurol.* **2011**, *69*, 292–302. [CrossRef]
30. Kurtzke, J.F. Rating neurologic impairment in multiple sclerosis: An expanded disability status scale (EDSS). *Neurology* **1983**, *33*, 1444–1452. [CrossRef]
31. Marsh, S.G. Nomenclature for factors of the HLA system, update June 2012. *Tissue Antigens* **2012**, *80*, 289–293. [CrossRef]
32. Lancaster, A.K.; Single, R.M.; Solberg, O.D.; Nelson, M.P.; Thomson, G. PyPop update—A software pipeline for large-scale multilocus population genomics. *Tissue Antigens* **2007**, *69* (Suppl. 1), 192–197. [CrossRef]
33. Papassavas, E.C.; Spyropoulou-Vlachou, M.; Papassavas, A.C.; Schipper, R.F.; Doxiadis, I.N.; Stavropoulos-Giokas, C. MHC class I and class II phenotype, gene, and haplotype frequencies in Greeks using molecular typing data. *Hum. Immunol.* **2000**, *61*, 615–623. [CrossRef]
34. Benjamini, Y.; Drai, D.; Elmer, G.; Kafkafi, N.; Golani, I. Controlling the false discovery rate in behavior genetics research. *Behav. Brain Res.* **2001**, *125*, 279–284. [CrossRef]
35. Narum, S.R. Beyond Bonferroni: Less conservative analyses for conservation genetics. *Conserv. Genet.* **2006**, *7*, 783–787. [CrossRef]
36. Hadley, D.; Hagopian, W.; Liu, E.; She, J.X.; Simell, O.; Akolkar, B.; Ziegler, A.G.; Rewers, M.; Krischer, J.P.; Chen, W.M.; et al. HLA-DPB1*04:01 Protects Genetically Susceptible Children from Celiac Disease Autoimmunity in the TEDDY Study. *Am. J. Gastroenterol.* **2015**, *110*, 915–920. [CrossRef]

37. Ollila, H.M.; Ravel, J.M.; Han, F.; Faraco, J.; Lin, L.; Zheng, X.; Plazzi, G.; Dauvilliers, Y.; Pizza, F.; Hong, S.C.; et al. HLA-DPB1 and HLA class I confer risk of and protection from narcolepsy. *Am. J. Hum. Genet.* **2015**, *96*, 852. [CrossRef]
38. Misicka, E.; Sept, C.; Briggs, F.B.S. Predicting onset of secondary-progressive multiple sclerosis using genetic and non-genetic factors. *J. Neurol.* **2020**. [CrossRef]
39. Gontika, M.P.; Anagnostouli, M.C. Anti-Myelin Oligodendrocyte Glycoprotein and Human Leukocyte Antigens as Markers in Pediatric and Adolescent Multiple Sclerosis: On Diagnosis, Clinical Phenotypes, and Therapeutic Responses. *Mult. Scler. Int.* **2018**, *2018*, 8487471. [CrossRef]
40. Uher, T.; McComb, M.; Galkin, S.; Srpova, B.; Oechtering, J.; Barro, C.; Tyblova, M.; Bergsland, N.; Krasensky, J.; Dwyer, M.; et al. Neurofilament levels are associated with blood-brain barrier integrity, lymphocyte extravasation, and risk factors following the first demyelinating event in multiple sclerosis. *Mult. Scler.* **2020**. [CrossRef]
41. Warabi, Y.; Matsumoto, Y.; Hayashi, H. Interferon beta1b exacerbates multiple sclerosis with severe optic nerve and spinal cord demyelination. *J. Neurol. Sci.* **2007**, *252*, 57–61. [CrossRef]
42. Werneck, L.C.; Lorenzoni, P.J.; Kay, C.S.K.; Scola, R.H. Multiple sclerosis: Disease modifying therapy and the human leukocyte antigen. *Arq. Neuropsiquiatr.* **2018**, *76*, 697–704. [CrossRef] [PubMed]

11

Impaired Expression of Tetraspanin 32 (TSPAN32) in Memory T Cells of Patients with Multiple Sclerosis

Maria Sofia Basile [1], Emanuela Mazzon [2], Katia Mangano [1], Manuela Pennisi [1], Maria Cristina Petralia [2], Salvo Danilo Lombardo [1], Ferdinando Nicoletti [1], Paolo Fagone [1,*] and Eugenio Cavalli [2]

1 Department of Biomedical and Biotechnological Sciences, University of Catania, Via S. Sofia 89, 95123 Catania, Italy; sofiabasile@hotmail.it (M.S.B.); kmangano@unict.it (K.M.); manuela.pennisi@unict.it (M.P.); salvo.lombardo.sdl@gmail.com (S.D.L.); ferdinic@unict.it (F.N.)

2 IRCCS Centro Neurolesi "Bonino-Pulejo", Via Provinciale Palermo, Contrada Casazza, 98124 Messina, Italy; emanuela.mazzon@irccsme.it (E.M.); m.cristinapetralia@gmail.com (M.C.P.); eugenio.cavalli@irccsme.it (E.C.)

* Correspondence: paolofagone@yahoo.it

Abstract: Tetraspanins are a conserved family of proteins involved in a number of biological processes. We have previously shown that Tetraspanin-32 (TSPAN32) is significantly downregulated upon activation of T helper cells via anti-CD3/CD28 stimulation. On the other hand, TSPAN32 is marginally modulated in activated Treg cells. A role for TSPAN32 in controlling the development of autoimmune responses is consistent with our observation that encephalitogenic T cells from myelin oligodendrocyte glycoprotein (MOG)-induced experimental autoimmune encephalomyelitis (EAE) mice exhibit significantly lower levels of TSPAN32 as compared to naïve T cells. In the present study, by making use of ex vivo and in silico analysis, we aimed to better characterize the pathophysiological and diagnostic/prognostic role of TSPAN32 in T cell immunity and in multiple sclerosis (MS). We first show that TSPAN32 is significantly downregulated in memory T cells as compared to naïve T cells, and that it is further diminished upon ex vivo restimulation. Accordingly, following antigenic stimulation, myelin-specific memory T cells from MS patients showed significantly lower expression of TSPAN32 as compared to memory T cells from healthy donors (HD). The expression levels of TSPAN32 was significantly downregulated in peripheral blood mononuclear cells (PBMCs) from drug-naïve MS patients as compared to HD, irrespective of the disease state. Finally, when comparing patients undergoing early relapses in comparison to patients with longer stable disease, moderate but significantly lower levels of TSPAN32 expression were observed in PBMCs from the former group. Our data suggest a role for TSPAN32 in the immune responses underlying the pathophysiology of MS and represent a proof-of-concept for additional studies aiming at dissecting the eventual contribution of TSPAN32 in other autoimmune diseases and its possible use of TSPAN32 as a diagnostic factor and therapeutic target.

Keywords: TSPAN32; tetraspanins; multiple sclerosis; cellular immunity; memory T cells

1. Introduction

Tetraspanins are a conserved family of proteins involved in several biological processes, such as the regulation of cellular adhesion, motility, cancer metastasis, signal transduction, and activation [1,2]. Tetraspanins comprise four transmembrane (TM) domains. TM domains 1 and 2 flank a small extracellular loop (SEL), while TM3 and TM4 flank a large extracellular loop (LEL). TM domains are typically involved in the interaction with non-tetraspanin molecules. The juxtamembrane cysteine residues in the cytoplasmic domains contribute to the formation of tetraspanin-enriched microdomains

(TEMs), while the cytoplasmic regions provide links to cytoskeletal and signaling molecules [3]. Several immune-related proteins take part in TEMs, including pattern recognition receptors, co-stimulatory molecules, Major Histocompatibility Complex molecules and T cell receptor-associated proteins (reviewed in [2]). The tetraspanins Cluster of Differentiation 82 (CD82), CD9, CD63, CD81, and CD53 exert a co-stimulatory role in T cells [4,5], whereas cells deficient for CD37, CD151, and CD81 have been shown to be hyperproliferative following stimulation [6–8]. Tarrant and colleagues [9] have shown that T cells from Tssc6 Tetraspanin-32 (TSPAN32)-deficient mice have increased responses upon stimulation, and have proposed that TSPAN32 may negatively regulate peripheral T-lymphocyte activation. Along the same lines, we have previously shown that TSPAN32 expression is significantly reduced upon cell activation, although in Treg cells, TSPAN32 levels undergo minor changes. Moreover, significantly lower levels of TSPAN32 were found in encephalitogenic T cells from myelin oligodendrocyte glycoprotein (MOG)-Induced experimental autoimmune encephalomyelitis (EAE) mice. Finally, ex vivo-activated circulating CD4 T cells from MS patients showed lower levels of TSPAN32 as compared to cells from healthy donors [10].

Multiple sclerosis (MS) is the most frequent immuno-inflammatory disorder of the central nervous system, characterized by immune cell infiltration, microglia activation and progressive demyelination, with consequent neurological deficits. It is well-known that increased conversion from naïve to memory cells can be observed in MS [11] and that most of the myelin-reactive T cells are present in the memory T cell subset [12]. It has been also shown that memory T cells are activated independently of CD28 co-stimulation [13,14]. In the present paper, we aimed to better characterize the pathophysiological role of TSPAN32 in cellular immunity and in MS. To this aim, by making use of ex vivo and in silico analysis, we have evaluated the expression levels of TSPAN32 in memory T cells from healthy donors and MS patients, both in inactive state and upon activation. Next, we determined the diagnostic and prognostic value of TSPAN32 in the peripheral blood mononuclear cells (PBMCs) of MS patients. Our analysis demonstrates that TSPAN32 is significantly downregulated in memory T cells as compared to naïve T cells, and that it is further diminished upon ex vivo restimulation. In addition, following antigenic stimulation, myelin-specific memory T cells from MS patients exhibited significantly lower expression of TSPAN32 as compared to memory T cells from healthy donors (HD). Further, the expression levels of TSPAN32 was significantly downregulated in PBMCs from drug-naïve MS patients as compared to HD, irrespective of the disease state. Finally, we observed a moderate but significantly reduced expression of TSPAN32 in PBMCs from MS patients undergoing early relapses in comparison to those from patients with a longer course of stable disease.

2. Materials and Methods

2.1. Ex Vivo Study

2.1.1. Cell Isolation and Real-Time PCR

Mononuclear cells were obtained from the peripheral blood of healthy donors (HD) ($n = 7$) by step-gradient centrifugation, using the Ficoll–Hypaque medium (Sigma Aldrich, Milano, Italy), as per manufacturer's instructions. CD4 + CD45RA + CD45RO − CD25 + CD127^{low} cells (naive Treg cells), CD4 + CD45RA − CD45RO + CD25 + CD127^{low} cells (memory Treg cells), CD4 + CD45RA − CD45RO + CD25 − CD127 + cells (memory Teff cells), and CD4 + CD45RA + CD45RO − CD25 − CD127 + cells (naive Teff cells) were enriched by magnetic beads sorting, obtaining a cell purity of at least 95%. In another set of experiments, memory Teff cells from 3 healthy donors were activated by plate-bound anti-CD3 (10 μg/mL) and anti-CD28 (5 μg/mL) for 12 h.

2.1.2. Real-Time PCR

Total RNA was extracted and gene expression levels were determined by real-time PCR. 2 μg of total RNA were reverse-transcribed with a High-Capacity cDNA Reverse Transcription Kit (Applied

Biosystems, Monza, Italy) in a 20 μL reaction volume, and real-time PCR was performed using the SYBR Green PCR Master Mix (Applied Biosystems, Monza, Italy), 200 nM forward and 200 nM reverse primers, and 20 μg cDNA. Relative gene expression levels were obtained using the formula: $2^{-\Delta\Delta Ct}$, where $\Delta\Delta Ct = (Ct_{\text{target gene}} - Ct_{\text{beta-actin}})$ stimulated cells – $(Ct_{\text{target gene}} - Ct_{\text{beta-actin}})$ control cells.

2.2. *In Silico Analysis*

The Gene Expression Omnibus (GEO; https://www.ncbi.nlm.nih.gov/gds) browser was interrogated using the MeSH (Medical Subject Headings) term "Multiple Sclerosis". Datasets were manually excluded if the studies were not performed on human subjects, if the patients enrolled were under immunosuppressive/immunomodulatory treatment, and if the cell types analyzed were not immune cells. For the evaluation of the expression levels of TSPAN32 in encephalitogenic memory T cells, and the evaluation of the diagnostic role of TSPAN32, datasets carried out only on one cohort of subjects (i.e., MS patients and healthy donors) were excluded. For the afore-mentioned reasons, the analysis was then carried out on the GSE66763 and the GSE138064, respectively. For the determination of the prognostic properties of TSPAN32 in predicting MS relapses, the GSE15245 was selected as it is the only dataset including prospective data on disease evolution. A flowchart of the in silico study design is provided as Figure 1. The characteristics of the datasets used are described in the following sections.

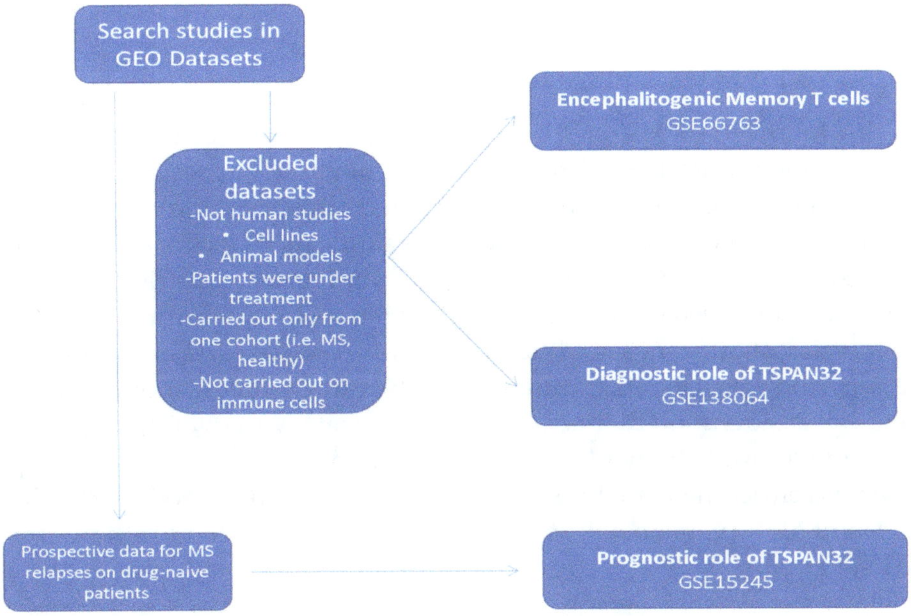

Figure 1. Flowchart of the in silico study.

2.2.1. TSPAN32 in Memory T Cells from MS Patients

The GSE66763 dataset was used to investigate the expression levels of TSPAN32 in circulating memory T cells from MS patients [15]. The dataset included whole-genome RNA sequencing data of C-C Motif Chemokine Receptor 6 $(CCR6)^+$ memory (CD45RA – CD45RO + CD25 – CCR6+) CD4+ T from 3 Human Leukocyte Antigen – DR isotype (HLA-DR)4+ healthy subjects and 5 HLA-DR4+ MS patients. Cells were amplified by PhytoHaemAgglutinin (PHA) and Interleukin (IL)-2 and stimulated by irradiated autologous monocytes and DR4 myelin peptides Myelin Oligodendrocyte Glycoprotein $((MOG)_{97-109}$ and ProteoLipid Protein $(PLP)_{180-199})$. Patients were immunotherapeutic naïve or had not received treatment for at least 12 months. Cell proliferation was determined and the highest proliferated wells were chosen for DR4 tetramers staining (MOG_{97-109}-tetramers and $PLP_{180-199}$-tetramers). Then, myelin tetramer+ and tetramer– cells were sorted and lysed for the extraction of RNA and subsequent

RNA sequencing. Gene expression is shown as log_2 Fragments Per Kilobase of transcript per Million mapped (FPKM) values.

2.2.2. TSPAN32 in PBMCs from MS Patients

In order to investigate the expression levels of TSPAN32 in PBMCs from MS patients in both stable and active disease, as compared to healthy donors, we interrogated the GSE138064 dataset [16]. The dataset included transcriptomic data from therapy-naïve Relapse-Remitting (RR) MS patients (10 with stable MS, age 45.2 ± 2.6, 8/2 female/male, and 9 during relapse, age 46.3 ± 3.5, 8/2 female/male). Eight healthy controls were included, age 42.3 ± 4.8, 5/3 female/male.

2.2.3. Predictive Analysis of TSPAN32 in MS

In order to evaluate the relationship between expression levels of TSPAN32 and the time to relapse in MS patients, we interrogated the GSE15245 dataset that included whole-genome transcriptomic profiles of PMBCs from 51 drug-naïve MS patients [17]. The patient's age was 38.5 ± 1.4, with a mean Expanded Disability Status Scale (EDSS) score of 2.4 ± 0.2. The Affymetrix Human Genome U133A 2.0 Array was used for the generation of the dataset and raw data were preprocessed using the robust multi-array average (RMA) algorithm. Sample population was sorted based on the expression levels of TSPAN32 and log-rank test was applied to evaluate differences in the percentage of patients developing acute relapses in a 1500-day time frame.

2.3. Statistical Analysis

Data are shown as mean ± SD and statistical analysis was performed using either a Student's *t*-test or one-way ANOVA followed by Fisher's Least Significant Difference test. Correlation analysis was performed using the non-parametric Spearman's test. Hierarchical clustering was used to determine the relative distance of samples using Pearson's correlation as similarity comparison. The self organizing map (SOM) algorithm was used for the unsupervised identification of clusters of commonly modulated genes [18]. Distance metric for SOM was Pearson's correlation, with random genes initialization, Gaussian neighborhood, and 2000 iterations. The linear model for microarray (LIMMA) algorithm was used to evaluate statistical significance for differences in RNA sequencing data [19]. As the experimental design and the information provided are different for the three whole-genome transcriptomic datasets here analyzed, and in consideration that no additional datasets with overlapping experimental layouts are currently available in publicly available databases, a meta-analysis cannot be performed. Gene ontology and gene term enrichment analysis was conducted using the web-based utility, Metascape [20]. GraphPad Prism 8 and MeV (version 4.9) software programs were used for the statistical analysis and the generation of the graphs.

3. Results

3.1. TSPAN32 in Memory T Cells

When analyzing the expression levels of TSPAN32 in memory CD4+ T cells from healthy donors, we observed significantly lower levels of TSPAN32 in memory T effector cells as compared to naïve T cells ($p < 0.01$) (Figure 2A). On the other hand, no modulation was observed in memory Treg cells (Figure 2A). We also wanted to determine whether a modulation of TSPAN32 could be found upon restimulation. As shown in Figure 2B, restimulation of memory T cells is associated to a significant down regulation in TSPAN32 levels ($p < 0.001$) (Figure 2B). Similar data have been obtained from the analysis of the GSE22886 dataset (Table S1).

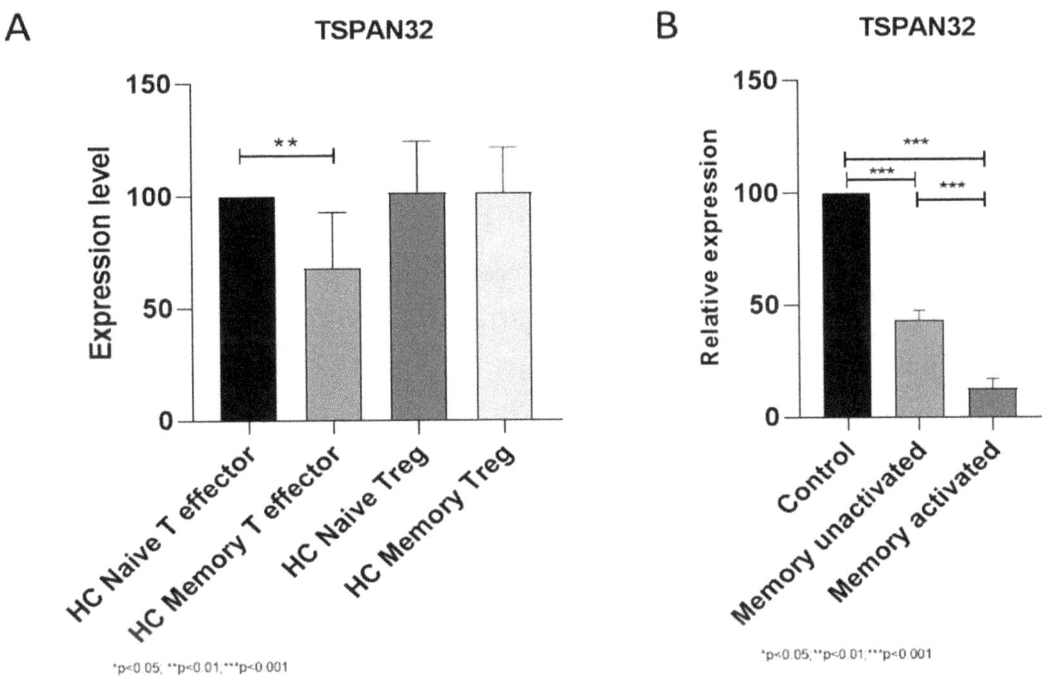

Figure 2. (**A**) Basal expression levels of Tetraspanin-32 (TSPAN32) in naïve T effector, Treg, memory T effector, and memory Treg cells from healthy donors; (**B**) modulation of TSPAN32 expression in memory T cells upon reactivation. ** $p < 0.01$, *** $p < 0.001$.

Next, we wanted to determine the expression of TSPAN32 in memory CD4+ T cells from HLA-DR4+ MS patients, following amplification by PHA and IL-2 and stimulation by irradiated autologous monocytes and DR4 myelin peptides. As shown in Figure 3A, significant lower levels of TSPAN32 were observed in tetramer+ memory T cells from MS patients as compared to tetramer- memory T cells from HD ($p < 0.05$). Similarly, comparable levels of TSPAN32 were observed in tetramer+ memory T cells from HD (Figure 3A). SOM analysis identified 599 genes that clustered together with TSPAN32 (Cluster 5) (Figure 3B). Gene ontology revealed that the most significant enriched terms were "Small GTPase-mediated signal transduction", "Meiosis", "DNA repair", "BARD1 pathway" and "Membrane lipid biosynthetic process" (Figure 3B–D). Interestingly, significantly lower TSPAN32 levels were also observed in tetramer- memory T cells from MS patients (Figure 3A). As LIMMA analysis revealed significant transcriptomic differences between tetramer- MS memory T cells and tetramer- HD memory T cells, with enrichment of several immune-related biological processes (Figure S1A,B), and HCL analysis clustered together tetramer- and tetramer+ memory T cells from MS patients (Figure S1C), the reduced TSPAN32 levels may be associated to a reduced activation threshold of memory T cells from MS patients, and could explain the underlying autoimmune process.

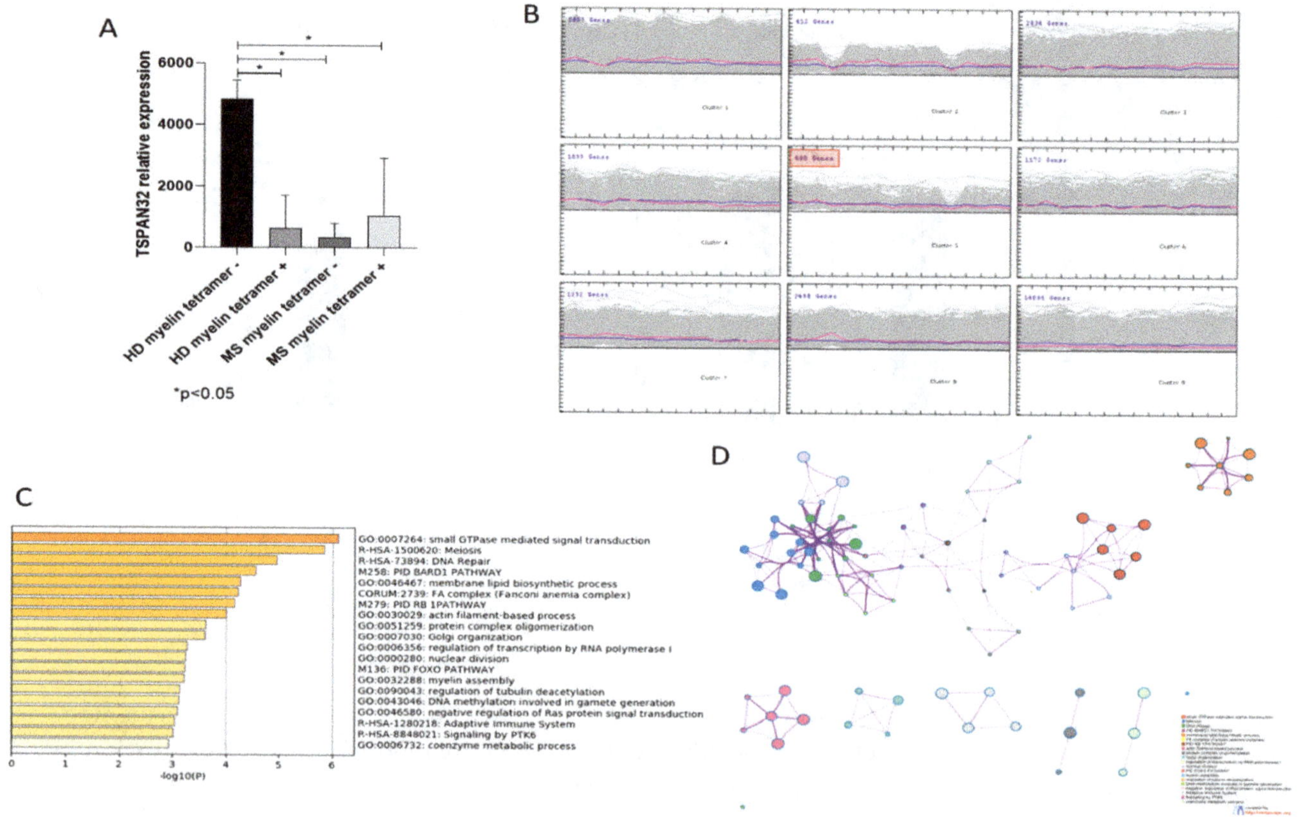

Figure 3. (**A**) TSPAN32 expression in memory T cells from healthy donors and multiple sclerosis (MS) patients; * $p < 0.05$; (**B**) clusters of genes obtained from the self organizing map (SOM) analysis; (**C**) most enriched biological processes by genes commonly regulated with TSPAN32, as obtained from SOM analysis; (**D**) network showing the interconnection among the most enriched biological processes by genes commonly regulated with TSPAN32, obtained from SOM analysis.

3.2. TSPAN32 Expression in PBMCs from MS Patients

In order to evaluate whether a modulation in TSPAN32 levels could be observed in peripheral immune cells from MS patients, we interrogated the GSE138064 dataset. As shown in Figure 4A, a significant reduction in TSPAN32 expression was observed in PBMCs from MS patients in both stable and relapsing disease ($p < 0.001$) (Figure 4A). Receiver operating characteristic (ROC) analysis confirmed the diagnostic ability of TSPAN32 to discriminate MS from HD, entailing a $p < 0.001$ (Figure 4B,C). No significant differences were instead observed when comparing TSPAN32 levels in PBMCs from patients in stable disease as compared to PBMCs from patients in exacerbation (Figure 4A). Accordingly, ROC curve area was 0.6889, entailing a $p = 0.1651$ (Figure 4D). This is in accordance with data from the GSE19224 dataset, that show an adjusted p value > 0.99 and a $\log_2$(fold) change of 0.276 for TSPAN32 expression levels when comparing PBMCs from MS patients in stable versus relapsing disease (https://www.ncbi.nlm.nih.gov/geo/geo2r/?acc=GSE19224).

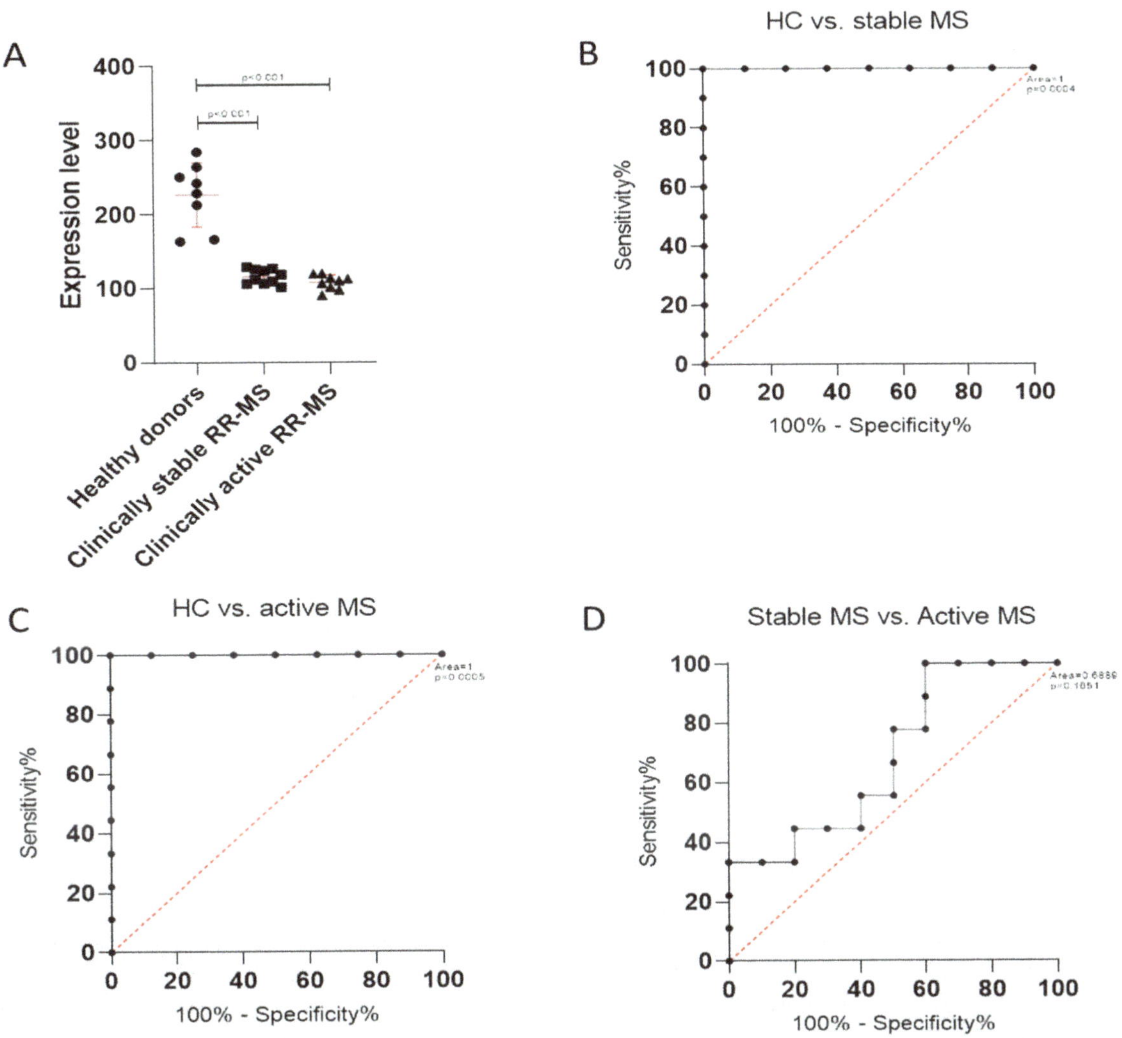

Figure 4. (**A**) TSPAN32 in peripheral blood mononuclear cells (PBMCs) from healthy donors and RRMS patients in stable and relapsing disease; (**B**) receiver operating characteristic (ROC) curve for TSPAN32 in healthy controls (HC) and multiple sclerosis patients in stable disease; (**C**) receiver operating characteristic (ROC) curve for TSPAN32 in healthy controls (HC) and multiple sclerosis patients in active disease; (**D**) receiver operating characteristic (ROC) curve for TSPAN32 in multiple sclerosis patients in stable and active disease.

Finally, we evaluated whether the different transcriptional levels of TSPAN32 in PBMCs from MS patients could promote disease exacerbation or protect MS patients from acute relapses. Non-parametric correlation between TSPAN32 and the time-to-relapse revealed a trend of direct correlation, which did not reach the statistical significance ($p = 0.0856$) (Figure 5A). ROC curve area was 0.6036, entailing a $p = 0.3695$ (Figure 5B). However, Log-rank analysis performed on patients divided into two groups based on the expression level of TSPAN32 in PBMCs (referred as High and Low TSPAN32) showed that a trend of protection from acute relapses was observed in patients expressing higher TSPAN32 levels (Figure 5C). In addition, significantly lower levels of TSPAN32 were found in PBMCs from MS patients developing exacerbation of the disease before 300 days as compared with patients who underwent relapses later than 1500 days (Figure 5D).

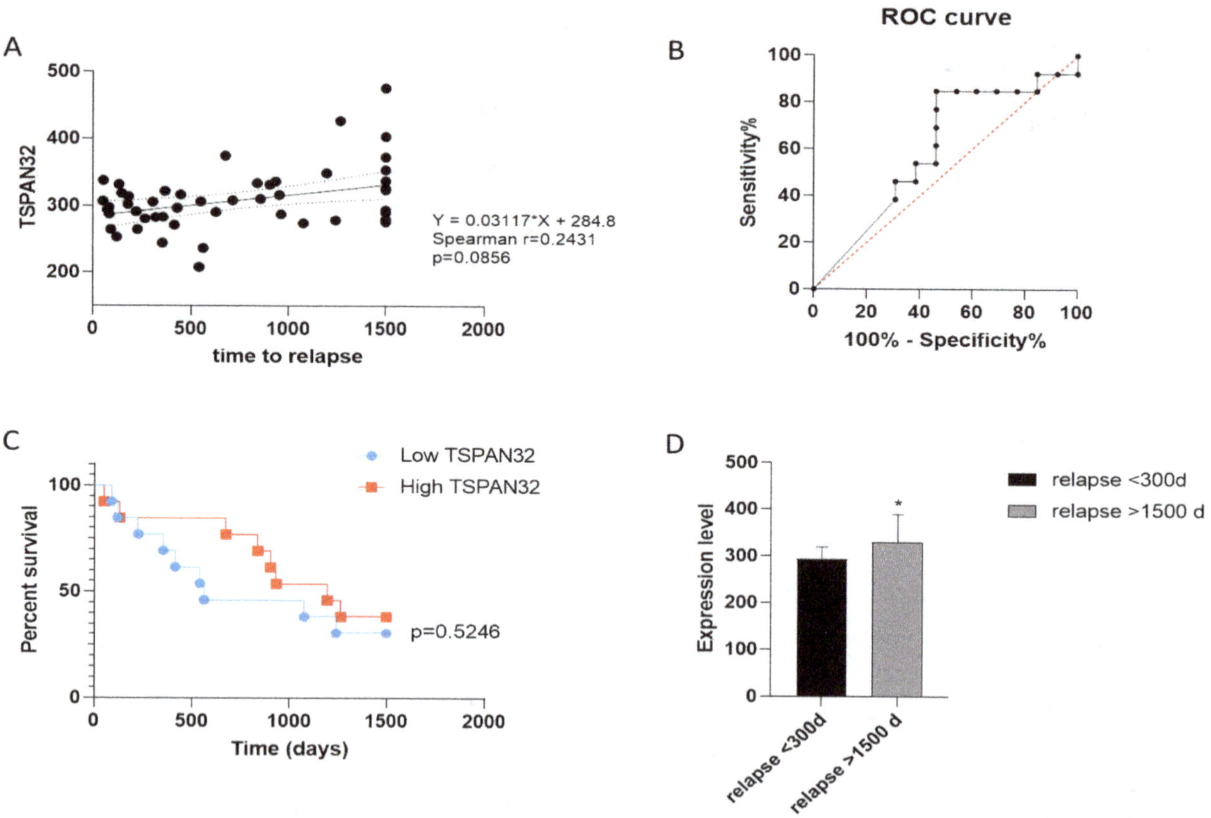

Figure 5. (**A**) Correlation between TSPAN32 expression in PBMCs from drug-naïve MS patients and the time-to-relapse; Spearman correlation value (r) and p value (p) are indicated. (**B**) receiver operating characteristic (ROC) curve for the evaluation of the prognostic value of TSPAN32 in predicting relapses in MS patients; (**C**) log-rank analysis for time-to-relapse in patients expressing low and high levels of TSPAN32 in PBMCs, respectively; (**D**) expression levels of TSPAN32 in MS patients undergoing early exacerbation of the disease (<300 days) or with longer stable disease (relapse > 1500 days).

4. Discussion

Diverse members of the TSPAN family have been shown to be involved in the regulation of both the innate and adaptive immune responses. For instance, CD81 is involved in the formation of the immune synapse, providing a link between the Antigen Presenting Cells and the T cells [21,22], while CD37 and CD151 promote antigen presentation and regulate the costimulatory signaling pathways [23].

In a TSPAN32 (Tssc6)-deficient mouse model, despite normal hemopoiesis, T cell proliferation and responses are significantly augmented [9]. It has also been observed that the activity of T cells from mice double knockout for CD37 and TSPAN32 are upregulated, and that the dendritic cell stimulation capacity is increased as compared to single knockout, suggesting a cooperative role for these two tetraspanins in controlling T cell-mediated immunity [24]. These findings suggest that TSPAN32 might contribute to shape cellular immunity. In our previous work, we have described that T cells express a baseline level of TSPAN32, favoring the maintenance of an inactive state, which is decreased following CD3-mediated signaling [10].

By means of in silico and ex vivo analyses, in this study we wanted to gain further insights into the role of TSPAN in the biology and physiology of memory T cells and evaluated whether its expression was altered in memory T cells from MS patients as compared to HD. We also studied the possible diagnostic and prognostic value of TSPAN32 expression in PBMC of MS patients, on the course of the disease. The use of whole-genome expression databases has been largely exploited [25–28] for the characterization of pathogenic pathways and to identify therapeutic targets for a variety of disorders, including immunoinflammatory and autoimmune diseases [29–36], cancer [37–39], and has allowed dismantling pathogenetic pathways [40–42], along with the identification of novel tailored therapeutic targets [43–46].

MS is an autoimmune/immunoinflammatory disorder sustained by activated, myelin-specific T cells that migrate into the central nervous system (CNS), promoting inflammation. The characterization of the phenotype of myelin-specific immune cells is, therefore, crucial for the elucidation of MS pathogenesis [47–49].

In the present study, we have first analyzed the expression levels of TSPAN32 in circulating memory T cells from HD and we show that significantly lower levels of TSPAN32 can be observed in memory T effector cells but not in memory Treg cells. This is in line with our previous observation that only a marginal downregulation of TSPAN32 occurs in Treg cells, upon activation [10]. Interestingly, following the in vitro reactivation of memory T effector cells, TSPAN32 expression levels further decreased. The differential pattern of expression and modulation of TSPAN32 in Treg cells has yet to be deciphered.

Next, we analyzed the expression of TSPAN32 in autoreactive T cells from MS patients. As shown by Cao et al., myelin-reactive T cells from MS patients are prevalently from the memory CCR6+ T cell population, and are characterized by the secretion of larger amounts of proinflammatory cytokines as compared to T cells from HD. As expected, the expression levels of TSPAN32 in myelin-reactive MS tetramer-positive T cells resulted significantly lower than those in tetramer-negative memory T cells from HD. On the other hand, a significant lower expression of TSPAN32 was found in MS tetramer-negative memory T cells, comparable to that of MS tetramer-positive T cells. Although this may be counterintuitive, the observation that the transcriptomic features of the MS tetramer-negative memory T cells are more closely related to those of the MS tetramer-positive memory T cells than those of HD tetramer-negative memory T cells suggests that a lower activation threshold characterizes memory T cells from MS patients. Notably, a similar trend of reduced TSPAN32 levels was also observed in myelin-reactive HD tetramer-positive T cells. It is already known that MS patients and healthy subjects share a similar number of circulating myelin-reactive T cells. The lower levels of TSPAN32 in these cells suggest that regardless of the activation state of the T cells, the engagement of the TCR with the cognate ligand is sufficient to modulate the expression of TSPAN32. This is in accordance with our previous data, showing that the CD3-mediated signaling is sufficient to downregulate TSPAN32 gene expression.

Finally, we found diminished TSPAN32 levels in PBMCs from MS patients, both in stable and active disease, as compared to HD. No differences were however found between patients in stable versus relapsing disease. In addition, only a moderate reduction in the time-to-relapse was observed in patients expressing higher levels of TSPAN32 when MS patients were divided into two groups on the basis of their level of TSPAN32 expression in PBMC (referred as High and Low TSPAN32).

However, it was possible to observe that those with high expression had a moderate but significant protection from acute relapses. In agreement with this observation, significantly lower levels of TSPAN32 were found in PBMCs from MS patients developing exacerbation of the disease before 300 days, as compared with patients who underwent relapses later than 1500 days. Overall, our data suggest that the defective expression of TSPAN32 may characterize different T cell subsets of MS patients, including memory T cells, and that this may contribute to trigger anti-myelin immune responses. Along with our previous publication [10], this new transcriptomic analysis strengthens our hypothesis that defective TSPAN32 expression may represent an additional important immunopathogenetic abnormality that may play a role in the pathogenesis of at least some cases of MS.

It should also be pointed out that, although all of the in silico data have been generated from third-party reanalysis of whole-genome transcriptomic datasets previously validated by the respective original authors, the number of biological replicates in each of these datasets is relatively low. Therefore, although statistical significance has been achieved in most cases of our analyses, the data warrant to be confirmed from a larger population of MS patients. Along this line of research, it will be interesting to study if and how the current disease modifying therapies influence the course of the disease by modulating TSPAN32 expression. In a similar manner, the expression profile of TSPAN32 in secondary progressive and primary progressive MS seems of interest. Additional studies may also be warranted to dismantle whether defective expression of TSPAN32 is also observed in other T cell-mediated autoimmune diseases.

Moreover, further effort is required to understand the molecular pathways involved in the regulation of the immune responses exerted by TSPAN32. Up to now, no drugs targeting tetraspanins have received approval for the use in the clinical setting, but many strategies have been explored, including the use of monoclonal antibodies, recombinant soluble large extracellular loops or RNA interference (RNAi) (reviewed in [50]). Therefore, it is reasonable that several chances for tailored-specific intervention will be available in the future. Additionally, a deeper understanding of the mechanisms that control TSPAN32 expression could be pursued for their possible efficacy in patients suffering from MS.

5. Conclusions

Our data suggest a role for TSPAN32 in the immune responses underlying the pathophysiology of MS and represent a proof-of-concept for additional studies aiming at dissecting the eventual contribution of TSPAN32 in other autoimmune diseases and its possible use of TSPAN32 as a diagnostic factor and therapeutic target.

Author Contributions: Conceptualization, M.S.B., F.N., P.F., and E.C.; methodology, P.F.; formal analysis, K.M., M.P., M.C.P., and E.C.; investigation, M.S.B., K.M., S.D.L., M.C.P.; resources, E.M., and F.N.; writing—original draft preparation, M.S.B., M.P., S.D.L, P.F., E.C.; writing—review and editing, E.M., K.M., and F.N.; visualization, M.S.B., M.C.P., and P.F.; supervision, P.F. and F.N.; project administration, F.N.; funding acquisition, E.M. All authors have read and agreed to the published version of the manuscript.

References

1. Termini, C.M.; Gillette, J.M. Tetraspanins Function as Regulators of Cellular Signaling. *Front. Cell Dev. Biol.* **2017**, *5*, 34. [CrossRef] [PubMed]
2. Charrin, S.; Jouannet, S.; Boucheix, C.; Rubinstein, E. Tetraspanins at a glance. *J. Cell Sci.* **2014**, *127*, 3641–3648. [CrossRef] [PubMed]
3. Levy, S.; Shoham, T. The tetraspanin web modulates immune-signalling complexes. *Nat. Rev. Immunol.* **2005**, *5*, 136–148. [CrossRef] [PubMed]
4. Lebel-Binay, S.; Lagaudrière, C.; Fradelizi, D.; Conjeaud, H. CD82, member of the tetra-span-transmembrane protein family, is a costimulatory protein for T cell activation. *J. Immunol.* **1995**, *155*, 101–110.
5. Tai, X.G.; Yashiro, Y.; Abe, R.; Toyooka, K.; Wood, C.R.; Morris, J.; Long, A.; Ono, S.; Kobayashi, M.; Hamaoka, T.; et al. A role for CD9 molecules in T cell activation. *J. Exp. Med.* **1996**, *184*, 753–758. [CrossRef]
6. van Spriel, A.B.; Puls, K.L.; Sofi, M.; Pouniotis, D.; Hochrein, H.; Orinska, Z.; Knobeloch, K.-P.; Plebanski, M.; Wright, M.D. A regulatory role for CD37 in T cell proliferation. *J. Immunol.* **2004**, *172*, 2953–2961. [CrossRef]
7. Miyazaki, T.; Müller, U.; Campbell, K.S. Normal development but differentially altered proliferative responses of lymphocytes in mice lacking CD81. *EMBO J.* **1997**, *16*, 4217–4225. [CrossRef]
8. Wright, M.D.; Geary, S.M.; Fitter, S.; Moseley, G.W.; Lau, L.-M.; Sheng, K.-C.; Apostolopoulos, V.; Stanley, E.G.; Jackson, D.E.; Ashman, L.K. Characterization of mice lacking the tetraspanin superfamily member CD151. *Mol. Cell. Biol.* **2004**, *24*, 5978–5988. [CrossRef]
9. Tarrant, J.M.; Groom, J.; Metcalf, D.; Li, R.; Borobokas, B.; Wright, M.D.; Tarlinton, D.; Robb, L. The absence of Tssc6, a member of the tetraspanin superfamily, does not affect lymphoid development but enhances in vitro T-cell proliferative responses. *Mol. Cell. Biol.* **2002**, *22*, 5006–5018. [CrossRef]
10. Lombardo, S.D.; Mazzon, E.; Basile, M.S.; Campo, G.; Corsico, F.; Presti, M.; Bramanti, P.; Mangano, K.; Petralia, M.C.; Nicoletti, F.; et al. Modulation of Tetraspanin 32 (TSPAN32) Expression in T Cell-Mediated Immune Responses and in Multiple Sclerosis. *Int. J. Mol. Sci.* **2019**, *20*, 4323. [CrossRef]
11. Zaffaroni, M.; Rossini, S.; Ghezzi, A.; Parma, R.; Cazzullo, C.L. Decrease of CD4+ CD45+ T-cells in chronic-progressive multiple sclerosis. *J. Neurol.* **1990**, *237*, 1–4. [CrossRef] [PubMed]
12. Burns, J.; Bartholomew, B.; Lobo, S. Isolation of myelin basic protein-specific T cells predominantly from the memory T-cell compartment in multiple sclerosis. *Ann. Neurol.* **1999**, *45*, 33–39. [CrossRef]

13. Perrin, P.J.; Lovett-Racke, A.; Phillips, S.M.; Racke, M.K. Differential requirements of naïve and memory T cells for CD28 costimulation in autoimmune pathogenesis. *Histol. Histopathol.* **1999**, *14*, 1269–1276. [PubMed]
14. Lovett-Racke, A.E.; Trotter, J.L.; Lauber, J.; Perrin, P.J.; June, C.H.; Racke, M.K. Decreased dependence of myelin basic protein-reactive T cells on CD28-mediated costimulation in multiple sclerosis patients. A marker of activated/memory T cells. *J. Clin. Invest.* **1998**, *101*, 725–730. [CrossRef] [PubMed]
15. Cao, Y.; Goods, B.A.; Raddassi, K.; Nepom, G.T.; Kwok, W.W.; Love, J.C.; Hafler, D.A. Functional inflammatory profiles distinguish myelin-reactive T cells from patients with multiple sclerosis. *Sci. Transl. Med.* **2015**, *7*, 287ra74. [CrossRef]
16. Feng, X.; Bao, R.; Li, L.; Deisenhammer, F.; Arnason, B.G.W.; Reder, A.T. Interferon-β corrects massive gene dysregulation in multiple sclerosis: Short-term and long-term effects on immune regulation and neuroprotection. *EBioMedicine* **2019**, *49*, 269–283. [CrossRef]
17. Gurevich, M.; Tuller, T.; Rubinstein, U.; Or-Bach, R.; Achiron, A. Prediction of acute multiple sclerosis relapses by transcription levels of peripheral blood cells. *BMC Med. Genom.* **2009**, *2*, 46. [CrossRef]
18. Jansen, C.; Ramirez, R.N.; El-Ali, N.C.; Gomez-Cabrero, D.; Tegner, J.; Merkenschlager, M.; Conesa, A.; Mortazavi, A. Building gene regulatory networks from scATAC-seq and scRNA-seq using Linked Self Organizing Maps. *PLoS Comput. Biol.* **2019**, *15*, e1006555. [CrossRef]
19. Ritchie, M.E.; Phipson, B.; Wu, D.; Hu, Y.; Law, C.W.; Shi, W.; Smyth, G.K. limma powers differential expression analyses for RNA-sequencing and microarray studies. *Nucleic Acids Res.* **2015**, *43*, e47. [CrossRef]
20. Zhou, Y.; Zhou, B.; Pache, L.; Chang, M.; Khodabakhshi, A.H.; Tanaseichuk, O.; Benner, C.; Chanda, S.K. Metascape provides a biologist-oriented resource for the analysis of systems-level datasets. *Nat. Commun.* **2019**, *10*, 1523. [CrossRef]
21. Unternaehrer, J.J.; Chow, A.; Pypaert, M.; Inaba, K.; Mellman, I. The tetraspanin CD9 mediates lateral association of MHC class II molecules on the dendritic cell surface. *Proc. Natl. Acad. Sci. USA* **2007**, *104*, 234–239. [CrossRef] [PubMed]
22. Mittelbrunn, M.; Yanez-Mo, M.; Sancho, D.; Ursa, A.; Sanchez-Madrid, F. Cutting Edge: Dynamic Redistribution of Tetraspanin CD81 at the Central Zone of the Immune Synapse in Both T Lymphocytes and APC. *J. Immunol.* **2002**, *169*, 6691–6695. [CrossRef]
23. Sheng, K.-C.; van Spriel, A.B.; Gartlan, K.H.; Sofi, M.; Apostolopoulos, V.; Ashman, L.; Wright, M.D. Tetraspanins CD37 and CD151 differentially regulate Ag presentation and T-cell co-stimulation by DC. *Eur. J. Immunol.* **2009**, *39*, 50–55. [CrossRef] [PubMed]
24. Gartlan, K.H.; Belz, G.T.; Tarrant, J.M.; Minigo, G.; Katsara, M.; Sheng, K.-C.; Sofi, M.; van Spriel, A.B.; Apostolopoulos, V.; Plebanski, M.; et al. A Complementary Role for the Tetraspanins CD37 and Tssc6 in Cellular Immunity. *J. Immunol.* **2010**, *185*, 3158–3166. [CrossRef] [PubMed]
25. Gustafsson, M.; Edström, M.; Gawel, D.; Nestor, C.E.; Wang, H.; Zhang, H.; Barrenäs, F.; Tojo, J.; Kockum, I.; Olsson, T.; et al. Integrated genomic and prospective clinical studies show the importance of modular pleiotropy for disease susceptibility, diagnosis and treatment. *Genome Med.* **2014**, *6*, 17. [CrossRef] [PubMed]
26. Falzone, L.; Scola, L.; Zanghì, A.; Biondi, A.; Di Cataldo, A.; Libra, M.; Candido, S. Integrated analysis of colorectal cancer microRNA datasets: Identification of microRNAs associated with tumor development. *Aging* **2018**, *10*, 1000–1014. [CrossRef] [PubMed]
27. Candido, S.; Lupo, G.; Pennisi, M.; Basile, M.; Anfuso, C.; Petralia, M.; Gattuso, G.; Vivarelli, S.; Spandidos, D.; Libra, M.; et al. The analysis of miRNA expression profiling datasets reveals inverse microRNA patterns in glioblastoma and Alzheimer's disease. *Oncol. Rep.* **2019**, *42*, 911–922. [CrossRef]
28. Lombardo, S.D.; Mazzon, E.; Mangano, K.; Basile, M.S.; Cavalli, E.; Mammana, S.; Fagone, P.; Nicoletti, F.; Petralia, M.C. Transcriptomic Analysis Reveals Involvement of the Macrophage Migration Inhibitory Factor Gene Network in Duchenne Muscular Dystrophy. *Genes* **2019**, *10*, 939. [CrossRef]
29. Lombardo, S.D.; Mazzon, E.; Basile, M.S.; Cavalli, E.; Bramanti, P.; Nania, R.; Fagone, P.; Nicoletti, F.; Petralia, M.C. Upregulation of IL-1 Receptor Antagonist in a Mouse Model of Migraine. *Brain Sci.* **2019**, *9*, 172. [CrossRef]
30. Petralia, M.C.; Mazzon, E.; Fagone, P.; Falzone, L.; Bramanti, P.; Nicoletti, F.; Basile, M.S. Retrospective follow-up analysis of the transcriptomic patterns of cytokines, cytokine receptors and chemokines at preconception and during pregnancy, in women with post-partum depression. *Exp. Ther. Med.* **2019**, *18*, 2055–2062. [CrossRef]

31. Fagone, P.; Mazzon, E.; Cavalli, E.; Bramanti, A.; Petralia, M.C.; Mangano, K.; Al-Abed, Y.; Bramati, P.; Nicoletti, F. Contribution of the macrophage migration inhibitory factor superfamily of cytokines in the pathogenesis of preclinical and human multiple sclerosis: In silico and in vivo evidences. *J. Neuroimmunol.* **2018**, *322*, 46–56. [CrossRef]
32. Nicoletti, F.; Mazzon, E.; Fagone, P.; Mangano, K.; Mammana, S.; Cavalli, E.; Basile, M.S.; Bramanti, P.; Scalabrino, G.; Lange, A.; et al. Prevention of clinical and histological signs of MOG-induced experimental allergic encephalomyelitis by prolonged treatment with recombinant human EGF. *J. Neuroimmunol.* **2019**, *332*, 224–232. [CrossRef]
33. Cavalli, E.; Mazzon, E.; Basile, M.S.; Mangano, K.; Di Marco, R.; Bramanti, P.; Nicoletti, F.; Fagone, P.; Petralia, M.C. Upregulated Expression of Macrophage Migration Inhibitory Factor, Its Analogue D-Dopachrome Tautomerase, and the CD44 Receptor in Peripheral CD4 T Cells from Clinically Isolated Syndrome Patients with Rapid Conversion to Clinical Defined Multiple Sclerosis. *Medicina* **2019**, *55*, 667. [CrossRef]
34. Fagone, P.; Mazzon, E.; Mammana, S.; Di Marco, R.; Spinasanta, F.; Basile, M.S.; Petralia, M.C.; Bramanti, P.; Nicoletti, F.; Mangano, K. Identification of CD4+ T cell biomarkers for predicting the response of patients with relapsing-remitting multiple sclerosis to natalizumab treatment. *Mol. Med. Rep.* **2019**, *20*, 678–684. [CrossRef]
35. Cavalli, E.; Mazzon, E.; Basile, M.S.; Mammana, S.; Pennisi, M.; Fagone, P.; Kalfin, R.; Martinovic, V.; Ivanovic, J.; Andabaka, M.; et al. In Silico and In Vivo Analysis of IL37 in Multiple Sclerosis Reveals Its Probable Homeostatic Role on the Clinical Activity, Disability, and Treatment with Fingolimod. *Molecules* **2019**, *25*, 20. [CrossRef]
36. Petralia, M.C.; Mazzon, E.; Basile, M.S.; Cutuli, M.; Di Marco, R.; Scandurra, F.; Saraceno, A.; Fagone, P.; Nicoletti, F.; Mangano, K. Effects of Treatment with the Hypomethylating Agent 5-aza-2′-deoxycytidine in Murine Type II Collagen-Induced Arthritis. *Pharmaceuticals* **2019**, *12*, E174. [CrossRef]
37. Cavalli, E.; Mazzon, E.; Mammana, S.; Basile, M.S.; Lombardo, S.D.; Mangano, K.; Bramanti, P.; Nicoletti, F.; Fagone, P.; Petralia, M.C. Overexpression of Macrophage Migration Inhibitory Factor and Its Homologue D-Dopachrome Tautomerase as Negative Prognostic Factor in Neuroblastoma. *Brain Sci.* **2019**, *9*, 284. [CrossRef]
38. Petralia, M.C.; Mazzon, E.; Fagone, P.; Russo, A.; Longo, A.; Avitabile, T.; Nicoletti, F.; Reibaldi, M.; Basile, M.S. Characterization of the Pathophysiological Role of CD47 in Uveal Melanoma. *Molecules* **2019**, *24*, 2450. [CrossRef]
39. Lombardo, S.D.; Presti, M.; Mangano, K.; Petralia, M.C.; Basile, M.S.; Libra, M.; Candido, S.; Fagone, P.; Mazzon, E.; Nicoletti, F.; et al. Prediction of PD-L1 Expression in Neuroblastoma via Computational Modeling. *Brain Sci.* **2019**, *9*, 221. [CrossRef]
40. Mangano, K.; Mazzon, E.; Basile, M.S.; Di Marco, R.; Bramanti, P.; Mammana, S.; Petralia, M.C.; Fagone, P.; Nicoletti, F. Pathogenic role for macrophage migration inhibitory factor in glioblastoma and its targeting with specific inhibitors as novel tailored therapeutic approach. *Oncotarget* **2018**, *9*, 17951–17970. [CrossRef]
41. Mammana, S.; Fagone, P.; Cavalli, E.; Basile, M.; Petralia, M.; Nicoletti, F.; Bramanti, P.; Mazzon, E. The Role of Macrophages in Neuroinflammatory and Neurodegenerative Pathways of Alzheimer's Disease, Amyotrophic Lateral Sclerosis, and Multiple Sclerosis: Pathogenetic Cellular Effectors and Potential Therapeutic Targets. *Int. J. Mol. Sci.* **2018**, *19*, 831. [CrossRef]
42. Mammana, S.; Bramanti, P.; Mazzon, E.; Cavalli, E.; Basile, M.S.; Fagone, P.; Petralia, M.C.; McCubrey, J.A.; Nicoletti, F.; Mangano, K. Preclinical evaluation of the PI3K/Akt/mTOR pathway in animal models of multiple sclerosis. *Oncotarget* **2018**, *9*, 8263–8277. [CrossRef]
43. Fagone, P.; Mangano, K.; Quattrocchi, C.; Cavalli, E.; Mammana, S.; Lombardo, G.A.G.; Pennisi, V.; Zocca, M.-B.; He, M.; Al-Abed, Y.; et al. Effects of NO-Hybridization on the Immunomodulatory Properties of the HIV Protease Inhibitors Lopinavir and Ritonavir. *Basic Clin. Pharmacol. Toxicol.* **2015**, *117*, 306–315. [CrossRef]
44. Paskas, S.; Mazzon, E.; Basile, M.S.; Cavalli, E.; Al-Abed, Y.; He, M.; Rakocevic, S.; Nicoletti, F.; Mijatovic, S.; Maksimovic-Ivanic, D. Lopinavir-NO, a nitric oxide-releasing HIV protease inhibitor, suppresses the growth of melanoma cells in vitro and in vivo. *Invest. New Drugs* **2019**, *37*, 1014–1028. [CrossRef]
45. Basile, M.; Mazzon, E.; Krajnovic, T.; Draca, D.; Cavalli, E.; Al-Abed, Y.; Bramanti, P.; Nicoletti, F.; Mijatovic, S.; Maksimovic-Ivanic, D. Anticancer and Differentiation Properties of the Nitric Oxide Derivative of Lopinavir in Human Glioblastoma Cells. *Molecules* **2018**, *23*, 2463. [CrossRef]

46. Lazarević, M.; Mazzon, E.; Momčilović, M.; Basile, M.S.; Colletti, G.; Petralia, M.C.; Bramanti, P.; Nicoletti, F.; Miljković, Đ. The H_2S Donor GYY4137 Stimulates Reactive Oxygen Species Generation in BV2 Cells While Suppressing the Secretion of TNF and Nitric Oxide. *Molecules* **2018**, *23*, 2966. [CrossRef]
47. McFarland, H.F.; Martin, R. Multiple sclerosis: A complicated picture of autoimmunity. *Nat. Immunol.* **2007**, *8*, 913–919. [CrossRef]
48. Goverman, J. Autoimmune T cell responses in the central nervous system. *Nat. Rev. Immunol.* **2009**, *9*, 393–407. [CrossRef]
49. Nylander, A.; Hafler, D.A. Multiple sclerosis. *J. Clin. Invest.* **2012**, *122*, 1180–1188. [CrossRef]
50. Hemler, M.E. Targeting of tetraspanin proteins–potential benefits and strategies. *Nat. Rev. Drug Discov.* **2008**, *7*, 747–758. [CrossRef]

12

Women's Health: Contemporary Management of MS in Pregnancy and Post-Partum

Kelly Tisovic and Lilyana Amezcua *

Department of Neurology, Keck School of Medicine, University of Southern California, Los Angeles, CA 90033, USA; tisovic@usc.edu

* Correspondence: lamezcua@usc.edu;

Abstract: Multiple sclerosis (MS) primarily affects women in childbearing age and is associated with an increased risk of adverse post-partum outcomes. Relapses and now fetal exposure to disease modifying treatments in the early phase of pregnancy and thereafter are of concern. Safe and effective contraception is required for women who wish to delay or avoid pregnancy while on disease-modifying treatments. Counseling and planning is essential to assess the risk of both fetal and maternal complications, particularly now in the era of highly efficient and riskier therapies. The purpose of this review is to provide a practical framework using the available data surrounding pregnancy in MS with the goal of optimizing outcomes during this phase in MS.

Keywords: multiple sclerosis; pregnancy; post-partum; treatment

1. Introduction

Multiple sclerosis (MS) is an autoimmune disease of the central nervous system (CNS) characterized by inflammation and demyelination with almost 1 million affected in the US [1]. The disease predominantly affects females and often starts in childbearing age [1], making this period a particularly important stage for treatment decisions. Evidence supporting a reduction of disease activity during pregnancy [2] is likely contributing to the recent observation that more women with MS are considering pregnancy [3]. Because most disease-modifying treatments (DMT) are contraindicated during pregnancy, understanding the risk behind discontinuation and early pregnancy exposure is important. In the current era, a neurologist can now be faced with concerns relating to pregnancy, including contraception, fertility, relapses during pregnancy and post-partum, and breastfeeding.

The purpose of this paper is to provide a practical clinical framework to assist physicians in the treatment of women with MS surrounding pregnancy by reviewing the most recent data surrounding pre-conception care, pregnancy and the post-partum phase in MS with the goal of facilitating informed decisions.

2. Methods

We performed a literature search in Pubmed using the search term "multiple sclerosis," with additional search terms of "pregnancy," "breastfeeding," "contraception," "fertility," "disease modifying therapy," "pregnancy outcomes," "guidelines," and "counseling" in the last 10 years. The studies felt to be most relevant for clinical practice were selected for inclusion in this review.

3. Pre-Pregnancy

3.1. *Family Planning and Counseling*

The rates of pregnancies in MS patients has increased in the US from 2006 to 2014, from 7.91% to 9.47%, while the rate of women without MS decreased from 8.83% to 7.75% over this time [3]. Because there is a high rate of unintentional pregnancies [4] and safety concerns surrounding certain MS DMTs in pregnancy [5], counseling should be performed for all women with MS of reproductive age. In addition, the neurologist should be aware of other related issues such as contraception, fertility, and the low risk of transmission of MS to offspring (2–3% if one parent is affected and about 20% if both parents are affected) [5]. Once a patient has decided to become pregnant, a number of steps can be taken in an effort to achieve optimal outcomes. These are described below, and are outlined in Figure 1.

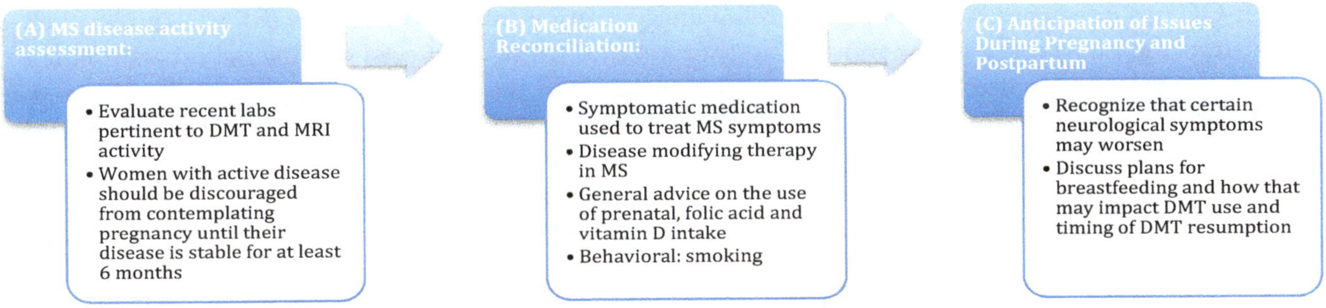

Figure 1. Pre-pregnancy care. (**A**) Multiple sclerosis (MS) disease activity assessment, (**B**) medication reconciliation, (**C**) anticipation of issues during pregnancy and post-partum.

3.1.1. MS Disease Activity Assessment

The current MS disease activity should be evaluated. Appropriate laboratory analysis and MRIs should be included in this assessment. For those with active MS disease activity, postponing attempted conception until disease is stable for at least six months is recommended.

3.1.2. Medication Reconciliation

The current symptomatic MS medications a patient is taking and their safety in pregnancy should be evaluated. This should be performed with the assistance of a patient's obstetrician-gynecologist whenever possible. Current DMT use should be discussed in regards to safety and optimal discontinuation timing, which is typically 5 maximal half lives of the DMT, but this time frame may vary in specific circumstances [6]. Standard prenatal medications including prenatal vitamins and folic acid supplementation is advised [6]. Optimal Vitamin D supplementation is important to maintain throughout pregnancy, as an increased risk of MS was seen in offspring of women with low gestational Vitamin D (25(OH)D) levels of less than 30nmol/L in a Finnish study [7]. Smoking cessation is recommended for all patients, given its impact on both MS disease activity and on pregnancy [6].

3.1.3. Anticipation of Issues Encountered during Pregnancy and Post-partum

Physicians should discuss the potential for MS symptoms to worsen or for new MS symptoms to appear, especially during the less-protective phases of pregnancy and especially in patients with highly active disease or on DMTs with risk for rebound activity. Plans regarding breastfeeding should also be discussed pre-conception, as this will affect the timing of DMT resumption.

3.2. *Oral Contraceptives and Multiple Sclerosis (MS) Disease Activity*

Estrogen has known anti-inflammatory properties and has shown to be neuroprotective in preclinical studies [8]. The reduction in disease activity observed during pregnancy is thought to be related to high levels of estriol, especially in the third trimester [9]. In experimental autoimmune encephalomyelitis (EAE) models, administration of estriol improved EAE, which correlated with a decrease in the number of CNS inflammatory cells [8]. However, retrospective and prospective studies have reported mixed results regarding oral contraceptive (OC) use and MS risk [10–12] and have reported a positive influence on relapse rates [13]. While Hellwig et al. found that OC use was associated with a slightly increased risk of MS/clinically isolated syndrome (CIS) (adjusted odds ratio

(OR) = 1.52, 95% CI = 1.21–1.91; $p < 0.001$) [12], the risk did not change with duration of OC use, suggesting non-causal association. Other studies have supported a positive effect. Rejali et al. found a statistically significant relationship between history of OC use (OR = 0.492, $p = 0.002$) and MS risk and in the duration of OC use (OR = 0.881, $p = 0.008$) and MS risk [11]. Holmqvist et al. found the mean age of MS onset was significantly higher in patients with OC use prior to MS onset than those without OC use (26 years old vs. 19 years old, $p < 0.001$). Additionally, age of MS onset increased with increasing time of OC use prior to MS onset [10]. Bove et al. evaluated effects of past-, current- or never-OC use in women with new onset relapsing remitting multiple sclerosis (RRMS) or CIS started on a first-line injectable disease-modifying therapy and found that past OC users had a statistically significant lower annualized relapse rate (ARR) compared to never OC users (Relative Risk (RR) = 0.64, $p = 0.031$) and that current OC users had a non-statistically significant lower ARR compared to never OC users (RR = 0.97, $p = 0.91$) [13].

The anti-inflammatory effects of estradiol in combination with injectable MS therapies have been demonstrated in preliminary studies [9,14]. Pozzilli et al. combined low-dose and high-dose oral contraceptives with interferon beta and evaluated disease activity via cumulative number of combined unique active (CUA) lesions on magnetic resonance imagining (MRI) at 96 weeks. There was a 26.5% ($p = 0.04$) reduction in CUA lesions in the high dose OC group compared to interferon beta alone and a non-significant reduction in the low dose OC group compared to interferon beta alone [14]. Voskuhl et al. published a randomized, double-blind, placebo controlled phase 2 trial to assess the safety and efficacy of estriol and progesterone in combination to glatiramer acetate versus glatiramer acetate alone using a primary endpoint of annualized confirmed relapse rate at 24 months, and using a significance level of $p = 0.01$. Confirmed relapse rate was 0.25 (95% CI 0.17–0.37) relapses per year in the estriol treated group compared to 0.37 (95% CI 0.25–0.53) relapses per year in the placebo group with an adjusted rate ratio of 0.63 (95% CI 0.37–1.05, $p = 0.077$) [9]. Larger studies with longer treatment times are needed to better evaluate the effect of OC treatment and to help better stratify the risk-benefit of long term estrogen use.

Clinical considerations: reliable contraception is recommended for patients taking DMT. DMT-specific recommendations for contraceptive use are included in Table 1 [15–20], if provided specifically in the prescribing recommendations. Beyond the need for pregnancy protection while using DMT, oral contraceptive use is considered safe in MS [13], and potential additional benefits on disease activity may be seen with oral contraceptive use in combination with platform injectable therapy [9,14].

Table 1. Summary of prescribing contraception recommendations for MS disease-modifying treatments (DMTs).

Disease Modifying Treatment (DMT)	Prescribing Contraception Recommendations *
Interferon beta	N/A
Glatiramer acetate	N/A
Fingolimod	Effective contraception during treatment and two months following therapy [15]
Dimethyl fumarate	N/A
Teriflunomide	Effective contraception during treatment and until plasma concentrations of teriflunomide are less than 0.02 mg/L [16]

Table 1. *Cont.*

Disease Modifying Treatment (DMT)	Prescribing Contraception Recommendations *
Natalizumab	N/A
Alemtuzumab	Effective contraceptive measures during treatment and for 4 months following that course of treatment [17]
Ocrelizumab	Effective contraception during therapy and for 6 months after the last infusion [18]
Mitoxantrone	Women should not become pregnant during therapy [19]
Cyclophosphamide **	Effective contraception during therapy and for up to 1 year after completion of treatment [20]

* Contraception recommendations included if provided in the prescribing label. ** Not Food and Drug Administration (FDA) approved for use in MS.

3.3. *Fertility*

3.3.1. Effects of MS on Fertility

There are multiple observational studies supporting the argument that fertility may be influenced by MS [21–25]. An Italian study found that women with MS are more frequently childless compared to the general population, with reported rates of 22% vs. 13%, respectively [21]. However, it is unclear if childlessness is due to behavioral factors such as disability, fear or beliefs about caring for a newborn child or transmitting MS to her offspring, or actually a disease-related pathology [26]. Another important factor impacting fertility in MS patients includes sexual dysfunction, which is very common, reported in 30–70% of MS patients [26] and is beyond the scope of this paper.

Reassuringly, an observational study in a French cohort evaluated fecundity, defined as the time to become pregnant, in MS patients both before and after MS onset [22]. No differences in the time to conception prior to or after MS disease onset were found (on average <1 year). However, despite their normal fecundity, the mean number of children per women with MS was less than in the general French population (1.37 versus 1.99, respectively) [22]. It is important to note that infertility in Western populations is not uncommon, estimated at 10–20%, and because MS occurs at a fertile age, it is possible that infertility is not actually MS mediated [27]. Nevertheless, assisted reproductive techniques (ART) have been reported to be more common in women with MS [23].

Other studies have focused on evaluating hormonal differences, where higher levels of prolactin, luteinizing hormone (LH), and follicle-stimulating hormone (FSH) and lower levels of estrogen have been reported among MS women [24]. Elevated FSH in the early follicular phase is an indicator of low ovarian reserve [25]. Another marker of low ovarian reserve, Anti-Mullerian hormone (AMH), has been found to be decreased in reproductive-aged women with other autoimmune diseases and does not fluctuate with menstrual cycles as FSH and LH levels do. To better understand ovarian reserve in women with MS, serum AMH levels were examined in 76 RRMS patients and in 58 healthy controls and found serum AMH levels to be significantly lower in patients with RRMS than in healthy controls, and a higher proportion of RRMS patients showed very low AMH levels [25]. However, in a follow up study, no significant differences in AMH levels were found [28] indicating that larger studies are needed to better understand if lower ovarian reserve is found in reproductive-aged women with MS. Thus, the ability to conceive may be influenced by various factors which makes fertility a concern for many women affected with MS.

If a woman with MS does suffer from infertility, ART should be considered with caution. Gonadotropin-releasing hormone (GnRH) agonists and antagonists are used to suppress the influence of the hypothalamic-pituitary gland axis, preventing an LH surge and thus spontaneous ovulation. Subsequent ovarian hyperstimulation is accomplished by administration of gonadotropins. Following stimulation, controlled ovulation is accomplished by human choriongonadotropin (hCG), and administration of progesterone to support the luteal phase. Fertilization is completed by intrauterine insemination, in vitro fertilization, or intracytoplasmatic sperm injection [27].

There are no randomized control trials to evaluate the safety or changes in relapse rate in MS patients who are treated with ART. Despite the clinical improvements seen with the use of GnRH agonists in EAE models [29], their use in humans with MS have shown opposite effects [27]. ART therapy in MS patients may cause increased disease activity, and patients who plan to pursue these therapies should be counseled about this risk sufficiently. Hellwig et al. published a review of five small studies evaluating ART use in MS patients using various reproductive techniques. This collection of studies demonstrated an increase in relapse rate following unsuccessful ART and increased MRI activity. Downregulation of pituitary GnRH receptors via GnRH agonists might account for this increased relapse rate. Additional theories behind worsening MS activity following ART include discontinuation of DMT, stress related to infertility, rapidly changing hormone levels inducing pro-inflammatory changes, and ART-mediated increases in immune cell movement across the blood-brain-barrier via induction of interleukin-8 (IL-8), vascular endothelial growth factor (VEGF), and CXC chemokine ligand 12 (CXCL-12) [27].

3.3.2. Effects of Disease-Modifying Treatments (DMTs) on Fertility

In evaluating the potential influence of DMT use on fertility, information on humans is currently scarce. Table 2 summarizes reported effects of DMTs on fertility with special concerns to the following DMTs: interferon beta [30], natalizumab [31], alemtuzumab [17], mitoxantrone [31], and cyclophosphamide [31]. An additional concern exists for autologous stem cell transplant in combination with high-dose chemotherapy, which is an experimental MS treatment and may decrease fertility [32].

Table 2. Summary of reported MS DMT effects on fertility.

DMT	Fertility
Interferon beta	Reduced fertility in animals; no information in humans [30]
Glatiramer acetate	No effects
Fingolimod	No effects
Dimethyl Fumarate	No effects
Teriflunomide	No effects
Natalizumab	Reduced fertility in animals; no information in humans [31]
Alemtuzumab	Reduced fertility in animals; no information in humans [17]
Ocrelizumab	No effects
Mitoxantrone	Amenorrhea and transient azoospermia have been reported [31]
Cyclophosphamide *	Amenorrhea and transient azoospermia have been reported [31]

* Not FDA approved for the treatment of MS.

Clinical considerations: because it is prudent to optimize a patient's chance of conception off of DMT, strategies such as substituting barrier methods for OC, waiting for ovulation cycles to resume prior to discontinuing DMT, and referrals for evaluation of fertility if pregnancy does not result after 6 months of attempt should be considered [6].

4. Pregnancy

4.1. Pregnancy and the Risk of MS

There are multiple studies supporting the argument that pregnancy can be protective. Both a reduction in MS risk [10,11,33–35] and a delay in MS onset [10] has been reported. For example, Runmarker et al. found a higher risk of MS in nulliparous women compared to parous women, suggesting that pregnancy can be protective. This risk appeared to increase with older age [35]. Magyari et al. reported a 46% reduced risk of MS in Danish women during the five years following childbirth [33], while Ponsonby et al. found that a higher parity and a higher number of offspring was associated with reduced risk of a first clinical demyelinating event, and that each pregnancy conferred a decreased risk [34]. Similarly, in a case-controlled study, Rejali et al. found a significant relationship between the number of pregnancies and reduced risk of MS (OR = 0.586, 95% CI = 0.461–0.745), suggesting that higher parity also influences MS risk [11]. Holmqvist et al. found that pregnancy significantly delayed the mean age at MS onset in women who had given birth prior to disease onset. This increase in age was seen for each child born to a woman prior to MS onset, suggesting a protective effect of each pregnancy [10] which could be related to long-term epigenetic effects [36].

4.2. Pregnancy and Risk of Disease Activity

During pregnancy, the female's immune system is reported to be more immunotolerant due to a shift in the ratio of T helper 1 and 2 cells, mediated by high levels of estrogens, especially estradiol, in addition to other important hormones including progesterone and androgens [6,10]. Some of these changes support the clinical observation of decrease relapses during pregnancy and likely also support the return of disease activity observed in months post-partum.

One of the pivotal studies to support this was reported in 1998, where Confravreux et al. prospectively reported on the natural history of MS in pregnancy. A reduction in ARR during pregnancy of 70%, especially during the third trimester, compared with the year prior to pregnancy was reported and was followed by an increase in ARR during three months post-partum. The relapse rate subsequently returned to the pre-partum relapse rate [37]. Contrary to Poser's report [38], there was no negative effect of pregnancy on disability progression [37]. In 2004, a two-year post-partum follow up by Vukusic et al. noted that the risk of post-partum relapse was correlated to the number of relapses in the year prior to pregnancy, in the number of relapses during pregnancy, and in those with a higher Expanded Disability Status Scale (EDSS) at baseline [39]. Other studies [40,41] published worldwide have found similar trends in the pattern of relapse occurrence during pregnancy and post-partum which supports that the observations are more likely to be return of activity.

Clinical considerations: because there is the theoretical risk for relapses to occur in the early phases of pregnancy, it is important to provide a recommendation in the clinical setting concerning treatment. This risk of early relapses has become more apparent in patients who are becoming pregnant while on fingolimod and natalizumab.

Previous studies have reported on treatment effects with interferon beta or glatiramer acetate on relapse rates but little information is available concerning second-line therapies that are only more recently available and are not typically used during pregnancy due to safety concerns [42]. There is data to support the argument that the older treatments, such as glatiramer acetate or interferon beta had no effect [43]. There have been reports of rebound with newer and higher efficacy DMT with discontinuation of therapy prior to or during pregnancy [42]. A cross-sectional study of 99 pregnancies with nearly 90% of women treated with DMTs during the year prior to pregnancy showed a higher relapse occurrence during pregnancy than previously reported [42]. A four-fold increase in relapses during pregnancy occurred, mostly during the first and third trimesters. Relapses were primarily seen in patients treated with natalizumab and fingolimod before pregnancy. Longer DMT washout periods before pregnancy resulted in a higher probability of relapse (OR 3.9, 95% CI 1.4–10.6, $p = 0.008$), and were seen in patients previously treated with natalizumab and fingolimod who relapsed during the first trimester of pregnancy [42].

It is important to recognize that there are certain DMT's that can place a woman at risk for relapse prior to or during pregnancy. Discontinuing fingolimod has been reported to increase risk of rebound disease and a suggested washout of 2 months is recommended [15]. Women taking fingolimod should be counseled regarding the risk of rebound activity, and switching to a safer medication such as glatiramer acetate or interferon beta should be considered, based on newer data from postmarking studies [42,44–46]. Patients taking natalizumab may also be at increased risk of rebound disease activity and switching to glatiramer acetate or interferon beta may be similarly considered [42,46]. For women on natalizumab with highly active disease, Thone et al. [45] recommends a consideration of either shortening the washout period, continuing natalizumab until conception, or continuing natalizumab during pregnancy with extended interval dosing every 6 weeks through gestation week 30, with a pediatric check upon delivery for hematologic abnormalities. This should be done on a case-by-case basis and after a discussion about the risks with each patient [45]. Continuation of natalizumab during the entire pregnancy has also been suggested in those patients with high disease activity who are at high risk of rebound [47]. However, a full discussion between patient and physician needs to occur highlighting the potential risk of fetal hematologic abnormalities reported with natalizumab use [46,47]. If exposed, we recommend that women be under the care of a high-risk obstetrician and consider delivering in a hospital where a pediatrician is accessible to assess the newborn for potential complications [47]. Other considerations for these patients include discontinuation of DMT followed by empiric treatment with prophylactic monthly high-dose corticosteroids during attempted conception after a negative pregnancy test [6], switching treatment to alemtuzumab and waiting 4 months before attempted conception [17], or switching treatment to B-cell therapy and waiting 6 months before attempted conception [18]. These studies are part of the recommendations found in the joint European Committee of Treatment and Research in Multiple Sclerosis (ECTRIMS) and European Academy of Neurology (EAN) guidelines for treatment of women with MS who wish to become pregnant [48] (Table 3).

Table 3. European Committee of Treatment and Research in Multiple Sclerosis (ECTRIMS)/European Academy of Neurology (EAN) Guidelines for management of DMT in women with MS in pregnancy.

Only Glatiramer Acetate 20 mg/mL is Approved for Use during Pregnancy (Consensus) [48].
For women who are at risk of disease reactivation and planning pregnancy: ○ Consider switching the glatiramer acetate or interferon beta until conception is confirmed (weak) [48]. ○ For specific cases in women with active disease, consider continuing treatment throughout pregnancy (weak) [48].
Delaying pregnancy is advised for women with persistent, highly active disease. ○ Women who become pregnant unintentionally or despite recommendation, treatment with natalizumab during pregnancy can be considered after counseling about the potential consequences (weak) [48]. ○ For planned pregnancies with very active disease, alemtuzumab can be considered, but treatment must be followed by 4 months of effective contraception (weak) [48].

Relapses during pregnancy should have clinical and radiologic assessments when indicated. A brain MRI without contrast does not appear to be harmful to the fetus [49]. Treatment with prednisone, prednisolone, or methylprednisolone can be used to shorten symptom duration, as these medications are metabolized by the placenta by about 90% [50]. However, their use in the first trimester of pregnancy is considered teratogenic and an increased risk of cleft lip or palate has been reported [51].

4.3. Maternal and Delivery Complications

The effect of MS on pregnancy outcomes in the US and throughout the world has been previously described, with conflicting results [40,41,52–55]. A meta-analysis cited a relatively higher prevalence of abortions, cesarean sections, prematurity, and low birth weight in women with MS. However, due to the high heterogeneity between the studies, they felt the effects of regional, legal, and cultural differences could have hyper-inflated the abortion and cesarean section rates [40]. Studies using claims databases have mixed reports. A higher risk of both antenatal [53] or post-partum [52] hospitalization of mothers with MS were reported in two studies, whereas other studies found no increased risk [3,54,55]. Reports of maternal infections such as urinary tract infections (UTI) [54] and sexually transmitted diseases (STD) [3], cesarean section rates [53,54] and induction of labor [54] were increased in women with MS compared to controls. Risk of premature labor [3] and preterm delivery [55] have also been reported.

The conflicting evidence regarding pregnancy outcomes in women with MS may stem from ascertainment bias and other confounding variables. Both older age and an increased prevalence of co-morbidities in women with MS can independently affect pregnancy outcomes. There are several potential issues with using claims based databases, where coding and billing might simply reflect increased health care use in MS patients due to increased caution by their providers [41], where different databases capture differing MS subpopulations based on the health insurance included in that database, where reliance on hospital discharge summaries for identification of MS patients may not capture all patients if they are asymptomatic at the time of delivery and no code for MS is entered, and where a lack of vital background information including MS disease duration, disability, prior IV corticosteroid use during pregnancy, other medications used during pregnancy, and prior pregnancy outcomes limit interpretation of the results [3,52–55].

There is still much to be learned about MS and whether it is associated with adverse pregnancy outcomes. Well-designed analyses not reliant on recall, standardized and more detailed data collection, and increased participation in pregnancy registries are all vital to our future knowledge [3].

4.4. Fetal and Neonatal Complications

A majority of reported data regarding fetal and neonatal outcomes in women with MS has been reassuring [40,52–55]. Rates of malformations and neonatal deaths have been reported as low as 1.13–6.25%, which is similar to US reported rates [40,56]. Several US claims based studies have evaluated the rate of fetal malformations in newborns born to mothers with and without MS, and most [52–55], but not all [3], have not demonstrated an increased risk. Houtchens et al. alone found that a higher proportion of patients with MS than without MS had claims for acquired fetal damage (27.8% vs. 23.5% $p = 0.002$) and congenital fetal malformations (13.2% vs. 10.3% $p = 0.004$) [3]. Importantly, in this study, both MS and control groups had a higher rate of labor and delivery complications than reported in the general population [56]. Additional considerations include the fact that MS patients were older, were more likely to have other chronic medications conditions, and due to the study design, other pertinent health and pregnancy information was not available. Thus, independent predictors of adverse pregnancy outcomes were present, but were not able to be appropriately interpreted, again highlighting the need for additional information which could not be ascertained from the data [3,56].

Clinical considerations: none of the current US Food and Drug Administration (FDA) approved DMTs used to treat MS are specifically approved for women who are trying to conceive, who are currently pregnant, or who are breastfeeding. There are variations in DMT washout prior to pregnancy [15–19,57,58] which are summarized in Table 4 along with their associated FDA pregnancy categorization [46,59]. The recommendations differ in other countries from those in the US, especially for glatiramer acetate [48].

Table 4. FDA pregnancy categories and recommended washout periods for MS DMTs.

DMT	FDA Pregnancy Category	Recommended Washout Period
Interferon beta	Category C [46]	0–1 Menstrual cycles [57,58]
Glatiramer acetate	Category B [46]	0–1 Menstrual cycles [57,58]
Fingolimod	Category C [46]	2 Menstrual cycles [15]
Dimethyl Fumarate	Category C [46]	0–1 Menstrual cycles [57,58]
Teriflunomide	Category X [46]	Either: (1) Wait 24 Menstrual cycles, OR (2) Perform accelerated elimination until plasma concentration <0.02 mg/dL [16]

Table 4. *Cont.*

DMT	FDA Pregnancy Category	Recommended Washout Period
Natalizumab *	Category C [46]	1–3 Menstrual cycles [58]
Alemtuzumab	Category C [46]	4 Menstrual cycles [17]
Ocrelizumab	N/A	6 Menstrual cycles [18]
Mitoxantrone	Category D [46]	6 Menstrual cycles [19]

* Natalizumab: Case by case decision should be made in females with highly active disease or with history of severe natalizumab withdrawal relapse after full discussion of the risks and benefits with the patient.

A summary of prescribing recommendations in pregnancy can be found in the labels of MS DMTs, including a summary of their safety, lactation warnings, and contraception guidelines. Most FDA approved MS DMTs have established pregnancy registries, and providers should encourage patients with DMT exposures during pregnancy to enroll. Interestingly, a recent retrospective study using an international MS pregnancy database found an increasing percentage of MS patients becoming pregnant on DMTs, rising from 27% in 2006 to 62% in 2016, with a median exposure duration of one month. The proportion of pre-term births or miscarriages compared to the unexposed pregnancies were no different [60]. Updated information on the safety of DMT use during pregnancy based from the FDA label, registry data and other sources may be found in the Supplementary Materials, Table S1 [15–19,30,31,46,57,61–78].

5. Post-Partum

5.1. *Post-Partum and the Risk of Disease Activity*

Several studies have down that the post-partum period is a time of risk for increased disease activity [37,41,42]. In a cross-sectional study of 512 patients, Poser et al. found that women at six months post-partum were at increased risk of developing MS, disability progression, and of experiencing a higher number of relapses compared with during pregnancy [38]. Pregnancy may also increase the risk of conversion from radiologically isolated syndrome (RIS) to CIS [79]. In a small French cohort of 60 women with RIS, those who became pregnant developed a first neurologic event earlier or had more active MRI lesions than those who did not become pregnant [79]. Due to its small sample size and the rarity of RIS, larger studies are needed to better understand the influence of pregnancy on the risk of conversion from RIS to CIS.

As none of the current DMTs are FDA-approved for use during breastfeeding, it is important to discuss the appropriate time to resume DMT. To balance the risk of relapse to the mother with the benefit of breastfeeding to the baby in considering resuming DMT, the physician must consider a patient's likelihood to experience post-partum disease activity. Research supports that there is a relationship between post-partum relapse rates and prior disease activity the year before pregnancy [39]. The highest predictor of post-partum relapse was a higher annualized relapse rate in the 2 years prior to pregnancy [80]. For women at increased risk of relapse, a discussion regarding benefits of resuming DMT versus the risks of relapse with breastfeeding should occur. Women who chose to forego breastfeeding to resume DMT or who simply do not wish to breastfeed should resume DMT in 7–10 days post-partum [45].

5.2. *Breastfeeding and Disease Activity*

Breastfeeding has numerous health benefits to both the mother and infant. Exclusive breastfeeding for six months should be encouraged if possible, as recommended by the World Health Organization [81]. The reported effects of breastfeeding on post-partum relapse rate in MS have varied [6,37,82–84] and generally the patient is advised to make an informed decision.

Several prospective studies have found a benefit with breastfeeding and in particular exclusive breastfeeding on post-partum relapse rates [37,82,83] (Table 5). Exclusive breastfeeding is thought to provoke lactational amenorrhea and ovarian suppression, which may be important in the pathophysiology behind the observed benefit in MS [85]. In a small prospective study, women who exclusively breastfed were five times less likely to experience a relapse in the year following pregnancy compared to those who did not and exclusive breastfeeding was associated with protracted lactational amenorrhea. This study was limited by its small size, but showed a consistent benefit of exclusive breastfeeding when women with more highly active disease, a source of possible confounding, were excluded from analysis [82]. A meta-analysis of the effects of breastfeeding on relapse rate reported that women who breastfed were half as likely to have a post-partum relapse than women who did not [84]. Limitations included high heterogeneity between studies, exclusivity of breastfeeding was not always defined or was simplistically defined, and recall bias in the included retrospective studies. A larger prospective study was conducted using the German MS and Pregnancy Registry that enrolled pregnant MS women based on their intention to exclusively or non-exclusively breastfeed. A lower risk of relapse in the six months post-partum was seen in women who chose to breastfeed exclusively compared to those who did not, and compared to those who resumed DMT within 30 days [83].

Table 5. Annualized relapse rates (ARR) in breastfeeding.

Study	Breastfeeding	ARR Pre-Pregnancy	ARR During Pregnancy	ARR Post Partum
Confavreux et al. [37]	Yes	0.6	0.3	1–3 months: 1.2 4–6 months: 0.9
	No	0.8	0.5	1–3 months: 1.3 4–6 months: 1.0
Hellwig et al. [83]	Exclusive	N/A	0.22	0.48
	Non-Exclusive	N/A	0.36	0.77
Langer-Gould et al. [82]	Exclusive	0.57	0.19	0.36
	Non-Exclusive	0.83	0.18	0.87

A recent study examined the effects of breastfeeding on the risk of MS in the nursing mother. The authors hypothesized that breast-feeding leads to anovulation, which confers decreased MS risk. Interestingly, in this matched case-control study, a cumulative duration of breastfeeding for ≥15 months was associated with a reduced risk of developing MS (adjusted OR 0.47, 95% CI 0.28–0.77; $p = 0.003$) compared to <4 months of breastfeeding, concluding that longer breastfeeding confers protection of developing MS to the nursing mother. Interestingly, the authors did not find an association between ovulatory years and MS risk. Limitations of this study included recall bias, the lack of hypothesized association of ovulatory years with MS risk, and lack of information as to why women chose not to breastfeed [86]. The effect of breastfeeding on MS risk requires further evaluation.

Clinical considerations: when resuming DMT, it is important to consider that the patients with more highly active disease pre-pregnancy and/or during pregnancy are more likely to chose not to breastfeed and to resume DMT post-partum and thus confound the above results [6], although the authors did account for this as best they could [82,83]. A larger, prospective study evaluating the effects of exclusive breastfeeding on post-partum relapse is needed. At the least, breastfeeding appears to be safe in women with MS, and exclusive breastfeeding may be beneficial until food supplementation is introduced into the infant's diet. For women who wish to breastfeed, the data support greater benefit from exclusive and without supplementation.

In patients who wish to breastfeed but are at a high risk of post-partum relapse, a protective strategy is using monthly corticosteroids [87]. Although only about 10% of an infant's endogenous corticosteroid production is ingested from breast milk, the long-term risks are unknown. Thus, a four-hour period of delayed breastfeeding, or "pumping and dumping," is recommended [88]. For monitoring purposes, routine screening MRI with gadolinium after delivery, again followed by delayed breastfeeding for 24 h, in breastfeeding mothers is recommended to help identify subclinical MS activity, and those who may need DMT earlier than anticipated [6].

5.3. Newborn Care

Women with MS are faced with balancing their own needs with those of their newborn child during the post-partum period. Sleep management, rehabilitation (often in the form of pelvic floor exercises), and resumption of DMT are important maternal considerations. Family or paid assistance should be encouraged. Women should also be screened for post-partum depression due to its high overall prevalence in the population, with the strongest risk factor of having baseline depression [5].

6. Conclusions

Women with MS are becoming pregnant with increasing rates, while newer and more effective DMTs are used to treat MS patients. Knowledge about safe and effective DMT use and the pattern of disease activity around pregnancy is vital. Decisions regarding breastfeeding and DMT resumption post-partum are shared between patient and physician, but with appropriate discussion about risks and benefits. Special consideration should be taken with women who have highly active disease, or who take medications that might cause rebound disease activity. Generally speaking, women should feel reassured and confident about the management of their MS in the reproductive years.

Acknowledgments: Tisovic's Multiple Sclerosis Clinical Care Physician Fellowship is funded by the National Multiple Sclerosis Society.

References

1. Wallin, M.T.; Culpepper, W.J.; Campbell, J.D.; Nelson, L.M.; Langer-Gould, A.; Marrie, R.A.; Cutter, G.R.; Kaye, W.E.; Wagner, L.; Tremlett, H.; et al. The prevalence of MS in the United States: A population-based estimate using health claims data. *Neurology* **2019**, *92*, e1029–e1040. [CrossRef] [PubMed]
2. D'Hooghe, M.B.; Nagels, G.; Bissay, V.; De Keyser, J. Modifiable factors influencing relapses and disability in multiple sclerosis. *Mult. Scler.* **2010**, *16*, 773–785. [CrossRef]
3. Houtchens, M.K.; Edwards, N.C.; Schneider, G.; Stern, K.; Phillips, A.L. Pregnancy rates and outcomes in women with and without MS in the United States. *Neurology* **2018**, *91*, e1559–e1569. [CrossRef] [PubMed]
4. Finer, L.B.; Zolna, M.R. Unintended pregnancy in the United States: Incidence and disparities, 2006. *Contraception* **2011**, *84*, 478–485. [CrossRef]
5. Bove, R.; Alwan, S.; Friedman, J.M.; Hellwig, K.; Houtchens, M.; Koren, G.; Lu, E.; McElrath, T.F.; Smyth, P.; Tremlett, H.; et al. Management of multiple sclerosis during pregnancy and the reproductive years: A systematic review. *Obstet. Gynecol.* **2014**, *124*, 1157–1168. [CrossRef]
6. Rankin, K.; Bove, R. Caring for Women with Multiple Sclerosis Across the Lifespan. *Curr. Neurol. Neurosci. Rep.* **2018**, *18*, 36. [CrossRef] [PubMed]
7. Munger, K.L.; Aivo, J.; Hongell, K.; Soilu-Hanninen, M.; Surcel, H.M.; Ascherio, A. Vitamin D Status During Pregnancy and Risk of Multiple Sclerosis in Offspring of Women in the Finnish Maternity Cohort. *JAMA Neurol.* **2016**, *73*, 515–519. [CrossRef]
8. Spence, R.D.; Voskuhl, R.R. Neuroprotective effects of estrogens and androgens in CNS inflammation and neurodegeneration. *Front. Neuroendocrinol.* **2012**, *33*, 105–115. [CrossRef]
9. Voskuhl, R.R.; Wang, H.; Wu, T.C.; Sicotte, N.L.; Nakamura, K.; Kurth, F.; Itoh, N.; Bardens, J.; Bernard, J.T.; Corboy, J.R.; et al. Estriol combined with glatiramer acetate for women with relapsing-remitting multiple sclerosis: A randomised, placebo-controlled, phase 2 trial. *Lancet Neurol.* **2016**, *15*, 35–46. [CrossRef]
10. Holmqvist, P.; Hammar, M.; Landtblom, A.M.; Brynhildsen, J. Age at onset of multiple sclerosis is correlated to use of combined oral contraceptives and childbirth before diagnosis. *Fertil. Steril.* **2010**, *94*, 2835–2837. [CrossRef] [PubMed]
11. Rejali, M.; Hosseini, S.M.; Kazemi Tabaee, M.S.; Etemadifar, M. Assessing the Risk Factors for Multiple Sclerosis in Women of Reproductive Age Suffering the Disease in Isfahan Province. *Int. J. Prev. Med.* **2016**, *7*, 58. [CrossRef] [PubMed]

12. Hellwig, K.; Chen, L.H.; Stancyzk, F.Z.; Langer-Gould, A.M. Oral Contraceptives and Multiple Sclerosis/Clinically Isolated Syndrome Susceptibility. *PLoS ONE* **2016**, *11*, e0149094. [CrossRef]
13. Bove, R.; Rankin, K.; Chua, A.S.; Saraceno, T.; Sattarnezhad, N.; Greeke, E.; Stuart, F.; LaRussa, A.; Glanz, B.I.; Chitnis, T. Oral contraceptives and MS disease activity in a contemporary real-world cohort. *Mult. Scler.* **2018**, *24*, 227–230. [CrossRef] [PubMed]
14. Pozzilli, C.; De Giglio, L.; Barletta, V.T.; Marinelli, F.; Angelis, F.D.; Gallo, V.; Pagano, V.A.; Marini, S.; Piattella, M.C.; Tomassini, V.; et al. Oral contraceptives combined with interferon beta in multiple sclerosis. *Neurol. Neuroimmunol. Neuroinflamm.* **2015**, *2*, e120. [CrossRef] [PubMed]
15. Gilenya (Fingolimod) Capsules, for Oral Use. Highlights of Prescribing Information. Available online: https://www.pharma.us.novartis.com/sites/www.pharma.us.novartis.com/files/gilenya.pdf (accessed on 29 January 2019).
16. Aubagio (Teriflunomide) Tablets, for Oral Use. Highlights of Prescribing Information. Available online: http://products.sanofi.us/aubagio/aubagio.pdf (accessed on 28 January 2019).
17. Lemtrada (Alemtuzumab) Injection, for Intravenous Use. Highlights of Prescribing Information. Available online: http://products.sanofi.us/lemtrada/lemtrada.pdf?s_mcid=ps-LP-google-BRsitelink-pi (accessed on 28 January 2019).
18. Ocrevus (Ocrelizumab) Injection, for Intravenous Use. Highlights of Prescribing Information. Available online: https://www.gene.com/download/pdf/ocrevus_prescribing.pdf (accessed on 29 January 2019).
19. Novantrone, Mitoxantrone for Injection Concentrate. Available online: https://www.accessdata.fda.gov/drugsatfda_docs/label/2009/019297s030s031lbl.pdf (accessed on 29 January 2019).
20. yclophosphamide Injection, for Intravenous Use. Cyclophosphamide Tablets, for Oral Use. Highlights of prescribing information. Available online: https://www.accessdata.fda.gov/drugsatfda_docs/label/2013/012141s090,012142s112lbl.pdf (accessed on 29 January 2019).
21. Ferraro, D.; Simone, A.M.; Adani, G.; Vitetta, F.; Mauri, C.; Strumia, S.; Senesi, C.; Curti, E.; Baldi, E.; Santangelo, M.; et al. Definitive childlessness in women with multiple sclerosis: A multicenter study. *Neurol Sci* **2017**, *38*, 1453–1459. [CrossRef]
22. Roux, T.; Courtillot, C.; Debs, R.; Touraine, P.; Lubetzki, C.; Papeix, C. Fecundity in women with multiple sclerosis: An observational mono-centric study. *J. Neurol* **2015**, *262*, 957–960. [CrossRef] [PubMed]
23. Jalkanen, A.; Alanen, A.; Airas, L. Pregnancy outcome in women with multiple sclerosis: Results from a prospective nationwide study in Finland. *Mult. Scler.* **2010**, *16*, 950–955. [CrossRef]
24. Grinsted, L.; Heltberg, A.; Hagen, C.; Djursing, H. Serum sex hormone and gonadotropin concentrations in premenopausal women with multiple sclerosis. *J. Intern. Med.* **1989**, *226*, 241–244. [CrossRef]
25. Thone, J.; Kollar, S.; Nousome, D.; Ellrichmann, G.; Kleiter, I.; Gold, R.; Hellwig, K. Serum anti-Mullerian hormone levels in reproductive-age women with relapsing-remitting multiple sclerosis. *Mult. Scler.* **2015**, *21*, 41–47. [CrossRef]
26. Cavalla, P.; Rovei, V.; Masera, S.; Vercellino, M.; Massobrio, M.; Mutani, R.; Revelli, A. Fertility in patients with multiple sclerosis: Current knowledge and future perspectives. *Neurol. Sci.* **2006**, *27*, 231–239. [CrossRef]
27. Hellwig, K.; Correale, J. Artificial reproductive techniques in multiple sclerosis. *Clin. Immunol.* **2013**, *149*, 219–224. [CrossRef]
28. Sepulveda, M.; Ros, C.; Martinez-Lapiscina, E.H.; Sola-Valls, N.; Hervas, M.; Llufriu, S.; La Puma, D.; Casals, E.; Blanco, Y.; Villoslada, P.; et al. Pituitary-ovary axis and ovarian reserve in fertile women with multiple sclerosis: A pilot study. *Mult. Scler.* **2016**, *22*, 564–568. [CrossRef] [PubMed]
29. Guzman-Soto, I.; Salinas, E.; Hernandez-Jasso, I.; Quintanar, J.L. Leuprolide acetate, a GnRH agonist, improves experimental autoimmune encephalomyelitis: A possible therapy for multiple sclerosis. *Neurochem. Res.* **2012**, *37*, 2190–2197. [CrossRef] [PubMed]
30. AVONEX (Interferon beta-1a) Intramuscular Injection. Highlights of Prescribing Information. Available online: https://www.avonex.com/content/dam/commercial/multiple-sclerosis/avonex/pat/en_us/pdf/Avonex_US_Prescribing_Information.pdf (accessed on 29 January 2019).
31. Amato, M.P.; Portaccio, E. Fertility, pregnancy and childbirth in patients with multiple sclerosis: Impact of disease-modifying drugs. *CNS Drugs* **2015**, *29*, 207–220. [CrossRef] [PubMed]
32. Holmoy, T.; Torkildsen, O. Family planning, pregnancy and breastfeeding in multiple sclerosis. *Tidsskr. Nor. Laegeforen* **2016**, *136*, 1726–1729. [CrossRef]

33. Magyari, M. Role of socio-economic and reproductive factors in the risk of multiple sclerosis. *Acta Neurol. Scand.* **2015**, *132*, 20–23. [CrossRef]
34. Ponsonby, A.L.; Lucas, R.M.; van der Mei, I.A.; Dear, K.; Valery, P.C.; Pender, M.P.; Taylor, B.V.; Kilpatrick, T.J.; Coulthard, A.; Chapman, C.; et al. Offspring number, pregnancy, and risk of a first clinical demyelinating event: The AusImmune Study. *Neurology* **2012**, *78*, 867–874. [CrossRef]
35. Runmarker, B.; Andersen, O. Pregnancy is associated with a lower risk of onset and a better prognosis in multiple sclerosis. *Brain* **1995**, *118 Pt 1*, 253–261. [CrossRef]
36. Mehta, D.; Wani, S.; Wallace, L.; Henders, A.K.; Wray, N.R.; McCombe, P.A. Cumulative influence of parity-related genomic changes in multiple sclerosis. *J. Neuroimmunol* **2019**, *328*, 38–49. [CrossRef]
37. Confavreux, C.; Hutchinson, M.; Hours, M.M.; Cortinovis-Tourniaire, P.; Moreau, T. Rate of pregnancy-related relapse in multiple sclerosis. Pregnancy in Multiple Sclerosis Group. *N. Engl. J. Med.* **1998**, *339*, 285–291. [CrossRef]
38. Poser, S.; Poser, W. Multiple sclerosis and gestation. *Neurology* **1983**, *33*, 1422–1427. [CrossRef]
39. Vukusic, S.; Hutchinson, M.; Hours, M.; Moreau, T.; Cortinovis-Tourniaire, P.; Adeleine, P.; Confavreux, C. Pregnancy and multiple sclerosis (the PRIMS study): Clinical predictors of post-partum relapse. *Brain* **2004**, *127*, 1353–1360. [CrossRef]
40. Finkelsztejn, A.; Brooks, J.B.; Paschoal, F.M., Jr.; Fragoso, Y.D. What can we really tell women with multiple sclerosis regarding pregnancy? A systematic review and meta-analysis of the literature. *BJOG* **2011**, *118*, 790–797. [CrossRef]
41. Houtchens, M.K.; Edwards, N.C.; Phillips, A.L. Relapses and disease-modifying drug treatment in pregnancy and live birth in US women with MS. *Neurology* **2018**, *91*, e1570–e1578. [CrossRef]
42. Alroughani, R.; Alowayesh, M.S.; Ahmed, S.F.; Behbehani, R.; Al-Hashel, J. Relapse occurrence in women with multiple sclerosis during pregnancy in the new treatment era. *Neurology* **2018**, *90*, e840–e846. [CrossRef]
43. Fragoso, Y.D.; Boggild, M.; Macias-Islas, M.A.; Carra, A.; Schaerer, K.D.; Aguayo, A.; de Almeida, S.M.; Alvarenga, M.P.; Alvarenga, R.M.; Alves-Leon, S.V.; et al. The effects of long-term exposure to disease-modifying drugs during pregnancy in multiple sclerosis. *Clin. Neurol. Neurosurg.* **2013**, *115*, 154–159. [CrossRef]
44. Vukusic, S.; Marignier, R. Multiple sclerosis and pregnancy in the 'treatment era'. *Nat. Rev. Neurol.* **2015**, *11*, 280–289. [CrossRef]
45. Thone, J.; Thiel, S.; Gold, R.; Hellwig, K. Treatment of multiple sclerosis during pregnancy - safety considerations. *Expert Opin. Drug Saf.* **2017**, *16*, 523–534. [CrossRef] [PubMed]
46. Vaughn, C.; Bushra, A.; Kolb, C.; Weinstock-Guttman, B. An Update on the Use of Disease-Modifying Therapy in Pregnant Patients with Multiple Sclerosis. *CNS Drugs* **2018**, *32*, 161–178. [CrossRef] [PubMed]
47. Haghikia, A.; Langer-Gould, A.; Rellensmann, G.; Schneider, H.; Tenenbaum, T.; Elias-Hamp, B.; Menck, S.; Zimmermann, J.; Herbstritt, S.; Marziniak, M.; et al. Natalizumab use during the third trimester of pregnancy. *JAMA Neurol.* **2014**, *71*, 891–895. [CrossRef] [PubMed]
48. Montalban, X.; Gold, R.; Thompson, A.J.; Otero-Romero, S.; Amato, M.P.; Chandraratna, D.; Clanet, M.; Comi, G.; Derfuss, T.; Fazekas, F.; et al. ECTRIMS/EAN guideline on the pharmacological treatment of people with multiple sclerosis. *Eur. J. Neurol.* **2018**, *25*, 215–237. [CrossRef] [PubMed]
49. Kanal, E.; Barkovich, A.J.; Bell, C.; Borgstede, J.P.; Bradley, W.G., Jr.; Froelich, J.W.; Gimbel, J.R.; Gosbee, J.W.; Kuhni-Kaminski, E.; Larson, P.A.; et al. ACR guidance document on MR safe practices: 2013. *J. Magn. Reson. Imaging* **2013**, *37*, 501–530. [CrossRef] [PubMed]
50. Elliott, A.B.; Chakravarty, E.F. Immunosuppressive medications during pregnancy and lactation in women with autoimmune diseases. *Womens Health (Lond.)* **2010**, *6*, 431–442. [CrossRef]
51. Xiao, W.L.; Liu, X.Y.; Liu, Y.S.; Zhang, D.Z.; Xue, L.F. The relationship between maternal corticosteroid use and orofacial clefts-a meta-analysis. *Reprod. Toxicol.* **2017**, *69*, 99–105. [CrossRef]
52. Mueller, B.A.; Zhang, J.; Critchlow, C.W. Birth outcomes and need for hospitalization after delivery among women with multiple sclerosis. *Am. J. Obst. Gynecol.* **2002**, *186*, 446–452. [CrossRef]
53. Kelly, V.M.; Nelson, L.M.; Chakravarty, E.F. Obstetric outcomes in women with multiple sclerosis and epilepsy. *Neurology* **2009**, *73*, 1831–1836. [CrossRef] [PubMed]
54. Fong, A.; Chau, C.T.; Quant, C.; Duffy, J.; Pan, D.; Ogunyemi, D.A. Multiple sclerosis in pregnancy: Prevalence, sociodemographic features, and obstetrical outcomes. *J. Matern Fetal. Neonatal. Med.* **2018**, *31*, 382–387. [CrossRef] [PubMed]

55. MacDonald, S.C.; McElrath, T.F.; Hernandez-Diaz, S. Pregnancy Outcomes in Women With Multiple Sclerosis. *Am. J. Epidemiol.* **2019**, *188*, 57–66. [CrossRef] [PubMed]
56. Update on overall prevalence of major birth defects—Atlanta, Georgia, 1978–2005. *MMWR Morb. Mortal. Wkly. Rep.* **2008**, *57*, 1–5.
57. Voskuhl, R.; Momtazee, C. Pregnancy: Effect on Multiple Sclerosis, Treatment Considerations, and Breastfeeding. *Neurotherapeutics* **2017**, *14*, 974–984. [CrossRef]
58. Coyle, P.K. Multiple sclerosis and pregnancy prescriptions. *Expert Opin. Drug Saf.* **2014**, *13*, 1565–1568. [CrossRef] [PubMed]
59. Brucker, M.C.; King, T.L. The 2015 US Food and Drug Administration Pregnancy and Lactation Labeling Rule. *J. Midwifery Womens Health* **2017**, *62*, 308–316. [CrossRef]
60. Nguyen, A.L.; Havrdova, E.K.; Horakova, D.; Izquierdo, G.; Kalincik, T.; van der Walt, A.; Terzi, M.; Alroughani, R.; Duquette, P.; Girard, M.; et al. Incidence of pregnancy and disease-modifying therapy exposure trends in women with multiple sclerosis: A contemporary cohort study. *Mult. Scler. Relat. Disord.* **2019**, *28*, 235–243. [CrossRef]
61. Thiel, S.; Langer-Gould, A.; Rockhoff, M.; Haghikia, A.; Queisser-Wahrendorf, A.; Gold, R.; Hellwig, K. Interferon-beta exposure during first trimester is safe in women with multiple sclerosis-A prospective cohort study from the German Multiple Sclerosis and Pregnancy Registry. *Mult. Scler.* **2016**, *22*, 801–809. [CrossRef]
62. Coyle, P.K.; Sinclair, S.M.; Scheuerle, A.E.; Thorp, J.M., Jr.; Albano, J.D.; Rametta, M.J. Final results from the Betaseron (interferon beta-1b) Pregnancy Registry: A prospective observational study of birth defects and pregnancy-related adverse events. *BMJ Open* **2014**, *4*, e004536. [CrossRef]
63. Glatiramer Acetate (Glatiramer Acetate Injection) for Subcutaneous Use. Highlights of Prescribing Information. Available online: https://www.copaxone.com/Resources/pdfs/PrescribingInformation.pdf (accessed on 29 January 2019).
64. Herbstritt, S.; Langer-Gould, A.; Rockhoff, M.; Haghikia, A.; Queisser-Wahrendorf, A.; Gold, R.; Hellwig, K. Glatiramer acetate during early pregnancy: A prospective cohort study. *Mult. Scler.* **2016**, *22*, 810–816. [CrossRef]
65. Sandberg-Wollheim, M.; Neudorfer, O.; Grinspan, A.; Weinstock-Guttman, B.; Haas, J.; Izquierdo, G.; Riley, C.; Ross, A.P.; Baruch, P.; Drillman, T.; et al. Pregnancy Outcomes from the Branded Glatiramer Acetate Pregnancy Database. *Int. J. MS Care* **2018**, *20*, 9–14. [CrossRef] [PubMed]
66. Geissbuhler, Y.; Vile, J.; Koren, G.; Guennec, M.; Butzkueven, H.; Tilson, H.; MacDonald, T.M.; Hellwig, K. Evaluation of pregnancy outcomes in patients with multiple sclerosis after fingolimod exposure. *Ther. Adv. Neurol. Disord.* **2018**, *11*, 1756286418804760. [CrossRef] [PubMed]
67. Tecfidera (Dimethyl Fumarate) Delayed-Release Capsules, for Oral Use. Highlights of Prescribing Information. Available online: https://www.tecfidera.com/content/dam/commercial/multiple-sclerosis/tecfidera/pat/en_us/pdf/full-prescribing-info.pdf (accessed on 28 January 2019).
68. Kieseier, B.C.; Benamor, M. Pregnancy outcomes following maternal and paternal exposure to teriflunomide during treatment for relapsing-remitting multiple sclerosis. *Neurol. Ther.* **2014**, *3*, 133–138. [CrossRef] [PubMed]
69. Tysabri (Natalizumab) Injection, for Intravenous Use. Highlights of Prescribing Information. Available online: https://www.tysabri.com/content/dam/commercial/multiple-sclerosis/tysabri/pat/en_us/pdfs/tysabri_prescribing_information.pdf (accessed on 29 January 2019).
70. Ebrahimi, N.; Herbstritt, S.; Gold, R.; Amezcua, L.; Koren, G.; Hellwig, K. Pregnancy and fetal outcomes following natalizumab exposure in pregnancy. A prospective, controlled observational study. *Mult. Scler.* **2015**, *21*, 198–205. [CrossRef]
71. Friend, S.; Richman, S.; Bloomgren, G.; Cristiano, L.M.; Wenten, M. Evaluation of pregnancy outcomes from the Tysabri(R) (natalizumab) pregnancy exposure registry: A global, observational, follow-up study. *BMC Neurol.* **2016**, *16*, 150. [CrossRef] [PubMed]
72. Alroughani, R.; Altintas, A.; Al Jumah, M.; Sahraian, M.; Alsharoqi, I.; AlTahan, A.; Daif, A.; Dahdaleh, M.; Deleu, D.; Fernandez, O.; et al. Pregnancy and the Use of Disease-Modifying Therapies in Patients with Multiple Sclerosis: Benefits versus Risks. *Mult. Scler. Int.* **2016**, *2016*, 1034912. [CrossRef] [PubMed]
73. De Santis, M.; Straface, G.; Cavaliere, A.F.; Rosati, P.; Batocchi, A.P.; Caruso, A. The first case of mitoxantrone exposure in early pregnancy. *Neurotoxicology* **2007**, *28*, 696–697. [CrossRef] [PubMed]

74. Baumgartner, A.K.; Oberhoffer, R.; Jacobs, V.R.; Ostermayer, E.; Menzel, H.; Voigt, M.; Schneider, K.T.; Pildner von Steinburg, S. Reversible foetal cerebral ventriculomegaly and cardiomyopathy under chemotherapy for maternal AML. *Onkologie* **2009**, *32*, 40–43. [CrossRef] [PubMed]
75. Hellwig, K.; Schimrigk, S.; Chan, A.; Epplen, J.; Gold, R. A newborn with Pierre Robin sequence after preconceptional mitoxantrone exposure of a female with multiple sclerosis. *J. Neurol. Sci.* **2011**, *307*, 164–165. [CrossRef] [PubMed]
76. Rituxan (Rituximab) Injection, for Intravenous Use. Highlights of Prescribing Information. Available online: https://www.gene.com/download/pdf/rituxan_prescribing.pdf (accessed on 29 January 2019).
77. Chakravarty, E.F.; Murray, E.R.; Kelman, A.; Farmer, P. Pregnancy outcomes after maternal exposure to rituximab. *Blood* **2011**, *117*, 1499–1506. [CrossRef]
78. Das, G.; Damotte, V.; Gelfand, J.M.; Bevan, C.; Cree, B.A.C.; Do, L.; Green, A.J.; Hauser, S.L.; Bove, R. Rituximab before and during pregnancy: A systematic review, and a case series in MS and NMOSD. *Neurol. Neuroimmunol. Neuroinflamm.* **2018**, *5*, e453. [CrossRef] [PubMed]
79. Lebrun, C.; Le Page, E.; Kantarci, O.; Siva, A.; Pelletier, D.; Okuda, D.T. Impact of pregnancy on conversion to clinically isolated syndrome in a radiologically isolated syndrome cohort. *Mult. Scler.* **2012**, *18*, 1297–1302. [CrossRef]
80. Hughes, S.E.; Spelman, T.; Gray, O.M.; Boz, C.; Trojano, M.; Lugaresi, A.; Izquierdo, G.; Duquette, P.; Girard, M.; Grand'Maison, F.; et al. Predictors and dynamics of postpartum relapses in women with multiple sclerosis. *Mult. Scler.* **2014**, *20*, 739–746. [CrossRef] [PubMed]
81. Section on Breastfeeding. Breastfeeding and the use of human milk. *Pediatrics* **2012**, *129*, e827–e841. [CrossRef] [PubMed]
82. Langer-Gould, A.; Huang, S.M.; Gupta, R.; Leimpeter, A.D.; Greenwood, E.; Albers, K.B.; Van Den Eeden, S.K.; Nelson, L.M. Exclusive breastfeeding and the risk of postpartum relapses in women with multiple sclerosis. *Arch. Neurol.* **2009**, *66*, 958–963. [CrossRef] [PubMed]
83. Hellwig, K.; Rockhoff, M.; Herbstritt, S.; Borisow, N.; Haghikia, A.; Elias-Hamp, B.; Menck, S.; Gold, R.; Langer-Gould, A. Exclusive Breastfeeding and the Effect on Postpartum Multiple Sclerosis Relapses. *JAMA Neurol.* **2015**, *72*, 1132–1138. [CrossRef]
84. Pakpoor, J.; Disanto, G.; Lacey, M.V.; Hellwig, K.; Giovannoni, G.; Ramagopalan, S.V. Breastfeeding and multiple sclerosis relapses: A meta-analysis. *J. Neurol.* **2012**, *259*, 2246–2248. [CrossRef]
85. Howie, P.W.; McNeilly, A.S.; Houston, M.J.; Cook, A.; Boyle, H. Fertility after childbirth: Infant feeding patterns, basal PRL levels and post-partum ovulation. *Clin. Endocrinol (Oxf.)* **1982**, *17*, 315–322. [CrossRef] [PubMed]
86. Langer-Gould, A.; Smith, J.B.; Hellwig, K.; Gonzales, E.; Haraszti, S.; Koebnick, C.; Xiang, A. Breastfeeding, ovulatory years, and risk of multiple sclerosis. *Neurology* **2017**, *89*, 563–569. [CrossRef] [PubMed]
87. de Seze, J.; Chapelotte, M.; Delalande, S.; Ferriby, D.; Stojkovic, T.; Vermersch, P. Intravenous corticosteroids in the postpartum period for reduction of acute exacerbations in multiple sclerosis. *Mult Scler* **2004**, *10*, 596–597. [CrossRef] [PubMed]
88. Ost, L.; Wettrell, G.; Bjorkhem, I.; Rane, A. Prednisolone excretion in human milk. *J. Pediatr.* **1985**, *106*, 1008–1011. [CrossRef]

13

Cortical Excitability Measures May Predict Clinical Response to Fampridine in Patients with Multiple Sclerosis and Gait Impairment

Rechdi Ahdab [1,2,3], Madiha M. Shatila [1,3], Abed Rahman Shatila [4], George Khazen [1,5], Joumana Freiha [1,3], Maher Salem [1,3], Karim Makhoul [1,3], Rody El Nawar [1,3], Shaza El Nemr [1], Samar S. Ayache [6,7] and Naji Riachi [1,3,*]

1 Lebanese American University Gilbert and Rose Mary Chagoury School of Medicine, Byblos P.O. Box 36, Lebanon; chadahdab@gmail.com (R.A.); mado.shatila@gmail.com (M.M.S.); gkhazen@lau.edu.lb (G.K.); joumanafreiha@gmail.com (J.F.); Maher.Salem@lau.edu (M.S.); karim.makhoul@lau.edu (K.M.); roudynawar@hotmail.com (R.E.N.); shaza.el-nemr@hotmail.com (S.E.N.)

2 Hamidy Medical Center, Tripoli 1300, Lebanon

3 Neurology Division, Lebanese American University Medical Center Rizk Hospital, Beirut P.O Box 11-3288, Lebanon

4 Makassed General hospital, Beirut P.O. Box 11-6301, Lebanon; ashatila1@hotmail.com

5 Computer Science and Mathematics Department, Lebanese American University, Byblos P.O. Box 36 , Lebanon

6 Service de Physiologie-Explorations Fonctionnelles, Hôpital Henri Mondor, Assistance Publique—Hôpitaux de Paris, 51 avenue de Lattre de Tassigny, 94010 Créteil, France; samarayache@gmail.com

7 EA 4391, Excitabilité Nerveuse et Thérapeutique, Université Paris-Est-Créteil, 94010 Créteil, France

* Correspondence: naji.riachi@lau.edu.lb

Abstract: *Background:* Most multiple sclerosis (MS) patients will develop walking limitations during the disease. Sustained-release oral fampridine is the only approved drug that will improve gait in a subset of MS patients. *Objectives:* (1) Evaluate fampridine cortical excitability effect in MS patients with gait disability. (2) Investigate whether cortical excitability changes can predict the therapeutic response to fampridine. *Method:* This prospective observational study enrolled 20 adult patients with MS and gait impairment planned to receive fampridine 10 mg twice daily for two consecutive weeks. Exclusion criteria included: Recent relapse (<3 months), modification of disease modifying drugs (<6 months), or Expanded Disability Status Scale (EDSS) score >7. Neurological examination, timed 25-foot walk test (T25wt), EDSS, and cortical excitability studies were performed upon inclusion and 14 days after initiation of fampridine. *Results:* After treatment, the mean improvement of T25wt (ΔT25wt) was 4.9 s. Significant enhancement of intra-cortical facilitation was observed (139% versus 241%, $p = 0.01$) following treatment. A positive correlation was found between baseline resting motor threshold (rMT) and both EDSS ($r = 0.57$; $p < 0.01$) and ΔT25wt ($r = 0.57$, $p = 0.01$). rMT above 52% of the maximal stimulator output was found to be a good predictor of a favorable response to fampridine (accuracy: 75%). *Discussion:* Fampridine was found to have a significant modulatory effect on the cerebral cortex, demonstrated by an increase in excitatory intracortical processes as unveiled by paired-pulse transcranial magnetic stimulation. rMT could be useful in selecting patients likely to experience a favorable response to fampridine.

Keywords: short intracortical inhibition; intracortical facilitation; fampridine; multiple sclerosis; walking disability

1. Introduction

Most patients with multiple sclerosis (MS) will develop walking limitations at some point in the course of the disease [1]. The impact of such limitations on daily activities and quality of life is substantial [2]. Currently, sustained-release oral fampridine is the only approved drug for the symptomatic treatment of walking disability due to MS. Fampridine (4-aminopyridine) is a voltage-dependent potassium channel-blocker that restores action potential conduction in poorly myelinated central nerve fibers, with a positive impact on synaptic transmission and neuronal excitability [3,4]. Unfortunately, only a subset of patients with MS and walking disabilities are responders to fampridine [5]. Limited data suggest that more advanced walking disability [6,7] and prolonged central conduction times [6,8] are predictive of a favorable response to treatment. The predictive value of more advanced measurements of cortical dysfunction have not been studied.

Changes in cortical excitability are frequent in MS, especially in more advanced stages of the disease [9–12]. Such changes are influenced by several factors, including the clinical form, stage of the disease, and degree of disability. It has been suggested that some excitability parameters correlate with the level of disability. This concerns more particularly the short-interval intracortical inhibition (SICI), intracortical facilitation (ICF), and resting motor threshold (rMT) [9–12].

This study was designed to evaluate the effect of slow-release fampridine on cortical excitability in patients with MS and gait disabilities. In addition, we set out to investigate whether cortical excitability changes could serve as predictors of therapeutic response to fampridine.

2. Materials and Methods

2.1. *Study Design*

This prospective observational study included adult patients with MS and gait impairment. All patients planned to receive fampridine in the period between April 2016 and August 2017 were asked if they were willing to participate in the study. If so, the protocol was thoroughly explained and written informed consent was obtained. The study was approved by our institutional review board.

2.2. *Subjects*

Eligible patients were adults (aged 18 and above) with a definite diagnosis of MS according to the 2010 McDonald criteria [13]. All patients had gait disturbance and were planned to receive a 2-week fampridine trial to assess the clinical impact of the drug on walking speed. This is an essential step needed to secure approval for the treatment from third party payers in our country. Patients were required to have recordable motor evoked potentials (MEPs) in at least one hand. Those with a recent relapse (<3 months), a recent modification of disease modifying drugs (prior 6 months), or an EDSS above 7 were excluded. Patients with contraindication to fampridine (seizures, pregnancy, breastfeeding, and renal impairment) or transcranial magnetic stimulation (TMS) (seizure, pacemaker, or ferromagnetic material in the head area) were also excluded. Eligible patients received oral fampridine 10 mg twice daily for two consecutive weeks.

2.3. *Clinical and Neurophysiological Assessments*

Assessments were performed at baseline (T0) and 14 days after the commencement of fampridine (T1). The physicians performing the clinical assessment were blinded to the cortical excitability results and vice versa.

Clinical assessment was performed by N.R., S.E.N. and M.M.S.. At baseline (T0), a detailed medical history was obtained with particular emphasis on key MS related elements: Onset and type of MS, number and dates of clinical relapses, prior disease modifying drugs, comorbidities, and current medications. At the follow-up visit (T1), the interview was focused on drug side effects and subjective improvement. Particular attention was paid to the occurrence of any new symptom or any worsening of a pre-existing deficit that could be indicative of a new relapse. A thorough neurological examination and an assessment of disability status using the Kurtzke Expanded Disability Status Scale (EDSS) were done at baseline (T0) [14]. Cortical excitability assessment and a timed 25-foot walk test (T25wt) [15] were done during both visits (T0 and T1).

Decrease in T25wt was calculated as follows: ΔT25wt = T25wt at T0 − T25wt at T1. Then, the percentage of improvement was calculated as follows: % of improvement = $\frac{\Delta T25wt}{T25wtatT0} \times 100$.

Patients who showed a percentage of improvement greater than 20% were considered responders. This threshold was based on the finding that a 20% improvement in walking time is considered clinically meaningful for patients with MS [16].

Cortical excitability studies were performed by R.A. and included the resting motor threshold (rMT), short-interval cortical inhibition (SICI), intracortical facilitation (ICF), and cortical silent period (CSP). MEPs were recorded from the first dorsal interosseous muscle (FDI) using pre-gelled disposable surface electrodes in a tendon-belly montage (ref 019-400400, Natus, Pleasanton, CA, USA). Recording was done on the side affected least by MS or on the left side if both sides were normal or equally affected.

MEPs were filtered (20 Hz to 2 KHz), amplified, and stored for off-line analyses (Nicolet EDX, Natus, Pleasanton, CA, USA). Patients were seated in a comfortable chair with the arms at rest. Baseline muscle activity was continuously monitored to ascertain complete muscle relaxation (except for CSP measurement). A tight-fitting cap was placed on the patient's head to help mark the coil position. Magnetic stimulation was delivered using an eight-shaped coil with an inner diameter of 70 mm (M200^2 D70 double coil 3190-00, Magstim Co, Carmarthenshire, U.K.) placed tangentially to the scalp (handle pointing backwards) and connected to a Magstim Bistim^2 stimulator (Magstim Co, Carmarthenshire, U.K.).

The motor hot spot was determined by scanning the scalp for the coil position associated with the largest MEPs. This position was marked on the cap and used for all subsequent excitability measurements. It was determined in a fully relaxed FDI muscle and defined as the lowest stimulus intensity required to produce MEPs larger than 50 μV (peak-to-peak) in 5 out of 10 consecutive trials [17].

A paired stimulus paradigm was used to test SICI using interstimulus intervals (ISIs) of 2 and 4 ms (SICI2 and SICI4 respectively) [18]. ICF was tested using ISIs of 10 and 15 (ICF10 and ICF15, respectively) [18]. The conditioning stimulus was delivered at 80% of rMT and the test stimulus was delivered at 120% of rMT. Eight trials were performed for each condition. The average of eight trials of unconditioned TMS pulses delivered at 120% of rMT was used as control. The amplitudes of conditioned MEPs were expressed as the percentage of the mean unconditioned MEP amplitude. The mean degree of inhibition and facilitation from all tested ISIs were retained for analysis.

CSP was defined as the duration of electromyogram (EMG) activity interruption following a single TMS pulse delivered at 140% of the rMT. The degree of FDI activation was controlled by visual feedback. Five trials were performed and averaged. The minimal CSP duration was measured from the end of the MEP until the first reoccurrence of EMG activity on highly magnified traces [19].

This study was sponsored by an investigator-initiated trial grant from Biogen, who reviewed the protocol. Biogen did not participate in patient recruitment or study implementation, had no access to the data, and did not participate in the statistical analysis.

2.4. *Statistical Analysis*

The analysis was conducted using the R statistical program 3.5.3 (R Foundation for statistical computing, Vienna, Austria). Descriptive statistics are presented as mean ± standard deviation (SD) and median (interquartile range) for continuous variables.

The Wilcoxon rank sum paired test was used to assess changes in cortical excitability parameters (comparison between measurements at T0 and T1), and Pearson correlation coefficient was used to analyze the relationship between ΔT25wt and baseline cortical excitability measures (rMT, MEPs amplitude, SICI, ICF, CSP) and between ΔT25wt and EDSS scores. The relationship between EDSS and baseline excitability measures was also examined. A p-value <0.05 was considered significant.

A classification model using the C5.0 decision tree algorithm (Quinlan R (1993). C4.5: Programs for Machine Learning. Morgan Kaufmann Publishers [20] was used to classify the samples as fampridine responders and non-responders based on their rMT value. As stated previously, patients were considered responders if they had at least a 20% reduction in their T25wt at the follow-up visit (T1), and non-responders otherwise. A simple model was built using the formula "responder status ~ rMT" while keeping the default values for all the remaining parameters in the model. The C5.0 decision tree algorithm relies on the maximum information gain to identify the rMT cutoff value that best splits the samples as responders and non-responders to estimate a threshold value that discriminates between fampridine responders and non-responders. The model was built using the C5.0 from the C50 package in R.

3. Results

3.1. Clinical and Sociodemographic Data

A total of 20 patients (11 male) completed the study (Table 1). They had a mean age of 49.75 ± 11.36 (median interquartile range (IQR): 50.00 (18.00); overall range: 25–65) years. Thirteen had relapsing remitting, 6 had secondary progressive, and one had primary progressive MS. Mean disease duration was 13.75 ± 8.17 years (median (IQR): 12.50 [10]; overall range: 3–39). Their mean EDSS score was 4.70 ± 1.31 (median (IQR): 4.00 (1.88); overall range 2.5–7). Nineteen patients were on disease modifying treatment: 3 on interferon beta 1a, 12 on fingolimod, 3 on natalizumab, and 1 on dimethyl fumarate.

Table 1. Baseline characteristics of subjects.

Subjects	Age	Sex	Disease Duration	EDSS	MS Type	Present Medication
1	53	F	7 years	5	RRMS	Fingolimod
2	46	M	11 years	4	SPMS	Fingolimod
3	25	M	5 years	4	RRMS	Fingolimod
4	49	F	10 years	7	RRMS	Natalizumab
5	62	M	18 years	5	RRMS	Fingolimod
6	62	F	22 years	5.5	SPMS	Interferon β 1a
7	42	F	17 years	4	SPMS	Natalizumab
8	47	F	8 years	5.5	RRMS	Fingolimod
9	58	M	19 years	4	SPMS	Fingolimod
10	58	F	12 years	7	SPMS	Fingolimod
11	62	M	11 years	4	PPMS	None
12	51	F	13 years	6	SPMS	Dimethyl Fumarate
13	65	M	18 years	6	RRMS	Fingolimod
14	50	F	18 years	6.5	RRMS	Fingolimod
15	35	M	3 years	3.5	RRMS	Fingolimod
16	32	M	3 years	3	RRMS	Natalizumab
17	50	M	18 years	4	RRMS	Interferon β 1a
18	64	M	39 years	3.5	RRMS	Interferon β 1a
19	36	M	15 years	4	RRMS	Fingolimod
20	48	F	8 years	2.5	RRMS	Fingolimod

EDSS: Expanded Disability Status Scale; F: female; M: male; MS, Multiple sclerosis; PPMS: Primary progressive multiple sclerosis; RRMS: Relapsing remitting multiple sclerosis; SPMS: Secondary progressive multiple sclerosis.

3.2. Clinical Response to Fampridine

Significant improvement in T25wt was found following fampridine (21.5 ± 5.1 versus 16.64 ± 1.40 , $p < 0.001$). Mean ΔT25wt was 4.86 ± (range 0.04–17.62) seconds (s). Eleven patients (55%) were responders to fampridine, as defined previously.

The treatment was well tolerated, and no serious adverse effects were reported. Thirteen patients (65%) reported minor side effects, mostly nausea, abdominal pain, lumbar/cervical pain, and dizziness. There were no instances of patient withdrawal owing to treatment side effects.

3.3. *Effects of Fampridine on Cortical Excitability Measures*

As depicted in Table 2, the follow-up visit (T1) showed a statistically significant enhancement of ICF15 (139.17 ± 110.98% versus 241.69 ± 131.46%, $p = 0.01$). ICF10 also tended to increase, but this effect did not reach statistical significance (161.58 ± 154.12% versus 242.94 ± 125.79%, $p = 0.06$) (Table 2). No significant changes were observed for the rMT (60.95 ± 12.47% versus 62.45 ± 15.20%, $p = 0.81$), SICI2 (53.08 ± 68.24% versus 73.62 ± 69.95%, $p = 0.11$), SICI4 (88.18 ± 107.10% versus 121.51 ± 88.48%, $p = 0.15$), or CSP (132.15 ± 55.67 ms versus 138.60 ± 51.90 ms, $p = 0.92$).

Table 2. Observed measures of excitability parameters and timed 25-foot walk test (T25wt) at baseline in seconds (s) and after fampridine treatment.

Parameter	Baseline Mean ± SD Median (IQR)	After Fampridine Mean ± SD Median (IQR)	Wilcoxon Paired-Test *p*-Value
rMT	60.95 ± 12.47 57.50 (19.75)	62.45 ± 15.20 58.50 (30.50)	0.81
SICI2	53.08 ± 68.24 31.95 (53.22)	73.62 ± 69.95 50.00 (70.94)	0.11
SICI4	88.18 ± 107.10 47.05 (52.77)	121.51 ± 88.48 107.90 (150.17)	0.15
ICF10	161.58 ± 154.12 134.61 (172.06)	242.94 ± 125.79 217.67 (210.46)	0.06
ICF15	139.17 ± 110.98 114.75 (139.63)	241.69 ± 131.46 235.00 (182.49)	**0.01**
CSP	132.15 ± 55.67 119.00 (54.25)	138.60 ± 51.90 147.50 (71.25)	0.92
T25wt	21.5 ± 5.1	16.64 ± 1.40	**<0.001**

The short intracortical inhibition at interstimulus intervals (ISIs) of 2 and 4 ms (SICI2, SICI4), intracortical facilitation at ISIs of 10 and 15 ms (ICF10, ICF15) are expressed as the percentage of the unconditioned motor evoked potential (MEP) amplitude. The cortical silent period (CSP) is expressed in ms. The resting motor threshold (rMT) is expressed as percentage of the maximal stimulator output. *p*-values in bold reflect significant difference ($p < 0.05$). IQR, interquartile range.

3.4. *Relationship Between EDSS and Baseline Excitability Measures*

At baseline (T0), a positive correlation was found between EDSS and rMT ($r = 0.57$; $p < 0.01$) (Table 3). Conversely, no statistically significant correlation was found between EDSS and any of the other cortical excitability measures.

Table 3. Correlation between the Expanded Disability Status Scale (EDSS) and baseline measures of resting motor threshold (rMT), short-interval intracortical inhibition at interstimulus intervals (ISIs) of 2 and 4 ms (SICI2 and SICI4, respectively), intracortical facilitation at ISIs of 10 and 15 (ICF10 and ICF15, respectively), cortical silent period (CSP), and timed 25-foot walking test (T25wt).

	Variables	Correlation	*p*-Value
EDSS	rMT	0.57	<0.01
	SICI2	−0.24	0.30
	SICI4	−0.27	0.24
	ICF10	−0.18	0.42
	ICF15	0.007	0.97
	CSP	−0.08	0.71
	ΔT25wt	0.75	<0.01

3.5. Relationships Between Improvement of T25wt (ΔT25wt) and Each of EDSS and Baseline Cortical Excitability Measures

A statistically significant positive correlation was found between baseline rMT and improvement of walking speed at the follow-up visit ($r = 0.57$, $p = 0.01$). No correlation was found between ΔT25wt and other baseline excitability parameters.

A positive correlation was also found between ΔT25wt and EDSS. ($r = 0.75$; $p < 0.01$) (Table 3).

3.6. Predictors of a Favorable Response to Fampridine

The predictive value of baseline rMT in terms of response to fampridine was studied. The threshold to predict good response to fampridine was found to be 52 (with 14 patients with rMT above 52 were found to be good responders to the treatment). Mean ± SD of rMT in responder and non-responder groups were 64.10 ± 11.99 and 57.11 ± 12.62, respectively. The classification of responders and non-responders had an accuracy of 75% (specificity: 83.3% (5/6) and sensitivity 71.4% (10/14)).

4. Discussion

Three interesting findings emerged from our study. First, higher rMT at baseline was predictive of a favorable response to fampridine, translating clinically into improved gait speed. Conversely, the other excitability parameters were not found to have any predictive value. From a clinical standpoint, patients with higher EDSS showed enhanced drug effects compared to those with lower EDSS. At a more mechanistic level, fampridine was found to induce a significant increase in intracortical excitatory mechanisms as revealed by paired-pulse TMS, with no significant effect on the other excitability parameters.

The positive impact of fampridine on gait speed is now well established, but only 40% of patients are expected to experience a clinically meaningful improvement [15,21]. Proper selection of patients most likely to experience clinical benefits from fampridine has been the subject of rare dedicated studies [6–8]. It has been suggested that patients with more disability at baseline have the best outcome. This seems logical, since advanced ambulatory impairment in MS is associated with a higher amount of axonal demyelination within the neural locomotor networks, providing more targets for fampridine to reinforce gait function [6,8]. Filli and collaborates tested the predictive value of a set of demographic and clinical criteria including T25wt, walking endurance 6-min walk test (6MWT), and the 12-item multiple sclerosis walking scale (MSWS-12) [7]. Their findings suggest that walking function at baseline (6MWT and T25wt) accurately predicts the responder status. EDSS only weakly correlated with the outcome. In this study, reduced walking endurance as measured by the 6MWT was the best predictor of a good outcome with an accuracy of 80% [7]. In comparison, we found that EDSS correlated with improvement in T25wt; however, we did not test walking endurance, since we included patients with advanced gait impairment who were unable to complete the 6MWT.

At the physiological level, high rMT was found to be correlated with high EDSS score, and seemed to be a good predictor of outcome. rMT is a global measurement of excitability and membrane properties of cortical pyramidal cells [22,23]. It can be regarded as the electrophysiological signature of clinical impairment in MS patients. Higher rMT was found to correlate with clinical relapses [24], disease progression [25], secondary progressive disease [10,26], and the presence of fatigue [11]. Another neurophysiological measure of potential predictive value is prolonged motor central conduction [6,8]. The latter parameter was not evaluated in our study.

Studies of cortical excitability, a surrogate measure of ion channel and synaptic functions, have repeatedly shown significant excitability changes in patients with MS [10–12]. In the earlier stages of relapsing remitting MS, this state of altered excitability can be improved by immunomodulatory therapy [27]. As the disease progresses and the degenerative process takes place, excitability changes could become permanent [10,26]. At this stage, drugs having a more direct effect on cortical excitability are more likely to reverse these changes than those with immunomodulatory effects. Our study clearly demonstrates a cortico-modulatory effect of fampridine, a rather predictable finding given its putative mechanism of action. Cortical excitability measures are dependent on networks of interneurons (both excitatory and inhibitory) and their synaptic interaction with each other. SICI reflects the recruitment of inhibitory pathways with GABAergic mediation (GABA-A receptors) and ICF reflects the recruitment of excitatory pathways with glutamatergic mediation. Healthy excitatory and inhibitory systems are essential for proper functioning of brain circuits. Fampridine was found to increase ICF in our study but had no impact on the other excitability parameters. Such findings would indicate an increase in facilitatory intracortical mechanisms aiming to improve the clinical outcomes, as reflected by an increase in walking speed [28,29].

Our study has many shortcomings, including an open label design, small sample size, and short follow-up period. Another shortcoming is that cortical excitability changes were correlated to changes in walking speed, but not other cortical functions. Since cortical excitability studies are classically measured in the hand, correlations with hand function (i.e., nine-hole pegboard test) would have been more appropriate, especially as fampridine has been shown to have a positive impact on hand function [30]. Alternatively, we could have chosen a lower extremity muscle (rather than the FDI) to measure lower extremity cortical excitability. This choice of the FDI was based on the many challenges associated with measuring cortical excitability in lower extremities, such as the deeper location of the lower extremity motor areas (making them significantly more difficult to activate), the difficulty of targeting individual lower extremity muscles, and the paucity of studies investigating the reliability and reproducibility of lower extremity excitability studies. Yet another limitation is the short follow-up period, which was limited to 2 weeks. It has been demonstrated that walking speed can continue to improve up to 4 weeks after fampridine initiation [15,21]. As such, a longer period of assessment might have been required to more reliably define the responder status. These shortcomings were inevitable, given the observational nature of the study. Indeed, the inclusion criteria and follow-up period were dictated by our national guidelines for selecting candidates for fampridine therapy. As such, inclusion was restricted to patients with gait impairment, most of which had little or no baseline abnormalities in the hands, and the follow-up period was limited to 2 weeks. Our study could also be criticized for including 10 patients on fingolimod, which was found to reduce ICF [4]. Since no changes in disease modifying and symptomatic treatments were allowed during the period extending from 6 months prior to inclusion to the end of the follow-up, this drug would have mostly affected the baseline recordings rather than the changes observed after fampridine administration. Patients receiving high-dose intravenous steroids, on the other hand, were excluded from the study, given its significant impact on cortical excitability (reduction of SICI and enhancement ICF) [9]. Lastly, it is important to mention the limitations of EDSS as a disability measure in MS. The latter has well documented weaknesses in reliability and sensitivity to change [31].

5. Conclusions

In conclusion, our work suggests that fampridine has a significant modulatory effect on the cerebral cortex, demonstrated by an increase in excitatory intracortical mechanisms as unraveled by paired-pulse TMS paradigms. rMT could be useful in selecting patients more likely to experience a favorable response to fampridine. Larger studies with more reliable outcomes (i.e., hand function) are needed to better define the cortical excitability parameters that best discriminate between potential responders and non-responders.

Author Contributions: Conceptualization, R.A., S.S.A. and N.R.; Formal analysis, G.K.; Investigation, R.A., M.M.S., A.R.S., J.F., M.S., K.M., R.E.N., S.E.N. and N.R.; Methodology, R.A., S.S.A. and N.R.; Writing—original draft, R.A., M.M.S., A.R.S., G.K., J.F., M.S., K.M., R.E.N., S.E.N., S.S.A. and N.R.; Writing—review & editing, R.A. and N.R.

Acknowledgments: This study was supported by an investigator-initiated grant from Biogen.

References

1. Bethoux, F.; Bennett, S. Evaluating walking in patients with multiple sclerosis: Which assessment tools are useful in clinical practice? *Int. J. MS Care* **2011**, *13*, 4–14. [CrossRef]
2. Heesen, C.; Bohm, J.; Reich, C.; Kasper, J.; Goebel, M.; Gold, S.M. Patient perception of bodily functions in multiple sclerosis: Gait and visual function are the most valuable. *Mult. Scler.* **2008**, *14*, 988–991. [CrossRef]
3. Kaji, R.; Sumner, A.J. Effects of 4-aminopyridine in experimental CNS demyelination. *Neurology* **1988**, *38*, 1884–1887. [CrossRef]
4. Mainero, C.; Inghilleri, M.; Pantano, P.; Conte, A.; Lenzi, D.; Frasca, V.; Bozzao, L.; Pozzilli, C. Enhanced brain motor activity in patients with MS after a single dose of 3,4-diaminopyridine. *Neurology* **2004**, *62*, 2044–2050. [CrossRef]
5. Pikoulas, T.E.; Fuller, M.A. Dalfampridine: A medication to improve walking in patients with multiple sclerosis. *Ann. Pharmacother.* **2012**, *46*, 1010–1015. [CrossRef] [PubMed]
6. Brambilla, L.; Rossi Sebastiano, D.; Aquino, D.; Torri Clerici, V.; Brenna, G.; Moscatelli, M.; Frangiamore, R.; Giovannetti, A.M.; Antozzi, C.; Mantegazza, R.; et al. Early effect of dalfampridine in patients with MS: A multi-instrumental approach to better investigate responsiveness. *J. Neurol. Sci.* **2016**, *368*, 402–407. [CrossRef] [PubMed]
7. Filli, L.; Werner, J.; Beyer, G.; Reuter, K.; Petersen, J.A.; Weller, M.; Zorner, B.; Linnebank, M. Predicting responsiveness to fampridine in gait-impaired patients with multiple sclerosis. *Eur. J. Neurol.* **2019**, *26*(2), 281–289. [CrossRef] [PubMed]
8. Zeller, D.; Reiners, K.; Brauninger, S.; Buttmann, M. Central motor conduction time may predict response to fampridine in patients with multiple sclerosis. *J. Neurol. Neurosurg. Psychiatry* **2014**, *85*, 707–709. [CrossRef] [PubMed]
9. Ayache, S.S.; Creange, A.; Farhat, W.H.; Zouari, H.G.; Mylius, V.; Ahdab, R.; Abdellaoui, M.; Lefaucheur, J.P. Relapses in multiple sclerosis: Effects of high-dose steroids on cortical excitability. *Eur. J. Neurol.* **2014**, *21*, 630–636. [CrossRef]
10. Conte, A.; Lenzi, D.; Frasca, V.; Gilio, F.; Giacomelli, E.; Gabriele, M.; Bettolo, C.M.; Iacovelli, E.; Pantano, P.; Pozzilli, C.; et al. Intracortical excitability in patients with relapsing-remitting and secondary progressive multiple sclerosis. *J. Neurol.* **2009**, *256*, 933–938. [CrossRef]
11. Liepert, J.; Mingers, D.; Heesen, C.; Baumer, T.; Weiller, C. Motor cortex excitability and fatigue in multiple sclerosis: A transcranial magnetic stimulation study. *Mult. Scler.* **2005**, *11*, 316–321. [CrossRef] [PubMed]
12. Rossi, S.; Furlan, R.; De Chiara, V.; Motta, C.; Studer, V.; Mori, F.; Musella, A.; Bergami, A.; Muzio, L.; Bernardi, G.; et al. Interleukin-1beta causes synaptic hyperexcitability in multiple sclerosis. *Ann. Neurol.* **2012**, *71*, 76–83. [CrossRef] [PubMed]
13. Polman, C.H.; Reingold, S.C.; Banwell, B.; Clanet, M.; Cohen, J.A.; Filippi, M.; Fujihara, K.; Havrdova, E.; Hutchinson, M.; Kappos, L.; et al. Diagnostic criteria for multiple sclerosis: 2010 revisions to the McDonald criteria. *Ann. Neurol.* **2011**, *69*, 292–302. [CrossRef] [PubMed]
14. Kurtzke, J.F. Rating neurologic impairment in multiple sclerosis: An expanded disability status scale (EDSS). *Neurology* **1983**, *33*, 1444–1452. [CrossRef] [PubMed]
15. Goodman, A.D.; Brown, T.R.; Krupp, L.B.; Schapiro, R.T.; Schwid, S.R.; Cohen, R.; Marinucci, L.N.; Blight, A.R. Sustained-release oral fampridine in multiple sclerosis: A randomised, double-blind, controlled trial. *Lancet* **2009**, *373*, 732–738. [CrossRef]
16. Hobart, J.; Blight, A.R.; Goodman, A.; Lynn, F.; Putzki, N. Timed 25-foot walk: Direct evidence that improving 20% or greater is clinically meaningful in MS. *Neurology* **2013**, *80*, 1509–1517. [CrossRef]
17. Rossini, P.M.; Barker, A.T.; Berardelli, A.; Caramia, M.D.; Caruso, G.; Cracco, R.Q.; Dimitrijevic, M.R.; Hallett, M.; Katayama, Y.; Lucking, C.H.; et al. Non-invasive electrical and magnetic stimulation of the brain, spinal cord and roots: Basic principles and procedures for routine clinical application. Report of an IFCN committee. *Electroencephalogr. Clin. Neurophysiol.* **1994**, *91*, 79–92. [CrossRef]
18. Kujirai, T.; Caramia, M.D.; Rothwell, J.C.; Day, B.L.; Thompson, P.D.; Ferbert, A.; Wroe, S.; Asselman, P.; Marsden, C.D. Corticocortical inhibition in human motor cortex. *J. Physiol.* **1993**, *471*, 501–519. [CrossRef]
19. Lefaucheur, J.P.; Drouot, X.; Menard-Lefaucheur, I.; Keravel, Y.; Nguyen, J.P. Motor cortex rTMS restores defective intracortical inhibition in chronic neuropathic pain. *Neurology* **2006**, *67*, 1568–1574. [CrossRef]

20. Quinlan, J.R. *C4.5: programs for machine learning*; Morgan Kaufmann Publishers Inc.: San Francisco, CA, USA, 1993.
21. Goodman, A.D.; Brown, T.R.; Edwards, K.R.; Krupp, L.B.; Schapiro, R.T.; Cohen, R.; Marinucci, L.N.; Blight, A.R. A phase 3 trial of extended release oral dalfampridine in multiple sclerosis. *Ann. Neurol.* **2010**, *68*, 494–502. [CrossRef]
22. Chen, R.; Samii, A.; Canos, M.; Wassermann, E.M.; Hallett, M. Effects of phenytoin on cortical excitability in humans. *Neurology* **1997**, *49*, 881–883. [CrossRef] [PubMed]
23. Ziemann, U.; Lonnecker, S.; Steinhoff, B.J.; Paulus, W. Effects of antiepileptic drugs on motor cortex excitability in humans: A transcranial magnetic stimulation study. *Ann. Neurol.* **1996**, *40*, 367–378. [CrossRef] [PubMed]
24. Caramia, M.D.; Palmieri, M.G.; Desiato, M.T.; Boffa, L.; Galizia, P.; Rossini, P.M.; Centonze, D.; Bernardi, G. Brain excitability changes in the relapsing and remitting phases of multiple sclerosis: A study with transcranial magnetic stimulation. *Clin. Neurophysiol. Off. J. Int. Fed. Clin. Neurophysiol.* **2004**, *115*, 956–965. [CrossRef] [PubMed]
25. Ayache, S.S.; Créange, A.; Farhat, W.H.; Zouari, H.G.; Lesage, C.; Palm, U.; Abdellaoui, M.; Lefaucheur, J.P. Cortical excitability changes over time in progressive multiple sclerosis. *Funct. Neurol.* **2015**, *30*, 257–263. [CrossRef]
26. Vucic, S.; Burke, T.; Lenton, K.; Ramanathan, S.; Gomes, L.; Yannikas, C.; Kiernan, M.C. Cortical dysfunction underlies disability in multiple sclerosis. *Mult. Scler.* **2012**, *18*, 425–432. [CrossRef]
27. Mori, F.; Kusayanagi, H.; Buttari, F.; Centini, B.; Monteleone, F.; Nicoletti, C.G.; Bernardi, G.; Di Cantogno, E.V.; Marciani, M.G.; Centonze, D. Early treatment with high-dose interferon beta-1a reverses cognitive and cortical plasticity deficits in multiple sclerosis. *Funct. Neurol.* **2012**, *27*, 163–168.
28. Ayache, S.S.; Chalah, M.A. Cortical excitability changes: A mirror to the natural history of multiple sclerosis? *Neurophysiolie Clin.* **2017**, *47*, 221–223. [CrossRef]
29. Savin, Z.; Lejbkowicz, I.; Glass-Marmor, L.; Lavi, I.; Rosenblum, S.; Miller, A. Effect of Fampridine-PR (prolonged released 4-aminopyridine) on the manual functions of patients with Multiple Sclerosis. *J. Neurol. Sci.* **2016**, *360*, 102–109. [CrossRef]
30. Rizzo, V.; Quartarone, A.; Bagnato, S.; Battaglia, F.; Majorana, G.; Girlanda, P. Modification of cortical excitability induced by gabapentin: A study by transcranial magnetic stimulation. *Neurol. Sci.* **2001**, *22*, 229–232. [CrossRef]
31. Meyer-Moock, S.; Feng, Y.S.; Maeurer, M.; Dippel, F.W.; Kohlmann, T. Systematic literature review and validity evaluation of the Expanded Disability Status Scale (EDSS) and the Multiple Sclerosis Functional Composite (MSFC) in patients with multiple sclerosis. *BMC Neurol.* **2014**, *14*, 58. [CrossRef]

Permissions

All chapters in this book were first published by MDPI; hereby published with permission under the Creative Commons Attribution License or equivalent. Every chapter published in this book has been scrutinized by our experts. Their significance has been extensively debated. The topics covered herein carry significant findings which will fuel the growth of the discipline. They may even be implemented as practical applications or may be referred to as a beginning point for another development.

The contributors of this book come from diverse backgrounds, making this book a truly international effort. This book will bring forth new frontiers with its revolutionizing research information and detailed analysis of the nascent developments around the world.

We would like to thank all the contributing authors for lending their expertise to make the book truly unique. They have played a crucial role in the development of this book. Without their invaluable contributions this book wouldn't have been possible. They have made vital efforts to compile up to date information on the varied aspects of this subject to make this book a valuable addition to the collection of many professionals and students.

This book was conceptualized with the vision of imparting up-to-date information and advanced data in this field. To ensure the same, a matchless editorial board was set up. Every individual on the board went through rigorous rounds of assessment to prove their worth. After which they invested a large part of their time researching and compiling the most relevant data for our readers.

The editorial board has been involved in producing this book since its inception. They have spent rigorous hours researching and exploring the diverse topics which have resulted in the successful publishing of this book. They have passed on their knowledge of decades through this book. To expedite this challenging task, the publisher supported the team at every step. A small team of assistant editors was also appointed to further simplify the editing procedure and attain best results for the readers.

Apart from the editorial board, the designing team has also invested a significant amount of their time in understanding the subject and creating the most relevant covers. They scrutinized every image to scout for the most suitable representation of the subject and create an appropriate cover for the book.

The publishing team has been an ardent support to the editorial, designing and production team. Their endless efforts to recruit the best for this project, has resulted in the accomplishment of this book. They are a veteran in the field of academics and their pool of knowledge is as vast as their experience in printing. Their expertise and guidance has proved useful at every step. Their uncompromising quality standards have made this book an exceptional effort. Their encouragement from time to time has been an inspiration for everyone.

The publisher and the editorial board hope that this book will prove to be a valuable piece of knowledge for researchers, students, practitioners and scholars across the globe.

List of Contributors

Marco Castellaro, Agnese Tamanti, Anna Isabella Pisani and Francesco Crescenzo
Department of Neurosciences, Biomedicine and Movement Sciences, University of Verona, 37134 Verona, Italy

Francesca Benedetta Pizzini
Department of Diagnostics and Public Health, University of Verona, 37134 Verona, Italy

Elien Wouters, Elien Grajchen, Winde Jorissen, Tess Dierckx, Melanie Loix, Marie Paule Tulleners, Piet Stinissen, Mansour Haidar, Jeroen F.J. Bogie and Jerome J.A. Hendriks
Department of Immunology and Infection, Biomedical Research Institute, Hasselt University, 3590 Diepenbeek, Belgium

Suzan Wetzels
Department of Pathology, CARIM, Maastricht University Medical Center, 6229 HX Maastricht, The Netherlands

Bart Staels
University of Lille, Inserm, CHU Lille, Institut Pasteur de Lille, U1011-EGID, F-59000 Lille, France

Miguel Ángel Macías Islas
Department of Neurosciences, CUCS, University of Guadalajara and Mexico, Guadalajara 44160, Mexico

Ethel Ciampi
Neurology, Pontificia Universidad Católica de Chile, Neurology, Hospital Dr. Sótero del Río, Santiago 8320000, Chile

Rodolfo Thome, Alexandra Boehm, Larissa Lumi Watanabe Ishikawa, Giacomo Casella, Jaqueline Munhoz, Bogoljub Ciric, Guang-Xian Zhang and Abdolmohamad Rostami
Department of Neurology, Thomas Jefferson University, Philadelphia, PA 19107, USA

Francesca Nuti, Feliciana Real Fernandez, Barbara Mulinacci, Ilaria Paolini, Margherita Di Pisa and Caterina Tiberi
Interdepartmental Research Unit of Peptide and Protein Chemistry and Biology, Department of Chemistry "Ugo Schiff", University of Florence, Via della Lastruccia 13, 50019 Sesto Fiorentino, Italy

Giuseppina Sabatino
Interdepartmental Research Unit of Peptide and Protein Chemistry and Biology, Department of Chemistry "Ugo Schiff", University of Florence, Via della Lastruccia 13, 50019 Sesto Fiorentino, Italy
CNR-IC Istituto di Cristallografia, Via Paolo Gaifami 18, 95126 Catania, Italy

Elisa Peroni
Interdepartmental Research Unit of Peptide and Protein Chemistry and Biology, Department of Chemistry "Ugo Schiff", University of Florence, Via della Lastruccia 13, 50019 Sesto Fiorentino, Italy
UMR 8076 CNRS-BioCIS Team of Chemical Biology and PeptLab@UCP Platform of Peptide and Protein Chemistry and Biology, Neuville Campus, CY Cergy Paris Université, 5 mail Gay-Lussac, 95031 Cergy-Pontoise CEDEX, France

Francesco Lolli
Department of Clinical and Experimental Biomedical Sciences "Mario Serio" and Careggi University Hospital, University of Florence, Largo Brambilla 3, 50134 Florence, Italy

Paolo Rovero
CNR-IC Istituto di Cristallografia, Via Paolo Gaifami 18, 95126 Catania, Italy
Interdepartmental Research Unit of Peptide and Protein Chemistry and Biology, Department of Neurosciences, Psychology, Drug Research and Child Health–Section of Pharmaceutical Sciences and Nutraceutics, University of Florence, Via Ugo Schiff 6, 50019 Sesto Fiorentino, Italy

Anna Maria Papini
Interdepartmental Research Unit of Peptide and Protein Chemistry and Biology, Department of Chemistry "Ugo Schiff", University of Florence, Via della Lastruccia 13, 50019 Sesto Fiorentino, Italy
CNR-IC Istituto di Cristallografia, Via Paolo Gaifami 18, 95126 Catania, Italy
UMR 8076 CNRS-BioCIS Team of Chemical Biology and PeptLab@UCP Platform of Peptide and Protein Chemistry and Biology, Neuville Campus, CY Cergy Paris Université, 5 mail Gay-Lussac, 95031 Cergy-Pontoise CEDEX, France

Martina Petruzzo, Roberta Lanzillo and Vincenzo Brescia Morra
Multiple Sclerosis Clinical Care and Research Centre, Department of Neurosciences, Reproductive Sciences and Odontostomatology, Federico II University, Via Sergio Pansini 5, 80131 Naples, Italy

Leire Iparraguirre
Multiple Sclerosis Group, Neurosciences Area, Biodonostia Health Research Institute, 20014 San Sebastian, Spain

Danel Olaverri and Telmo Blasco
Multiple Sclerosis Group, Neurosciences Area, Biodonostia Health Research Institute, 20014 San Sebastian, Spain
Department of Biomedical Engineering and Sciences, Tecnun-Universidad de Navarra, Manuel de Lardizábal 15, 20018 San Sebastián, Spain

Lucía Sepúlveda, David Otaegui and Maider Muñoz-Culla
Multiple Sclerosis Group, Neurosciences Area, Biodonostia Health Research Institute, 20014 San Sebastian, Spain
Spanish Network of Multiple Sclerosis, 08028 Barcelona, Spain

Tamara Castillo-Triviño
Multiple Sclerosis Group, Neurosciences Area, Biodonostia Health Research Institute, Neurology Department, Basque Health Service, 20014 San Sebastian, Spain

Mercedes Espiño and Lucienne Costa-Frossard
Departments of Immunology and Neurology, Multiple Sclerosis Unit, Hospital Ramon y Cajal, (IRYCIS), 28034 Madrid, Spain

Álvaro Prada
Multiple Sclerosis Group, Neurosciences Area, Biodonostia Health Research Institute, Immunology Department, Basque Health Service, 20014 San Sebastian, Spain

Luisa María Villar
Spanish Network of Multiple Sclerosis, 08028 Barcelona, Spain
Departments of Immunology and Neurology, Multiple Sclerosis Unit, Hospital Ramon y Cajal, (IRYCIS), 28034 Madrid, Spain

Fernando X. Cuascut and George J. Hutton
Baylor College of Medicine, Maxine Mesigner Multiple Sclerosis Center, Houston, TX 77030, USA

Olga Kammona
Chemical Process and Energy Resources Institute, Centre for Research and Technology Hellas, 57001 Thessaloniki, Greece

Costas Kiparissides
Chemical Process and Energy Resources Institute, Centre for Research and Technology Hellas, 57001 Thessaloniki, Greece
Department of Chemical Engineering, Aristotle University of Thessaloniki, 54124 Thessaloniki, Greece

Marco Pitteri, Stefano Ziccardi, Caterina Dapor, Maddalena Guandalini and Massimiliano Calabrese
Neurology section, Department of Neurosciences, Biomedicine and Movement Sciences, University of Verona, 37134 Verona, Italy

Maria Anagnostouli
Faculty of Neurology in Demyelinating Disease Unit & Director of Immunogenetics Laboratory, 1st Department of Neurology, Medical School, National and Kapodistrian University of Athens, NKUA, Aeginition Hospital, 115 28 Athens, Greece
Immunogenetics Laboratory, 1st Department of Neurology, Medical School, National and Kapodistrian University of Athens, NKUA, Aeginition Hospital, 115 28 Athens, Greece

Artemios Artemiadis
Immunogenetics Laboratory, 1st Department of Neurology, Medical School, National and Kapodistrian University of Athens, NKUA, Aeginition Hospital, 115 28 Athens, Greece
Medical School, University of Cyprus, Nicosia 1678, Cyprus

Maria Gontika, Charalampos Skarlis, Nikolaos Markoglou and Serafeim Katsavos
Immunogenetics Laboratory, 1st Department of Neurology, Medical School, National and Kapodistrian University of Athens, NKUA, Aeginition Hospital, 115 28 Athens, Greece

Konstantinos Kilindireas
Demyelinating Diseases Unit, 1st Department of Neurology, Medical School, National and Kapodistrian University of Athens, NKUA, Aeginition Hospital, 115 28 Athens, Greece

Ilias Doxiadis
Transplantation Immunological Laboratory, Institute of Transfusion Medicine, University Hospital Leipzig, 04103 Leipzig, Germany

Leonidas Stefanis
1st Department of Neurology, Medical School, National and Kapodistrian University of Athens, NKUA, Aeginition Hospital, 115 28 Athens, Greece

Maria Sofia Basile, Katia Mangano, Manuela Pennisi, Salvo Danilo Lombardo, Ferdinando Nicoletti and Paolo Fagone
Department of Biomedical and Biotechnological Sciences, University of Catania, Via S. Sofia 89, 95123 Catania, Italy

Emanuela Mazzon, Maria Cristina Petralia and Eugenio Cavalli
IRCCS Centro Neurolesi "Bonino-Pulejo", Via Provinciale Palermo, Contrada Casazza, 98124 Messina, Italy

Kelly Tisovic and Lilyana Amezcua
Department of Neurology, Keck School of Medicine, University of Southern California, Los Angeles, CA 90033, USA

Rechdi Ahdab
Lebanese American University Gilbert and Rose Mary Chagoury School of Medicine, Byblos, Lebanon
Hamidy Medical Center, Tripoli 1300, Lebanon
Neurology Division, Lebanese American University Medical Center Rizk Hospital, Beirut, Lebanon

Madiha M. Shatila, Joumana Freiha, Maher Salem, Karim Makhoul, Rody El Nawar and Naji Riachi
Lebanese American University Gilbert and Rose Mary Chagoury School of Medicine, Byblos, Lebanon
Neurology Division, Lebanese American University Medical Center Rizk Hospital, Beirut, Lebanon

Abed Rahman Shatila
Makassed General hospital, Beirut, Lebanon

George Khazen
Lebanese American University Gilbert and Rose Mary Chagoury School of Medicine, Byblos, Lebanon
Computer Science and Mathematics Department, Lebanese American University, Byblos, Lebanon

Shaza El Nemr
Lebanese American University Gilbert and Rose Mary Chagoury School of Medicine, Byblos, Lebanon

Samar S. Ayache
Service de Physiologie-Explorations Fonctionnelles, Hôpital Henri Mondor, Assistance Publique—Hôpitaux de Paris, 51 avenue de Lattre de Tassigny, 94010 Créteil, France
EA 4391, Excitabilité Nerveuse et Thérapeutique, Université Paris-Est-Créteil, 94010 Créteil, France

Index

www.ingramcontent.com/pod-product-compliance
Lightning Source LLC
LaVergne TN
LVHW060527210926
848485LV00005B/1162